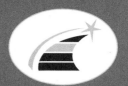

2016
FACILITY CODING
EXAM REVIEW
The Certification Step

Carol J. Buck
MS, CPC, CCS-P

Jackie L. Grass
CPC

Former Program Director
Medical Secretary Programs
Northwest Technical College
East Grand Forks, Minnesota

Lead Technical Collaborator
Coder III/Reimbursement Specialist
Grand Forks, North Dakota

ELSEVIER

ELSEVIER

3251 Riverport Lane
St. Louis, Missouri 63043

International Standard Book Number: 978-0-323-27982-6

Director, Private Sector Education & Professional/Reference: Jeanne R. Olson
Content Development Manager: Luke Held
Senior Content Development Specialist: Joshua S. Rapplean
Publishing Services Manager: Julie Eddy
Book Production Specialist: Celeste Clingan
Manager, Art & Design: Julia Dummitt

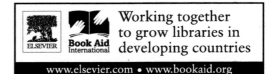

Dedication

*To coding instructors,
who each day strive to enhance the lives
of their students and provide the next generation
of knowledgeable medical coders.*

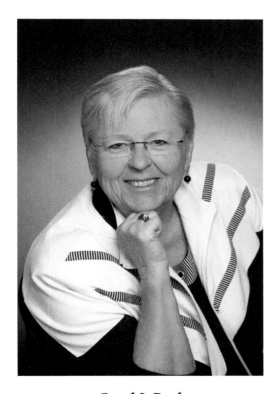

Carol J. Buck

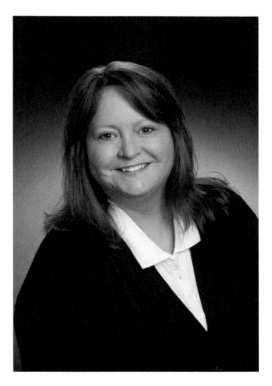

Jackie L. Grass

Acknowledgments

There are so many, many people who participated in the development of this text, and only through the effort of all of the team members has it been possible to publish this text. **Karla R. Lovaasen,** who has been a steady guiding presence through the development of the text and who never failed to keep the faith during the journey.

John W. Danaher, President, Education, who possesses great listening skills and the ability to ensure the publication of high-quality educational materials. **Jeanne R. Olson,** Director, Private Sector Education & Professional/Reference, who maintains an excellent sense of humor and is a valued member of the team who can always be depended upon for reasoned judgment. **Josh Rapplean,** Senior Content Development Specialist, who assumed the responsibility of shepherding this project to production with steady fortitude. **Mike Ederer and Ryan Yarber,** Project Managers at Graphic World, who assumed responsibility for many projects while maintaining a high degree of professionalism. The employees of Elsevier have participated in the publication of this text and demonstrated the highest levels of professionalism and competence.

Preface

Thank you for purchasing *Facility Coding Exam Review 2016: The Certification Step*. This 2016 edition has been carefully reviewed and updated with the latest content, making it the most current guide for your review. The author and publishers have made every effort to equip you with skills and tools you will need to succeed on the examination. To this end, this review guide endeavors to present essential information about all health care coding systems, anatomy, terminology, and pathophysiology, as well as sample examinations for practice. No other review guide on the market brings together such thorough coverage of all necessary examination material in one source.

Organization of This Textbook

Following a basic outline approach, this text takes a practical approach to assisting you with your examination preparations. The text is divided into five units—Anatomy, Terminology, and Pathophysiology; Reimbursement Issues and Data Quality; CPT and HCPCS Coding; ICD-10-CM/PCS Coding; Coding Challenge—and there are several appendices for your reference. Additionally, Unit 3 includes Practice Exercises, and examinations are provided on the companion Evolve website to help your progress.

ICD-9-CM versions of Units 4-5 and the Practice Examinations can be found in the Student Evolve Resources.

Some of the CPT code descriptions for physician services include physician extender services. Physician extenders, such as nurse practitioners, physician assistants, and nurse anesthetists, etc., provide medical services typically performed by a physician. Within this educational material the term "physician" may include "and other qualified health care professionals" depending on the code. Refer to the official CPT® code descriptions and guidelines to determine codes that are appropriate to report services provided by non-physician practitioners.

Unit 1, Anatomy, Terminology, and Pathophysiology
Covers all the essential body systems and terms you'll need to get certified. Organized by body systems, the sections also include illustrations to review each major anatomical area and quizzes to check your understanding and recall. (Answers are located in Appendix B.)

UNIT 1 Anatomy, Terminology, and Pathophysiology

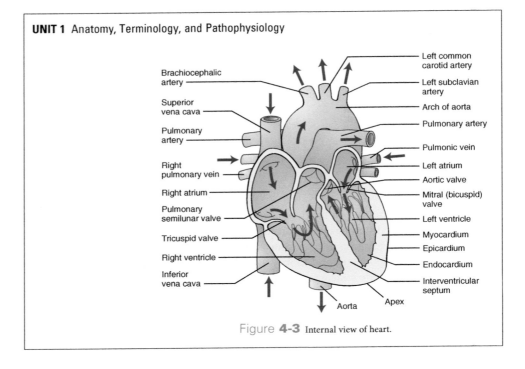

Figure **4-3** Internal view of heart.

Unit 2, Reimbursement Issues and Data Quality
Provides a review of important insurance and billing information to help you review the connections between medical coding, insurance, billing, and reimbursement.

Reimbursement Issues

■ Prospective Payment Systems (PPS)

For services provided to Medicare patients in inpatient or ambulatory surgical centers

Established by Tax Equity and Fiscal Responsibility Act (TEFRA) of 1982

Social Security amendments passed use of inpatient PPS in 1983

For services provided in

- Acute care hospitals
- Skilled nursing facilities
- Inpatient rehabilitation facilities
- Long-term care hospital settings
  - Psychiatric hospitals or exempt psychiatric units

Hospital/facility paid fixed amount for patient discharged in a treatment category

Excludes these hospitals:

- Children's
- Rehabilitation
- Cancer

Unit 3, CPT and HCPCS Coding and Unit 4, ICD-10-CM/PCS Coding.
Contain comprehensive coverage of the different coding systems and their applications, making other references unnecessary! Simplified text and clear examples are the highlights of these units, and illustrations are included to clarify difficult concepts.

Repair Arteriovenous Fistula (35180-35190)
Abnormal passage from artery or vein

Divided based on fistula type

- Congenital, acquired/traumatic, by site

Figure **17-7** Superior, inferior, and middle nasal turbinates.

NOTE: ICD-9-CM versions of Units 4 and 5 can be found in the Student Evolve Resources.

Unit 5, Coding Challenge
Contains directions for the examinations located on the Evolve website.

CHAPTER 26: EXAMINATIONS

You have three opportunities to practice taking an examination:

- Pre-Examination (before study)
- Post-Examination (after study)
- Final Examination (at the end of your complete program of study)

You should have the following manuals:

- 2016 ICD-10-CM, *(International Classification of Diseases, 10th Revision, Clinical Modification)*
- 2016 ICD-10-PCS *(International Classification of Disease, 10th Revision, Procedure Coding System)*
- 2016 HCPCS (Healthcare Common Procedure Coding System)
- On the certification examination, HCPCS questions are on the theory portion of the examination, not on the practical portion of the examination
- 2016 CPT *(Current Procedural Terminology)*

No other reference material, other than a medical dictionary, is allowed for any of the examinations.

- For the Pre-, Post-, and Final Examinations, you will need a computer that has Internet access and the four coding references listed above (ICD-10-CM, ICD-10-PCS, HCPCS, CPT).
- Each organization's certification examination has different scoring requirements, but as you take these examinations, you should strive for 80% to 90% on the Post-Examination and 65% as a minimum on the Final Examination.

  ICD-9-CM versions of the Pre-/Post- and Final Examinations can be found in the Student Evolve Resources.

NOTE: To enable the learner to calculate an examination score, minimums have been identified as "passing" within this text; however, this may or may not be the percentage identified by the certifying organization as a "passing" grade. It is your responsibility to review all certification information published by the certifying organization.

About the Practice Examinations

The companion Evolve website contains valuable resources to assist you with your preparation for the **Facility** coding certification examination. (See *Additional Evolve Resources* on page x for more information on how to access this website.) It includes two timed and scored 105-question examinations, contained in two major sections. The Pre-Examination must be completed at the start of your study. After your study is complete, the same examination is to be taken again as the Post-Examination. By comparing the results of both examinations, you can see your improvement after using the review guide. Once you check your scores, you are ready to take the Final Examination.

ICD-9-CM versions of the Practice Examinations can be found in the Student Evolve Resource.

Exam Sessions Screen

After choosing your exam format, the Exam Sessions screen serves as home base. Here you can find information relating to your progress and performance in different examination sections. From this screen, you can choose an examination mode (Pre-, Post-, or Final), submit an examination section, check your progress, or review your results.

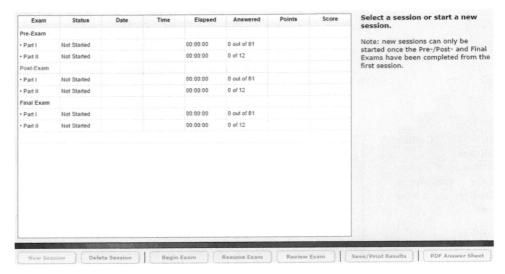

Exam	Status	Date	Time	Elapsed	Answered	Points	Score	
Pre-Exam								Select a session or start a new session.
• Part I	Not Started			00:00:00	0 out of 81			Note: new sessions can only be started once the Pre-/Post- and Final Exams have been completed from the first session.
• Part II	Not Started			00:00:00	0 of 12			
Post-Exam								
• Part I	Not Started			00:00:00	0 out of 81			
• Part II	Not Started			00:00:00	0 of 12			
Final Exam								
• Part I	Not Started			00:00:00	0 out of 81			
• Part II	Not Started			00:00:00	0 of 12			

New Session   Delete Session   Begin Exam   Resume Exam   Review Exam   Save/Print Results   PDF Answer Sheet

Exam Sessions screen.

In addition to displaying your scores for completed sections and tracking the total elapsed time, this screen also shows the answered, unanswered, and bookmarked questions in each subsection. You can return to the Exam Sessions screen at any point while taking or reviewing an examination, and all information related to your answers and position is saved.

Taking the Examination

The Practice Examinations are divided into two sections:

Part I: Multiple Choice Section—This section includes 97 single-response multiple-choice questions.

Part II: Fill in the Blank Section (Case Studies)—This section includes 8 case studies.

For Part I of the Pre-Exam, click on the letter to select answers and use the navigation buttons to move from question to question. For Part II, codes can be typed into the electronic answer sheet as you read through the provided case. Your answers will be saved when you close the answer sheet.

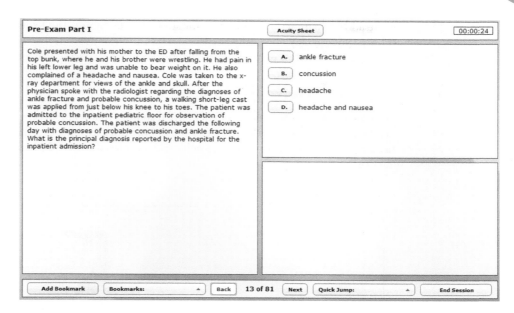

Question screen.

The screen also displays a Quick Jump feature, which is a pull-down menu that allows you to jump to any question in the current section. The Bookmark button at the bottom of the screen allows you to mark questions for later reference. Bookmarked questions can be reviewed using the dropdown menu labeled "Bookmarks."

Reviewing Your Results

Once you have taken the Post-Examination on the companion Evolve website, you have the option to review all the Pre- and Post-Examination questions with rationales, even the ones you answered correctly, by clicking the "Review Exam" button at the bottom of the screen. The correct answer is shown for each question, and a rationale is given for each answer option. Or, if you prefer, you can review the answers and rationales using a PDF answer sheet. You can also compare your results on the Pre- and Post-Examinations by clicking on each exam on the Exam Sessions screen and viewing your results in the "Completed Exams" on the right or by printing out your results.

Once you have completed the Final Examination, the software will then provide you with all the answers and rationales.

Supplemental Resources

However you decide to prepare for the certification examination, we have developed supplements designed to complement the *Facility Coding Exam Review 2016: The Certification Step*. Each of these supplements has been developed with the needs of both students and instructors in mind.

Instructor's Electronic Resource

No matter what your level of teaching experience, this total-teaching solution, located on the companion Evolve site, will help you plan your lessons with ease, and the author has developed all the curriculum materials necessary to use the textbook in the classroom. This includes additional unit quizzes, a course calendar and syllabus, lesson plans, ready-made tests for easy assessment, and PDF files with the questions and answers for the Pre-/Post- and Final Examinations. Also included is a comprehensive PowerPoint collection and ExamView test banks. The PowerPoint slides can be easily customized to support your lectures or formatted as overhead transparencies or handouts for student note-taking. The ExamView test generator will help you quickly and easily prepare quizzes and exams from the ready-made test questions, and the test banks can be customized to your specific teaching methods.

Additional Evolve Resources

The Evolve companion website offers many resources that will extend your studies beyond the classroom. Related WebLinks offer you the opportunity to expand your knowledge base and stay current with this ever-changing field, and additional material is available for help and practice.

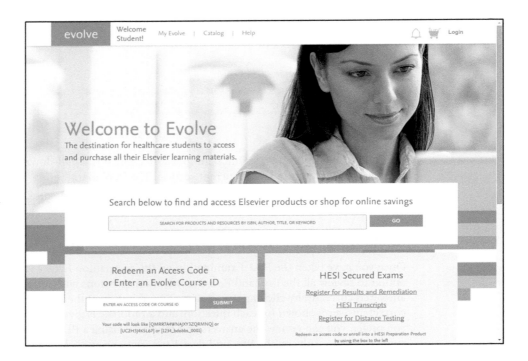

A Course Management System (CMS) is also available free to instructors who adopt this textbook. This web-based platform gives instructors yet another resource to facilitate learning and to make medical coding content accessible to students. In addition to the Evolve Resources available to both faculty and students, there is an entire suite of tools available that allows for communication between instructors and students. Students can log on through the Evolve portal to take online quizzes and practice examinations, participate in threaded discussions, post assignments to instructors, or chat with other classmates, and instructors can use the online grade book to follow class progress.

To access this comprehensive online resource, follow the instructions located on the inside front cover of this book. You will need the Course ID Number provided by your instructor. If your instructor has not set up a Course Management System, you can still access the free Evolve resources at http://evolve.elsevier.com/Buck/facilityexam/.

Development of This Edition

This book would not have been possible without a team of educators and professionals, including practicing coders and technical consultants. The combined efforts of the team members have made this text an incredible learning tool.

QUERY MANAGER

Patricia Cordy Henricksen, MS, CHCA, CPC-I, CPC, CCP-P, ACS-PM
AAPC-Approved ICD-10-CM Trainer
Auditing, Coding, and Education Specialist
Soterion Medical Services/Merrick Management
Lexington, Kentucky

SENIOR COLLABORATOR AND ICD-10-CM CONSULTANT

Nancy Maguire, ACS, CRT, PCS, FCS, HCS-D, APC, AFC
Physician Consultant for Auditing and Education
Palm Bay, Florida

CODING SPECIALISTS

Kathy Buchda, CPC, CPMA
Revenue Recognition
Forest City, Iowa

Letitia Patterson, MPA, CPC, CCS-P
Consultant
A Coder's Resource
Chicago, Illinois

EDITORIAL REVIEW BOARD

Julie Alles, MSCTE, RHIA
Assistant Professor/Program Director
Allendale, Michigan

Rolando Russell, MBA/HCM, CPC, CPAR
Program Director/Healthcare Consultant
Ultimate Medical Academy
Tampa, Florida

Katherine Sa, CMBS, CPC
Academic Advisor
Laguna Hills, California

Contents

Success Strategies

This review was developed to help you as you prepare for your certification examination. First, congratulations on your initiative. Preparing for a certification examination can seem like a daunting and formidable task. You have already taken the first and hardest step: you have made a commitment. Your steely determination and organizational skills are your best tools as you organize to complete this exciting journey successfully.

How do you prepare for a certification examination? The answers to that question are as varied as the persons preparing for a certification examination. Each person comes to the preparation with different educational, coding, and personal experiences. Therefore, each must develop a plan that meets his or her individual needs and preferences. Success Strategies will help you to develop your individual plan.

The Certification Examination

This text has been developed to serve as a tool in your preparation for the facility-based certification examination. For AHIMA, the CCS (Certified Coding Specialist) certification examination consists of a total of 105 questions: 97 multiple choice; and 8 open-ended coding scenarios. Questions cover medical terminology, anatomy, pathophysiology, pharmacology, CPT, ICD-10-CM, ICD-10-PCS, and HCPCS. You have 4 hours to complete the computer-based examination. Exam results are reported with score percentage for each "domain" tested, as well as the total possible score and the individual's score. Visit the AHIMA website (www.ahima.org/certification/ccs.aspx) for the latest information on the CCS exam.

To be successful on the certification examination, you will have to know how to assign medical codes to services and diagnoses. This textbook focuses on providing you with that coding practice as well as anatomy, terminology, pathophysiology, reimbursement, and coding concepts in preparation for the examination.

Date and Location

Although every journey begins with the first step, you have to know where you are going to make a plan to get there.

- Choose the **date and location** for taking the certification examination.
- The website www.ahima.org/certification/ccs.aspx contains detailed information about registering for the examination.
- AHIMA has a Candidate Guide that includes eligibility requirements, information on applying for the examination, test center restrictions and sample examination screens. The Candidate Guide can be downloaded from their website at www.ahima.org/~/media/AHIMA/Files/Certification/Candidate_Guide.ashx, or sent for by contacting:

American Health Information Management Association (AHIMA)

233 N. Michigan Avenue, 21st Floor

Chicago, IL 60601-5809

Telephone: (312) 233-1100

- After you have obtained the candidate guide and examination materials, read all the information carefully. Review all competencies outlined in the material to ensure that your study plan contains strategies to address each of these competencies. Check for the latest information on acceptable forms of identification, coding rules to follow, and passing scores.

- The questions within this textbook are not the same questions that are in the certification examination, but the skill and knowledge that you gain through analysis, coding, and recall will increase your ability to be successful on examination day.

Managing Your Time

Role strain! That is what you get when you have so many different roles in your life and you cannot find time for all of them. Know that feeling? Are you a daughter/son, mother/father, wife/husband, student, friend, worker, volunteer, hobbyist? The list is endless. Each takes time from your schedule, and somehow you now need to fit into the role of successful learner. Because you have only 24 hours in your day, being a successful learner requires a time-balancing act. Maybe you will have to be satisfied with dust bunnies under your bed, dishes in your kitchen sink, or fewer visits with your friends. Whatever you have to do to juggle the time around to give yourself ample time to devote to this important task of examination preparation, you must do and make a plan for in advance; otherwise, life just takes over and you find you do not have adequate study time.

If you are planning a big event in your life—moving, a trip, and so on—think about postponing it until after the examination. Your focus right now has to be on yourself. Make your motto **"It's All About Me!"** Sounds self-centered, I know, and most likely very different from who you are, but just this once, you need to carve out the time you need to accomplish this important goal. This time is for yourself. Make it happen for yourself. Move everything you can out of the way, focus on this preparation, and give this preparation your best effort.

Schedule

Each person has an individual learning style. The coding profession seems to attract those most influenced by logic and facts. The best way for a logical and factual person to learn is to problem-solve and apply the information. Hands-on practice is how you will build your skill and confidence for the examination.

- Choose a location to be your Study Central.
- Gather into Study Central the following study resources:
  - Certification information from www.ahima.org/certification/ccs.aspx
  - CPT, designated edition
  - ICD-10-CM, designated edition
  - ICD-10-PCS, designated edition
  - HCPCS, designated edition
  - *ICD-10-CM Official Guidelines for Coding and Reporting* (can be accessed by following the Evolve Resources link provided in Appendix A of this text)
  - *ICD-10-PCS Official Guidelines for Coding and Reporting* (can be accessed by following the Evolve Resources link provided in Appendix A of this text)
  - Medical dictionary
  - Coding textbooks, professional journals, and magazines
  - Terminology, anatomy, or pathology text, as needed
  - See Appendix H for Further Text Resources

Make Study Central your special place where you can get away from all other responsibilities. Make it a quiet, calm getaway, even if it is a corner of your bedroom. In this quiet place have a comfortable chair, adequate lighting, supplies, and sufficient desktop surface to use all your coding books. This is your place to focus all your attention on preparation for the examination, without distractions.

- Plan your **schedule** from now until the certification examination using a calendar. Make weekly goals so that you have definite tasks to accomplish each week and you can check the tasks off—a great feeling of accomplishment comes from being able to check off a task. In this way, you can see your progress on your countdown to success.

- Choose a specific **time** each day or several times a week when you are going to study, and mark them on your calendar. Make this commitment in writing. After each study session, you should check off that date on the calendar as a visual reminder that you are sticking to your plan and are one step closer to your goal.

- You should plan your study time in advance, know what you are going to be studying the next session, and **be prepared** for that upcoming study session. This will greatly increase the amount of material you are able to cover during the session. At the end of each session, decide what you are going to study next session and ensure that you have all the material and references you will need readily available. At the end of each session, you should be ready for the next study session.

- Your plan should **focus** on those areas where you know you will need improvement. For example, when is the last time you read, not referenced or reviewed, but really read, the CPT Surgery Guidelines? You may not code surgery services often, and as such are not familiar with the information in these guidelines. That is an area for improvement, and your plan should include a thorough reading of all the CPT section guidelines.

- DO THIS BEFORE YOU BEGIN YOUR STUDY: **Assess** your strengths and weaknesses. By making this assessment, you will know where to concentrate your efforts and where to focus your study schedule. You know those areas where you already have strong skills and knowledge and will not need to spend as much time preparing in these areas. The **Pre-Examination** is a 105-question examination that you can use as a tool to assess your current skill level. This examination should be taken before you begin your study and then again immediately after you have completed your entire study schedule. Do not analyze the questions by reviewing the rationales provided; rather, wait until after you have completed your studies and have taken this same examination a second time. If you review the rationales after the first time you take the examination, you will know the answers too well to provide a valid comparison between examinations.

- After you have completed your course of study, take the **Post-Examination.** You should plan to cover the examination in the same amount of time as will be given for the certification examination. Compare your scores with those from the first time you took this examination. Note the areas where you did not demonstrate sufficient skills and knowledge.

- Develop a **second plan** to improve the specific areas where you believe you need further study.

- You are now ready to take the **Final Examination.** Take the examination in the same amount of time that will be allocated for the certification examination. It is best if you complete this final in one sitting, thereby mimicking the actual examination. If your schedule does not allow for taking the examination in one sitting, plan to take it in several sessions, but always keep track of the time used to ensure that you take the examination in the same amount of time allowed for the official examination. Learning to work within the time allocated is part of the skill you are developing. Remember, the certification examinations assess not only your coding knowledge but also your efficiency in completing the test within the allocated time.

Using This Text

The text is divided into:

- Success Strategies
- Unit 1, Anatomy, Terminology, and Pathophysiology
- Unit 2, Reimbursement Issues
- Unit 3, CPT and HCPCS Coding
- Unit 4, ICD-10-CM/PCS Coding
- Unit 5, Coding Challenge

> **NOTE: ICD-9-CM versions of Units 4-5 and the Practice Evaluations can be found in the Student Evolve Resources.**

- Appendix A, Resources (Web-Based Information)
- Appendix B, Answers
- Appendix C, Medical Terminology
- Appendix D, Combining Forms
- Appendix E, Prefixes
- Appendix F, Suffixes
- Appendix G, Abbreviations
- Appendix H, Further Text Resources
- Appendix I, Pharmacology Review

Appendices C–G are combined lists of Medical Terminology, Combining Forms, Prefixes, Suffixes, and Abbreviations used within Unit 1, Anatomy, Terminology, and Pathophysiology.

The material in this review features the following:

- Comprehensive guide to areas of study
- Photos and drawings to illustrate key points
- Pre-/Post-Examination—105 questions (97 multiple-choice and 8 cases)
- Final Examination—105 questions (97 multiple-choice and 8 cases)
- **Unit 1** is a review of the anatomy, terminology, and pathophysiology by organ systems designed to provide you with a quick review of that organ system. In addition, there is a list of combining forms, prefixes, suffixes, and abbreviations that are often used in that organ system. At the end of each organ system, there is a quiz that will give you an opportunity to assess your knowledge of anatomy/terminology and pathophysiology. (Answers are located in Appendix B.)
- **Unit 2** is a review of reimbursement and data quality issues and terminology. A quiz is located at the end of the unit to assess your knowledge. (Answers are located in Appendix B.)
- **Unit 3 and Unit 4** review CPT, HCPCS, and ICD-10-CM/PCS. The CPT and ICD-10-CM/PCS material follows the order of the manuals. There is no quiz at the end of this unit because you will be applying this material in the practice examinations and in the Final Examination.
- **Unit 5** contains directions for the examinations. **ICD-9-CM versions of the Practice Examinations can be found in the Student Evolve Resources.** The Pre-/Post-Examination is a 105-question examination located on the companion Evolve website. The same examination should be taken twice—once before you begin your study and the second time after you have completed your study. You should allow 4 hours (240 minutes) to complete each examination. The computer software stores your scores and compares the results from the first and second time you took the examination; in this way, you can see not only your score on each section but also the improvement from the first to the second examination. The Final Examination is also a 105-question examination located on the companion Evolve

website, and you should allow 4 hours (240 minutes) to complete the examination (one hour for Parts I and three hours for Part II). Both examinations are divided into the following sections:

- **Parts I—97 questions**
  - Medical Terminology
  - Anatomy
  - ICD-10-CM/PCS
  - HCPCS
  - Concepts of Coding and Reimbursement, Information Technology, and Documentation
  - Pathophysiology
- **Part II—8 Case Studies**
  - Ambulatory surgery cases (outpatient)
  - Emergency department case (outpatient)
  - Outpatient surgery clinic
  - Inpatient

On the AHIMA examination some questions are beta test questions and do not contribute to your final score.

> NOTE: To enable the learner to calculate an examination score, minimums have been identified as "passing" within this text; however, this may or may not be the percentage identified by the certifying organization as a "passing" grade. It is your responsibility to review all certification information published by the certifying organization.

There are many ways you could use this text. Whichever way you decide to prepare, you should take the Pre-Examination before you begin your study to ensure that you develop a study plan that includes time and activities that will increase your knowledge in those areas where your test scores indicate areas of weakness. You could then take the units in the order in which they are presented, or you may want to review the anatomy, terminology, and pathophysiology for a body system and then review the CPT material for that body system. There is no one best way for approaching the use of this text because each individual will have a personal learning style and preferences that will direct how the material is used. Your skills may be very strong in one or more coding or knowledge areas, and you will want to delete those areas from your individual study plan.

This text is not meant to be the only study source; rather, it is just one tool among many that you will use. For example, if your terminology skills need a complete overhaul, the brief overview in this text may not meet your needs. You may want to supplement this text with a terminology text and an in-depth study of terminology.

- **Appendices** are a resource for you as you prepare your study plan.
  - **Appendix A,** Resources, is an Evolve Resources link (Web-Based) to the ICD-10-CM Official Guidelines for Coding and Reporting and the ICD-10-PCS Official Guidelines for Coding and Reporting. This link provides the rules for use of ICD-10-CM/PCS codes and will be referenced in Unit 4 during review of the use of ICD-10-CM/PCS codes. These can be utilized by following the Evolve Resources link provided.
  - **Appendix B,** Unit 1 and Unit 2 Quiz Answers, and Unit 3 Practice Exercises, Answers, and Rationales.
  - **Appendix C,** Medical Terminology, is a complete alphabetic list of all the medical terms listed in the Medical Terminology portion of the organ system reviews used in Unit 1.
  - **Appendix D,** Combining Forms, is a complete alphabetic list of the combining forms used in Unit 1.

- **Appendix E,** Prefixes, is a complete alphabetic list of the prefixes used in Unit 1.
- **Appendix F,** Suffixes, is a complete alphabetic list of the suffixes used in Unit 1.
- **Appendix G,** Abbreviations, is a complete list of the abbreviations referenced in Unit 1.
- **Appendix H,** Further Text References, is a list of texts that you may want to obtain to supplement your study plan.
- **Appendix I,** Pharmacology Review, is a list of commonly prescribed pharmaceuticals.

Day Before the Examination

- No cramming! Your study time is now over, and cramming the day before the test is not a good idea because it just increases your anxiety level. This day is your day to prepare yourself. Do some things that you enjoy. Take your mind off the examination. Pamper yourself: you deserve it.
- Be prepared and bring the following items with you on the day of the examination: Two forms of picture identification, CPT, ICD-10-CM, ICD-10-PCS, HCPCS code books, and optionally a medical dictionary, along with your examination admission ticket. It is your responsibility to refer to the certifying organization's website to be certain you have the correct identification and books necessary to take the examination.
- You cannot have excessive writing, sticky notes, labels, and so forth in your code books. Check the certifying organization's examination details to ensure that your books meet the specifications identified by the testing organization.
- Review the Candidate Guide one last time to ensure that you have all the required material.
- Listen to the weather and traffic reports. Plan your route to the examination site. If it is in a new location, drive to the location before the big day.
- Eat a light supper and get to bed early. Set the alarm in plenty of time to arrive at the site early. It is a good idea to have a friend or family member give you an early wake-up call to ensure that you do not oversleep.

Day of the Examination

- Wear comfortable clothes, and be prepared for any room temperature. A short-sleeved shirt with a sweater is a good plan. Dress in layers so you can ensure that you will be comfortable in any environment.
- Eat a good breakfast. Avoid caffeine because it initially stimulates you but will decrease your concentration in the long run.
- Arrive early. This is a day to be early.
- Ensure that you have the correct room for your examination. Often there are several examinations being administered at one time, so be certain you are in the correct room for your examination.

The Certification Examination

You are ready for this! You have planned your work and have worked your plan. Now it is time to reap the rewards for all that hard work.

- Place approved supplies on the table assigned to you.
- Have faith in yourself, and visualize yourself being successful. Say to yourself, "I can do this," and then take several deep breaths before you begin to help relax you.
- Some prefer to take the parts of the examination out of order, beginning with those questions about which they are most confident. Others prefer to start at the beginning and work through all questions in order. The approach that you use will depend on your individual test-taking style. For the AHIMA exam, one question appears on the computer screen at a time. Examinees are not able to move to the next question until the current question is answered.

- Attempt each question and flag those you are unsure of so that you can return to them when you have finished the entire examination. For the AHIMA exam, when an examinee is not confident of the answer, he or she is able to select a best guess, and then flag the question. Once the entire exam is completed, the examinee is allowed to return to flagged questions to review and change answers.

- Read the directions. This may sound too simple, but many persons do not completely read the directions, only to find that the directions gave specific directions about what or what not to code on a certain case (for example, "code only this certain portion of the procedure"). Yet the choices for answers included the full coding of the case as a selection; if you did not read all the directions, you would choose the response with codes for all the items listed in the report. For example, the question may have directed you to code the service only, not the diagnosis, and yet one of the choices would be the correct service and diagnosis codes, which of course would be an incorrect answer based on the directions. So read all of the directions.

- Your speed and accuracy are being tested. You do not have time to labor over each question for a long time if you intend to complete all the questions. Read the directions, read the question, put down your best assessment of the answer, and then move on to the next question.

- Words such as *always, every, never,* and *all* generally indicate broad terms that, with true/false questions, usually indicate a false question.

- If you do not know the answer to the question, first try eliminating those that you know are incorrect and then select the answer that seems most likely to be correct.

- Judge the time as you are moving through the examination. Keep assessing whether you are making sufficient progress or whether you can slow down or need to speed up.

- Answer all questions. Even if you have to guess, at least fill in an answer. The best situation is that you answer all questions and have time left over to go back over the questions about which you are in doubt. For the multiple-choice section of the CCS examination, the computer program has a feature that allows you to mark questions to be returned to later. When you have finished answering all the questions, the computer program gives you the option to return to just the marked questions or to all of the questions. So, fill in the answer with your best hunch and then mark the question to return to later.

- Use every minute of the test time, but it is not a good idea to begin second-guessing yourself. Do not return to those questions for which you did not have serious doubts about the correct answer. Usually, your first answer is the best.

- When the time is finished, pat yourself on the back. You have done an excellent job! Now it is time to go get a good supper and a good night's sleep.

- You will be given results to the test before you leave.

Days After the Examination

- You will miss the preparation! Okay, maybe not miss it exactly, but your life will be different now without that constant preparation.
- You have done your best. That is always good enough!
- **Be proud of yourself;** this was no small undertaking, and you did it!

My personal best wishes to you as you prepare for your certification. You can do this!

Best regards,

Carol J. Buck, MS, CPC, CCS-P

Our goals can only be reached through a vehicle of a plan, in which we must fervently believe, and upon which we must vigorously act. There is no other route to success.

Stephen A. Brennen

Course Syllabus and Student Calendar

The following documents are the syllabus and the course calendar that would be used in a classroom setting. It is suggested that these documents be used in development of your personal educational plan.

Course Syllabus

Course Description

The focus of this class is a review of terminology, anatomy, pathophysiology, reimbursement, and data quality as a preparation to take the **Facility** coding certification examination. A review of CPT, ICD-10-CM, ICD-10-PCS, and HCPCS coding will be an integral part of this review course. Two practice certification review examinations will be taken under timed conditions. The course assists the learner in establishing a personal plan for continued development in preparation for a certification examination.

Texts

Facility Coding Exam Review 2016: The Certification Step, by Carol J. Buck, Elsevier

2016 ICD-10-CM Standard Edition, by Carol J. Buck, Elsevier

2016 ICD-10-PCS Standard Edition, by Carol J. Buck, Elsevier

2016 HCPCS Level II, by Carol J. Buck, Elsevier

2016 CPT, American Medical Association

Medical dictionary

Performance Objectives

1. Write a personal plan for preparation for a certification examination.
2. Review the structure, function, terminology, pathophysiology, and abbreviations of the integumentary system.
3. Review the structure, function, terminology, pathophysiology, and abbreviations of the musculoskeletal system.
4. Review the structure, function, terminology, pathophysiology, and abbreviations of the respiratory system.
5. Review the structure, function, terminology, pathophysiology, and abbreviations of the cardiovascular system.
6. Review the structure, function, terminology, pathophysiology, and abbreviations of the female genital system and pregnancy.

7. Review the structure, function, terminology, pathophysiology, and abbreviations of the male genital system.
8. Review the structure, function, terminology, pathophysiology, and abbreviations of the urinary system.
9. Review the structure, function, terminology, pathophysiology, and abbreviations of the digestive system.
10. Review the structure, function, terminology, and abbreviations of the mediastinum and diaphragm.
11. Review the structure, function, terminology, pathophysiology, and abbreviations of the hemic and lymphatic systems.
12. Review the structure, function, terminology, pathophysiology, and abbreviations of the endocrine system.
13. Review the structure, function, terminology, pathophysiology, and abbreviations of the nervous system.
14. Review the structure, function, terminology, and abbreviations of the senses of the body.
15. Demonstrate knowledge of structure, function, terminology, pathophysiology, and abbreviations of organ systems.
16. Review medical reimbursement, documentation, information technology, and data quality issues.
17. Demonstrate knowledge of medical reimbursement issues.
18. Review CPT E/M section.
19. Review CPT Surgery section.
20. Review HCPCS.
21. Review format and conventions of ICD-10-CM/PCS.
22. Review assignment of ICD-10-CM/PCS codes.
23. Review ICD-10-CM/PCS Official Guidelines for Coding and Reporting.
24. Demonstrate coding ability by assigning CPT codes.
25. Demonstrate ability to assign E/M levels to facility outpatient services.
26. Demonstrate coding ability by assigning HCPCS codes.
27. Demonstrate coding ability by assigning ICD-10-CM/PCS codes.
28. Demonstrate ability to abstract information from the medical record.
29. Demonstrate coding abilities by completing Practice Exercises.

Personal Objectives

The student will:

- Attend class sessions.
- Prepare for class sessions.
- Complete assignments in a timely manner.
- Demonstrate a high level of responsibility.
- Display respect for other members of the class.
- Participate in class discussions.

Evaluation and Grading

- Evaluation is directly related to the performance objectives.
- Performance is measured by examination, assignments, and/or quizzes.

- The letter grade is based on the percentage of the total points earned throughout the semester based on the following scale:
  - A = 93% to 100%
  - B = 85% to 92%
  - C = 79% to 84%
  - D = 70% to 78%
  - F = 69% and below
- Examinations are scheduled in advance. To qualify for the total points on the examinations, the student must take the examination at the scheduled time. Five points will be deducted from each examination if the examination is not taken at the scheduled time. This rule reinforces the need for on-time performance. Any make-up examination must be completed within 3 days of the scheduled examination or no points will be awarded for the examination.
- Assignments are scheduled in advance. To qualify for the total points on the assignment, the student must submit the completed assignment at the scheduled time. Five points are deducted from each assignment if the assignment is not submitted at the scheduled time. This rule reinforces the need for on-time performance. Any late assignment must be completed within 3 days from the date the assignment was due or no points will be awarded for the assignment.
- Cases are due as indicated on the calendar to qualify for the total points for the case. No points will be awarded for late submission of cases.
- Quizzes are scheduled in advance. Quizzes cannot be made up, and no points are awarded for missed quizzes.
- There are a total of 35 Practice Exercises located in Unit 3, worth 2 points each for a total of 70 points.

Methods of Instruction

The instructional methods used include lecture, class discussion, and assignments.

Course Calendar

Lesson 1

Reading assignment(s):	Success Strategies, pages S1-S7
Assignment(s):	Complete the Pre-Examination on the companion Evolve website, and at **Lesson 3** class period, hand in your scores on the two sections for 73 points. The Pre-Examination is nongraded, each question attempted is worth ½ point, but award 3.07 points for each case attempted in Part II.
	Download certification examination information
	Print one page to hand in at **Lesson 2** to demonstrate successful access to certification information from website (10 points—nongraded)

Lesson 2

Student hands in:	One printed page to demonstrate successful access to certifying organization's information from website (10 points—nongraded)
Reading assignment(s):	Chapters 1-2 (pages 1-52)

Assignment(s): Develop a Personal Plan for preparation for Certification Review (20 points—graded) to be submitted at **Lesson 6** class period
Integumentary Quizzes (20 points)
Musculoskeletal Quizzes (20 points)
Prepare results of Pre-Examination for **Lesson 3**

Lesson 3

Student hands in: Integumentary Quizzes (20 points)
Musculoskeletal Quizzes (20 points)
Results of Pre-Examination (73 points—nongraded, each question attempted is worth ½ point, but award 3.07 points for each case attempted in Part II)
Reading assignment(s): Chapters 3-5 (pages 53-112)
Assignment(s): Respiratory Quizzes (20 points)
Cardiovascular Quizzes (20 points)
Female Genital System and Pregnancy Quizzes (20 points)

Lesson 4

Student hands in: Respiratory Quizzes (20 points)
Cardiovascular Quizzes (20 points)
Female Genital System and Pregnancy Quizzes (20 points)
Reading assignment(s): Chapters 6-9 (pages 113-177)
Assignment(s): Male Genital System Quizzes (20 points)
Urinary System Quizzes (20 points)
Digestive System Quiz (20 points)
Mediastinum and Diaphragm Quiz (10 points)
(There is NO pathophysiology quiz for Mediastinum and Diaphragm.)

Lesson 5

Student hands in: Male Genital System Quizzes (20 points)
Urinary System Quizzes (20 points)
Digestive System Quizzes (20 points)
Mediastinum and Diaphragm Quiz (10 points)
(There is no pathophysiology quiz for Mediastinum and Diaphragm.)
Reading assignment(s): Chapters 10-11 (pages 178-208)
Assignment(s): Hemic and Lymphatic Quizzes (20 points)
Endocrine Quizzes (20 points)
Prepare to submit Personal Plan for Preparation for Certification Examination

Lesson 6

Student hands in: Hemic and Lymphatic Quizzes (20 points)
Endocrine Quizzes (20 points)
Submit Personal Plan for Preparation for Certification Examination (20 points—graded)

Reading assignment(s):   Chapters 12-13 (pages 209-248)
Assignment(s):   Nervous System Quizzes (20 points)
      Senses Quizzes (20 points)
      Prepare for Unit 1, Anatomy, Terminology, and
          Pathophysiology, Test 1 (50 points, 25 questions, 15
          minutes)

Lesson 7

      **UNIT 1: ANATOMY, TERMINOLOGY, AND
      PATHOPHYSIOLOGY, TEST 1**
Student hands in: Nervous System Quizzes (20 points)
      Senses Quizzes (20 points)
Reading assignment(s):   Chapter 14 (pages 249-257, to Ambulatory Payment
          Classifications)
Assignment(s):   None

Lesson 8

Student hands in: None
Reading assignment(s):   Chapter 14 (pages 257-261, to -CA modifier)
Assignment(s):   None

Lesson 9

Student hands in: None
Reading assignment(s):   Chapter 14 (pages 261-271, to Post Acute Transfer)
Assignment(s):   None

Lesson 10

Student hands in: None
Reading assignment(s):   Chapter 14 (pages 272-285)
Assignment(s):   Reimbursement Quiz (10 points)

Lesson 11

Student hands in: None
Reading assignment(s):   Chapter 15 (pages 286-288, to ASC Modifiers)
      E/M Guidelines
Assignment(s):   Prepare for Unit 2, Reimbursement, Test 2 (24 points, 20
          minutes)

Lesson 12

      UNIT 2: REIMBURSEMENT, TEST 2
Student hands in: None
Reading assignment(s):   Chapters 15-16 (pages 288-302)
Assignment(s):   Complete Practice Exercises 16-1 through 16-5, pages 297-302
          (10 points)

Lesson 13

Student hands in: Practice Exercises 16-1 through 16-5, pages 297-302 (10 points)
Reading assignment(s):   Chapter 17 (pages 303-304, to General subsection)
      Read Surgery Guidelines
Assignment(s):   None

Lesson 14

Student hands in:	None
Reading assignment(s):	Chapter 17 (pages 304-312, to Musculoskeletal System subsection)
Assignment(s):	Complete Practice Exercises 17-1 through 17-5, pages 313-318 (10 points)

Lesson 15

Student hands in:	Practice Exercises 3-6 through 3-10, pages 313-318 (10 points)
Reading assignment(s):	Chapter 17 (pages 319-331, to Respiratory System subsection)
Assignment(s):	Complete Practice Exercises 17-6 through 17-10, pages 324-331 (10 points)

Lesson 16

Student hands in:	Practice Exercises 17-6 through 17-10, pages 324-331 (10 points)
Reading assignment(s):	Chapter 17 (pages 332-336, to Cardiovascular System subsection)
Assignment(s):	None

Lesson 17

Student hands in:	None
Reading assignment(s):	Chapter 17 (pages 336-343, to Hemic and Lymphatic System subsection)
Assignment(s):	Complete Practice Exercises 17-11 through 17-15, pages 345-350 (10 points)

Lesson 18

Student hands in:	Practice Exercises 17-11 through 17-15, pages 345-350 (10 points)
Reading assignment(s):	Chapter 17 (pages 351-361, to Female Genital System subsection)
Assignment(s):	Complete Practice Exercises 17-16 through 17-20, pages 353-358 (10 points)

Lesson 19

Student hands in:	Practice Exercises 3-21 through 3-25, pages 353-358 (10 points)
Reading assignment(s):	Chapter 17 (pages 361-371, to Endocrine System subsection)
Assignment(s):	Post-Examination (73 points—nongraded, each question attempted is worth ½ point, but award 3.07 points for each case attempted in Part II) Due at **Lesson 24** class period. Complete Practice Exercises 17-21 through 17-25, pages 366-371 (10 points)

Lesson 20

Student hands in:	Practice Exercises 17-21 through 17-25, pages 366-371 (10 points)
Reading assignment(s):	Chapters 17-18 (pages 372-384)
Assignment(s):	Prepare for Unit 3, Test 3, Surgery (26 points, 20 minutes); (requires ICD-10-CM/PCS and CPT manuals) Complete Practice Exercises 17-26 through 17-30, pages 376-382 (10 points)

Lesson 21

	UNIT 3: SURGERY, TEST 3
Student hands in:	Practice Exercises 17-26 through 17-30, pages 376-382 (10 points)
Reading assignment(s):	Chapter 19 (pages 385-391)
Assignment(s):	None

Lesson 22

Student hands in:	None
Reading assignment(s):	Chapter 20 (pages 391-395)
Assignment(s):	Prepare for Unit 4, Test 4 (16 points, 15 minutes) (requires ICD-10-CM/PCS and CPT manuals)

Lesson 23

	UNIT 4, TEST 4
Student hands in:	None
Reading assignment(s):	Chapter 21 (pages 395-402)
Assignment(s):	Prepare for Unit 4, Test 5 (15 points, 25 minutes) (requires ICD-10-CM and CPT manuals)
	Prepare Post-Examination for submission

Lesson 24

	UNIT 4, TEST 5
Student hands in:	Results of Post-Examination (as assigned in **Lesson 19**) (73 points—nongraded, each question attempted is worth ½ point, but award 3.07 points for each case attempted in Part II)
Reading assignment(s):	Chapters 22-23 (pages 402-410)
Assignment(s):	Prepare for Unit 4, Test 6 (15 points, 25 minutes) (requires ICD-10-CM/PCS and CPT manuals)
	Prepare to begin Final Examination

Lesson 25

	UNIT 4, TEST 6
	Begin Final Examination
Student hands in:	None
Reading assignment(s):	Chapter 24 (pages 410-412)
Assignment(s):	Prepare for Unit 4, Test 7 (20 points, 15 minutes) (requires ICD-10-CM/PCS and CPT manuals)

Lesson 26

	UNIT 4, TEST 7
	Final Examination continues
Student hands in:	None
Reading assignment(s):	Chapter 25 (pages 412-415)
Assignment(s):	None

Lesson 27

	Final Examination continues
Student hands in:	None
Reading assignment(s):	None
Assignment(s):	None

Lesson 28

	Final Examination continues
Student hands in:	None
Reading assignment(s):	None
Assignment(s):	None

Lesson 29

	Final Examination continues
Student hands in:	None
Reading assignment(s):	None
Assignment(s):	None

Lesson 30

	Final Examination continues
Student hands in:	None
Reading assignment(s):	None
Assignment(s):	None

Lesson 31

	Complete Final Examination (144 points)
Student hands in:	Final Examination results
Reading assignment(s):	None
Assignment(s):	None

Lesson 32

Final grade calculation
Final course evaluation

Anatomy, Terminology, and Pathophysiology

Some of the CPT code descriptions for physician services include physician extender services. Physician extenders, such as nurse practitioners, physician assistants, and nurse anesthetists, etc., provide medical services typically performed by a physician. Within this educational material the term "physician" may include "and other qualified health care professionals" depending on the code. Refer to the official CPT® code descriptions and guidelines to determine codes that are appropriate to report services provided by non-physician practitioners.

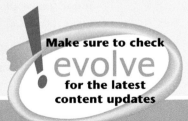

Make sure to check
evolve
for the latest
content updates

CHAPTER 1: INTEGUMENTARY SYSTEM

Anatomy and Terminology

The skin and accessory organs (nails, hair, and glands)

■ Layers (Fig. 1-1)

■ Two Layers Make Up Skin: Epidermis and Dermis

Epidermis. Outermost layer; containing keratin

Stratum corneum, most superficial layer of four layers called stratum

Basal layer, deepest region of epidermis (stratum germinativum or stratum basale), is growth layer

Dermis. The second layer of skin

Two layers are papillary and reticular and contain:

    Fibrous connective tissue or skin appendages

    Blood vessels

    Nerves

    Hair

    Nails

    Glands

Subcutaneous Tissue or Hypodermis. Not considered a layer of skin

Contains fat tissue and fibrous connective tissue

AKA: superficial fascia

Connects skin to underlying muscle

■ Nails

Keratin plates covering dorsal surface of each finger and toe

Lunula—semilunar or half-moon

    White area at base of nail plate is growth area

    Thickens and lengthens nail

Eponychium or cuticle: narrow band of epidermis at base and sides of nail

Paronychium: soft tissue around nail border

■ Glands

Sebaceous glands located in dermal layer

Secrete sebum that lubricates skin/hair

Influenced by sex hormones so they hypertrophy in adolescence and atrophy in old age

Sudoriferous glands originate in dermis. See Fig. 1-1.

AKA: sweat glands

Extend up through epidermis opening as pores

Secrete mostly water and salts to cool body

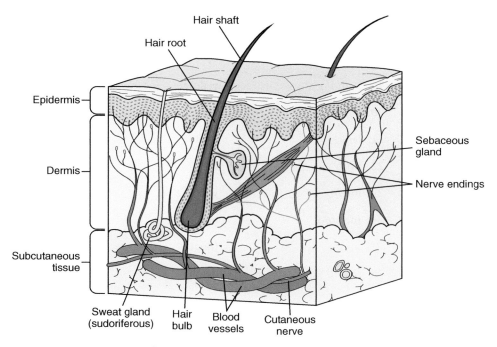

Figure **1-1** Integumentary system.

COMBINING FORMS

1.	aden/o	in relationship to a gland
2.	adip/o	fat
3.	albin/o	white
4.	aut/o	self
5.	bi/o	life
6.	caus/o	burning sensation
7.	cauter/o	burn
8.	crypt/o	hidden
9.	cutane/o	skin
10.	cyan/o	blue
11.	derm/o, dermat/o	skin
12.	diaphor/o	profuse sweating
13.	eosin/o	rosy
14.	erythem/o	red
15.	erythr/o	red
16.	heter/o	different

17. hidr/o	sweat
18. ichthy/o	dry/scaly
19. jaund/o	yellow
20. kerat/o	hard
21. leuk/o	white
22. lip/o	fat
23. lute/o	yellow
24. melan/o	black
25. myc/o	fungus
26. necr/o	death
27. onych/o	nail
28. pachy/o	thick
29. phyt/o	plant
30. pil/o	hair
31. poli/o	gray matter
32. py/o	pus
33. rhytid/o	wrinkle
34. rube/o	red
35. seb/o	sebum/oil
36. staphyl/o	clusters
37. steat/o	fat
38. strept/o	twisted chain
39. steat/o	fat
40. squam/o	flat/scalelike
41. trich/o	hair
42. ungu/o	nail
43. xanth/o	yellow
44. xer/o	dry

PREFIXES

1. epi-	on/upon
2. hyper-	over

3. hypo-	under
4. intra-	within
5. para-	beside
6. per-	through
7. peri-	surrounding
8. sub-	under

SUFFIXES

1. -coccus	spherical bacterium
2. -ectomy	removal
3. -ia	condition
4. -malacia	softening
5. -opsy	view of
6. -plasty	surgical repair
7. -rrhea	discharge
8. -tome	an instrument to cut
9. -tomy	to cut

MEDICAL ABBREVIATIONS

1. bx	biopsy
2. ca	cancer
3. derm	dermatology
4. I&D	incision and drainage
5. subcu, subq, SC, SQ	subcutaneous
6. PPD	tuberculin skin test

MEDICAL TERMS

Absence	Without
Adipose	Fatty
Albinism	Lack of color pigment
Allograft	Homograft, same species graft
Alopecia	Condition in which hair falls out
Anhidrosis	Deficiency of sweat

Autograft	From patient's own body
Avulsion	Ripping or tearing away of part either surgically or accidentally
Biopsy	Removal of a small piece of living tissue for diagnostic purposes
Causalgia	Burning pain
Collagen	Protein substance of skin
Debridement	Cleansing of or removal of dead tissue from a wound
Delayed flap	Pedicle of skin with blood supply that is separated from origin over time
Dermabrasion	Planing of skin by means of sander, brush, or sandpaper
Dermatologist	Physician who treats conditions of skin
Dermatoplasty	Surgical repair of skin
Electrocautery	Cauterization by means of heated instrument
Epidermolysis	Loosening of epidermis
Epidermomycosis	Superficial fungal infection
Epithelium	Surface covering of internal and external organs of body
Erythema	Redness of skin
Escharotomy	Surgical incision into necrotic (dead) tissue
Fissure	Cleft or groove
Free full-thickness graft	Graft of epidermis and dermis that is completely removed from donor area
Furuncle	Nodule in skin caused by *Staphylococcus* entering through hair follicle
Hematoma	A localized collection of blood, usually result of a break in a blood vessel
Homograft	Allograft, same species graft
Ichthyosis	Skin disorder characterized by scaling
Incise	To cut into
Island pedicle flap	Contains a single artery and vein that remains attached to origin temporarily or permanently
Leukoderma	Depigmentation of skin
Leukoplakia	White patch on mucous membrane
Lipocyte	Fat cell
Lipoma	Fatty tumor
Melanin	Dark pigment of skin
Melanoma	Tumor of epidermis, malignant and black in color

Mohs surgery or Mohs micrographic surgery	Removal of skin cancer in layers by a surgeon who also acts as a pathologist during surgery
Muscle flap	Transfer of muscle from origin to recipient site
Neurovascular flap	Contains artery, vein, and nerve
Pedicle	Growth attached with a stem
Pilosebaceous	Pertains to hair follicles and sebaceous glands
Sebaceous gland	Secretes sebum
Seborrhea	Excess sebum secretion
Sebum	Oily substance
Split-thickness graft	All epidermis and some of dermis
Steatoma	Fat mass in sebaceous gland
Stratified	Layered
Stratum (strata)	Layer
Subungual	Beneath nail
Xanthoma	Tumor composed of cells containing lipid material, yellow in color
Xenograft	Different species graft
Xeroderma	Dry, discolored, scaly skin

CHAPTER 1: ANATOMY AND TERMINOLOGY QUIZ

(Quiz answers are located in Appendix B)

1. This is the outermost layer of skin:
   a. basal
   b. dermis
   c. epidermis
   d. subcutaneous

2. Which of the following is/are NOT a part of skin or accessory organs?
   a. sudoriferous glands
   b. sebaceous gland
   c. nail
   d. arterioles

3. This prefix means beside:
   a. para-
   b. intra-
   c. per-
   d. epi-

4. This combining form means hair:
   a. xanth/o
   b. trich/o
   c. ichthy/o
   d. kerat/o

5. Lunula is the:
   a. narrow band of epidermis at base of nail
   b. opening of pores
   c. outermost layer of epidermis
   d. white area at base of nail plate

6. Subcutaneous tissue is also known as:
   a. dermal
   b. adipose
   c. hypodermis
   d. stratum corneum

7. Which of the following combining forms does NOT refer to a color?
   a. cyan/o
   b. jaund/o
   c. eosin/o
   d. pachy/o

8. This medical term means surgical incision into dead tissue:
   a. onychomycosis
   b. escharotomy
   c. keratotomy
   d. curettage

9. This suffix means surgical repair:
   a. -opsy
   b. -rrhea
   c. -plasty
   d. -tome

10. Soft tissue around nail border is the:
    a. cuticle
    b. lunula
    c. paronychium
    d. corium

Integumentary System—Pathophysiology

■ Lesions and Other Abnormalities (Fig. 1-2)

Macule
Flat area of color change (mostly reddened)

No elevation or depression

Example: flat moles, freckles

Papule
Solid elevation

Less than 1.0 cm in diameter

May run together and form plaques

Example: warts, lichen planus, elevated mole

Nodule
Solid elevation 1-2 cm in diameter

Extends deeper into dermis than papule

Example: lipoma, erythema nodosum, enlarged lymph nodes

Pustule
Elevated area

Filled with purulent fluid

Example: pimple, impetigo, abscess

Tumor
Solid mass

Uncontrolled, progressive growth of cells

Example: hemangioma, neoplasm, lipoma

Plaque
Flat, elevated surface

Equal or greater than 1.0 cm

Example: psoriasis, seborrheic keratosis

Wheal
Temporary localized elevation of skin

Results in transient edema in dermis

Example: insect bite, allergic reaction

Vesicle
Small blister

Less than 1 cm in diameter

Filled with serous fluid in epidermis

Example: herpes zoster (shingles), varicella (chickenpox)

Bulla
Large blister

Greater than 1.0 cm in diameter

Example: blister

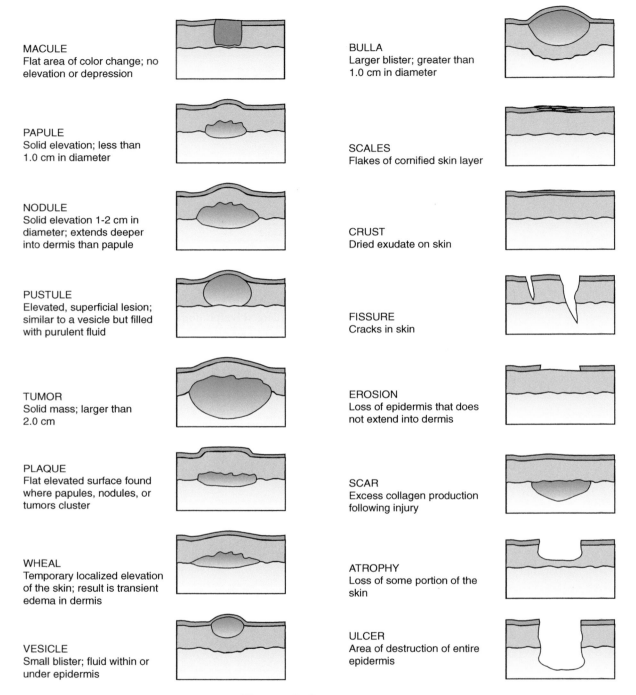

MACULE
Flat area of color change; no elevation or depression

PAPULE
Solid elevation; less than 1.0 cm in diameter

NODULE
Solid elevation 1-2 cm in diameter; extends deeper into dermis than papule

PUSTULE
Elevated, superficial lesion; similar to a vesicle but filled with purulent fluid

TUMOR
Solid mass; larger than 2.0 cm

PLAQUE
Flat elevated surface found where papules, nodules, or tumors cluster

WHEAL
Temporary localized elevation of the skin; result is transient edema in dermis

VESICLE
Small blister; fluid within or under epidermis

BULLA
Larger blister; greater than 1.0 cm in diameter

SCALES
Flakes of cornified skin layer

CRUST
Dried exudate on skin

FISSURE
Cracks in skin

EROSION
Loss of epidermis that does not extend into dermis

SCAR
Excess collagen production following injury

ATROPHY
Loss of some portion of the skin

ULCER
Area of destruction of entire epidermis

Figure **1-2** Lesions of skin.

Scales

Flakes of cornified skin layer

Example: dry skin

Crust

Dried exudate on skin

Example: scab

Fissure

Cracks in skin

Example: athlete's foot, openings in corners of mouth

Erosion

Loss of epidermis

Does not extend into dermis

Example: blisters

Scar

Excess collagen production following surgery or trauma

Example: healed surgical wound

Atrophy

Loss of some portion of skin and appears translucent

Example: aged skin

- Not a lesion, but a physiologic response in aging process

Ulcer

Area of destruction of entire epidermis

Example: missing tissue on heel, decubitus bedsore (pressure sore)

Pressure Ulcer (Decubitus Ulcer) (Fig. 1-3)

Result of Pressure or Force

Occludes blood flow, causing ischemia and tissue death

Develops over bony prominence

Locations

- Coccygeal (end of spine)
- Sacral (between hips)
- Heel
- Elbow
- Ischial (lower hip)
- Trochanteric (outer hip)

Staging or Classification System

- Stage 1: erythema (redness) of skin
- Stage 2: partial loss of skin (epidermis or dermis)
- Stage 3: full-thickness loss of skin (up to but not through fascia)
- Stage 4: full-thickness loss (extensive destruction and necrosis)

Deep ulcers may require surgical debridement

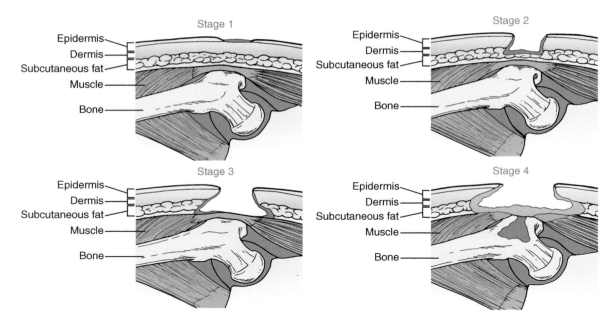

Figure **1-3** Stages 1, 2, 3, and 4 of pressure ulcers.

Keloids

Sharply elevated, irregularly shaped scars that progressively enlarge

Due to excessive collagen in corneum during connective tissue repair

Result of tissue repair or trauma

Familial tendency for formation

Cicatrix

Normal scar left after wound healing

■ Inflammatory Disorders

Atopic Dermatitis

Unknown etiology

Exogenous (External) Causes Include

Irritant dermatitis

Allergic contact dermatitis

Endogenous (Internal) Cause Includes

Seborrheic dermatitis

Results in Activation of

- Mast cells
- Eosinophils
- T lymphocytes
- Monocytes

Greater in Those with Family History of

- Asthma
- Dry skin

- Eczema
- Allergic rhinitis

Common in
- Children
- Infants

Results in
- Chronic inflammation
- Scratching
- Erythema
- Thickened, leathery skin (lichenification)
- Secondary *Staphylococcus aureus* infection

Treatment
- Topical steroid
- Antibiotic for secondary infection
- Antihistamines

Allergic Contact Dermatitis
Most common in infants and children

Potential Causes
- Hypersensitivity to allergens
  - Microorganisms
  - Drugs
  - Foreign proteins
  - Chemicals
  - Latex
  - Metals
  - Plants

Manifestations
- Scaling
- Lichenification (leathery, thickened skin)
- Erythema
- Itching (pruritus)
- Vesicular lesions
- Edema

Diagnosis and Treatment
- Check medical history
- Patch test
- Avoidance of irritant
- Skin lubrication and hydration
- Steroids
  - Topical
  - Systemic
- Topical tacrolimus (immunosuppressive agent)

Irritant Contact Dermatitis
Response to
- Chemical
- Exposure to irritant

Treatment
- Removal of irritant
- Topical agents

Stasis Dermatitis
Usually on the legs from venous stasis

Associated with
- Phlebitis
- Vascular trauma
- Varicosities

Progress
- Begins with erythema and pruritus
- Progresses to scaling, hyperpigmentation, petechiae (small hemorrhagic areas)
- Lesion becomes ulcerated

Treatment
- Elevate legs
- Reduce standing
- No constricting clothes
- Eliminate external compression
- Antibiotics for acute lesions
- Silver nitrate or Burow's solution dressings for chronic lesions

Seborrheic Dermatitis
Common chronic inflammation of sebaceous glands—cause unknown

Periods of remission and exacerbation

Commonly Occurs on
- Scalp (cradle cap in infants)
- Ear canals
- Eyelids
- Eyebrow
- Nose
- Axillae
- Chest
- Groin

Lesions are
- Scaly (dry or greasy)
- White or yellowish
- Mildly pruritic

Treatment of Mild Cases

- Soap/shampoo of
  - Coal tar
  - Sulfur
  - Salicylic acid

Treatment of More Severe Cases

- Corticosteroid

Papulosquamous Disorders

Conditions Associated with

- Scales
- Papules
- Plaque
- Erythema

Three Types

- Psoriasis
- Pityriasis
- Lichen planus

Psoriasis

Chronic, relapsing, proliferating skin disorder

Usually begins by age 20

Cause Unknown, Suggested to be

- Exacerbated by anxiety; appears to run in families
- Immunologic
- Biochemical alterations
- Triggering agent

Commonly Occurs on

- Face
- Scalp
- Forearms and elbows
- Knees and legs

Results in

- Thickened dermis and epidermis
- Well-demarcated plaque
- Cell hyperproliferation/scaly
- Inflammation (pruritus)
- Deep red lesions

Treatment

- Only palliative (treatment of symptoms)

Mild cases

- Keratolytic agents
- Corticosteroids
- Emollients

Moderate cases

- Interleukin-2 inhibitors
- Psoralens and ultraviolet A (PUVA) light therapy
- Coal tar
- Cyclosporin
- Vitamin D analogs

Severe cases

- Topical agents
- Systemic corticosteroids
- Antimetabolic
- Hospitalization

Pityriasis Rosea

Unknown cause

Self-limiting inflammatory disorder

Occurs most often in young adults

Primary Lesion

- Begins with herald patch 3 to 4 cm
- Salmon-pink colored
- Circular and well-defined lesions

Secondary Lesions

- 14 to 21 days

Trunk and upper extremities

- Oval lesions
- Severe pruritus

Diagnosis

May be confused with

- Secondary syphilis
- Seborrheic dermatitis
- Psoriasis

Treatment

- Antipruritics
- Antihistamines
- Corticosteroids
- Ultraviolet light
- Sunlight

Lichen Planus

Occurs on skin and mucous membranes

Unknown cause (idiopathic)

Autoimmune inflammatory disorder

Onset ages 30 to 70

Lesions

- Begin as pink lesions that turn into violet-colored pruritic papules
- Result in hyperpigmentation
- 2- to 10-mm flat lesions with central depression
- Last 12 to 18 months
- Tend to reoccur

Treatment

- Antihistamines
- Corticosteroids
  Topical
  Systemic

Acne Vulgaris

Site of lesion is sebaceous (pilosebaceous) follicles

Primarily on face and upper trunk

Occurs in 85% of the population between the ages of 12 and 25

Exact cause: unknown

Causative factor: sebum accumulation/inflammation in pores of skin

Types

Noninflammatory acne

- Whiteheads
- Blackheads

Inflammatory acne

- Follicle walls rupture
- Sebum expels into dermis
- Inflammation begins
  - Pustules, cysts, and papules result

Cause

Unknown

Treatment

Topical

- Antibiotics
- Salicylic acid
- Benzoyl peroxide
- Tretinoin

Systemic

- Antibiotic
- Hormones
- Corticosteroids
- Isotretinoin

Diaper Dermatitis

Variety of disorders

Causes

   Urine

   Feces

   Plastic diaper cover

   Allergic reaction

   Secondary *Candida albicans* infection

Treatment

   Clean, dry area

   Expose to air

   Topical antifungal medications

   Topical steroids

Pruritus (Itching)

Symptom of skin disorder/dermatitis

Can be localized or generalized and is a condition not an inflammation

Results from stimulation of nerves of skin reacting to an allergen or irritation from substances in blood or foreign bodies

Causes

Primary skin disorder

   Example: eczema or lice

Systemic disease

   Example: chronic renal failure

Opiates

Allergic reaction

Treatment is for Underlying Condition

   Antihistamines

   Minor tranquilizers

   Application of emollients (lotions)

   Topical steroids

▪ Skin Infections

Bacterial

Impetigo

Most common in infants and children

   Usually on face and begins as small vesicles

   Caused primarily by *Staphylococcus*

   • Sometimes by group A beta-hemolytic *Streptococcus*

It is a highly contagious pyoderma

Treatment in Mild Cases

   Topical antibiotics

   Topical antiseptics

Treatment in Moderate Cases
Systemic antibiotics

Local compresses

Analgesics

Cellulitis
Caused primarily by *Staphylococcus*

Often secondary to an injury

Results in
Erythema, usually of lower trunk and legs

Fever

Localized pain

Lymphangitis

Treatment
Systemic antibiotics

Burow's soaks for pain relief

Furuncles (Boils)
Infected hair follicle

Usually caused by *Staphylococcus*

Developed boil drains pus and necrotic tissue

Squeezing spreads infection

Collection of furuncles that have merged is a carbuncle

Folliculitis
Infection of hair follicles

Results in
Erythema

Pustules

Causes
Skin trauma, such as irritation or friction

Poor hygiene

Excessive skin moisture

Treatment
Cleansing of area

Topical antibiotics

Erysipelas
Infection of skin

Cause
Group A beta-hemolytic *Streptococcus*

Common occurrence: face, ears, lower legs

Prior to outbreak, presents with

- Fever
- Malaise
- Chills

Lesions Appear as

Bright red and hot

- Develop raised borders
- Itching
- Burning
- Tenderness

Acute Necrotizing Fasciitis

Flesh-Eating Disease

Virulent strain of gram-positive, group A beta-hemolytic *Streptococcus*

Mortality rate of over 40%

Causes

Skin trauma

Skin infection

Areas Secrete Tissue-Destroying Enzyme, Proteases

Extreme inflammation and pain

Rapidly increasing

Dermal gangrene develops

Systemic Toxicity May Develop with

Fever

Disorientation

Hypotension

Tachycardia (fast heart rate)

May lead to organ failure

Treatment

Antimicrobial therapy

Fluid replacement

Removal of areas of infection

Viral

Herpes Simplex (Cold Sores)

Causes

Herpes simplex virus type 1 (HSV-1)

- Most common type
- Results in fever blisters or cold sores on or near lips or canker sores of the mouth

Herpes simplex virus type 2 (HSV-2)

- Genital and oral type
- Prominent sexually transmitted disease

Primary infections may show no symptoms (asymptomatic)

Virus remains in nerve tissue to later reactivate

Reactivation May be Triggered by

Stress

Common cold

Exposure to sun

Presents with

Burning or tingling

Develops Painful Vesicles that Rupture

Causes spreading

May cause secondary infection of eye

- Episode lasts several weeks
- Treatment may include antiviral medication
  - No permanent cure exists

Herpes Zoster (Shingles)

Usually older adult

Caused by Varicella-Zoster Virus (VZV)

Virus was dormant and then reactivates

Result of varicella or chickenpox, usually in childhood

Affects

One cranial nerve or one dermatome (an area of skin supplied with afferent nerve fibers by a posterior spinal root)

Results in

Pain

Rash (unilateral)

Paresthesia (abnormal touch sensation, such as burning)

Course

Several weeks

Pain may continue even after lesion disappears

Treatment

Clears spontaneously

Antiviral medications provide symptomatic relief

Sedatives

Analgesic

Antipruritics

Warts (Verrucae)

Verruca vulgaris (common wart)

Caused by human papillomavirus (HPV)

- Numerous types of HPV

Spread by contact

Appear anywhere on body

Present with a grayish appearance

Variety of shapes and sizes

Transmitted by touch

Plantar warts (verrucae) are located on pressure points of body (such as feet; *plantar* means the bottom surface of foot)

Painful when pressure is applied

Juvenile warts occur on feet and hands of children

Venereal warts occur on genitals/anus

Treatment

Liquid nitrogen

Topical keratolytics

Laser

Electrocautery

Often persist even with treatment

Fungal (Mycoses)

Usually superficial dermatophytes (fungus)

Fungus lives off dead cells

Tinea

Superficial skin infections

Tinea capitis

- Infection of scalp
- Common in children
- Treatment with oral antifungal medication

Tinea corporis (ringworm)

- Infection of body
- Presents as a red ring
- Produces burning sensation and pruritus
- Treatment with topical antifungal medication

Tinea pedis (athlete's foot)

- Involves feet and toes
- Produces pain, inflammation, fissures, and foul odor
- Treatment with topical antifungal medication

Tinea unguium (onychomycosis)

- Nail infection
  - Usually toenails
- Nail turns white then brown, thickens and cracks
- Spreads to other nails

Candidiasis

Caused by *Candida albicans*

Normally on mucous membranes of gastrointestinal tract and vagina

Poor health and certain conditions predispose individuals to overarching infection by *Candida*

- Antibiotic therapy, which changes the balance of the normal flora in the body

Treatment is topical or oral antifungal medications

Tumors of Skin

Benign Tumors

Keratosis(es)

Seborrheic Keratosis

Proliferation of basal cells

Dark-colored lesion

Found on trunk and face

Actinic Keratosis

Pigmented, scaly patch

Often caused by exposure to sun

Often in fair-skinned individuals

Premalignant lesion

May develop into squamous cell carcinoma

Treatment with cryosurgery (freezing area) or excision

Keratoacanthoma

Occurs in hair follicles

Usually in those over 60

Often on face, neck, back of hands, and other locations exposed to the sun

Resolve spontaneously or are excised

Moles (Nevi)

Located on any body part

Various shapes and sizes

May become malignant

- Especially if located in area of continual irritation

Malignant Tumors

Squamous Cell Carcinoma

Similar to basal cell carcinoma

Grows wherever squamous epithelium is located (skin, mouth, pharynx, esophagus, lungs, bladder)

Most often appears in areas exposed to sun (actinic keratosis—precancerous)

Scaly appearance

Rarely metastatic (spreading)

Easily treated with good prognosis

Surgical excision

Cryotherapy

Curettage

Electrodesiccation

Radiotherapy

Basal Cell Carcinoma

Common type of skin cancer

Developed in deeper skin layers (basal cells) than squamous cell carcinoma

Often occurs with sun exposure in fair-skinned individuals

Shiny appearance and slow growing

Easily treated with good prognosis

Malignant Melanoma

Originates in cells that produce pigment (melanocytes) or nevi

Increased Incidence with

Sun exposure

Fair hair and skin, freckles

Genetic predisposition

Skin nevus (mole) often brown and evenly colored with irregular borders

Grow downward into tissues

- Metastasize quickly

Treatment is removal with extensive border excision

- Depending on extent, chemotherapy or radiation therapy may be used

Kaposi's Sarcoma

Rare form of vascular skin cancer

Associated with

Human immunodeficiency virus (HIV)

Acquired immunodeficiency syndrome (AIDS)

Herpes virus may be found in lesions

Cells originate from endothelium in small blood vessels

Painful lesions develop rapidly, appearing as purple papules; spread quickly to lymph nodes and internal organs

Treatment

Radiation

Chemotherapy

Merkel Cell Carcinoma

Neuroendocrine carcinoma of skin

Rare and very aggressive

Associated with

Sun-exposed skin in elderly patients

Treatment with excision, radiation, and chemotherapy

CHAPTER 1: PATHOPHYSIOLOGY QUIZ

(Quiz answers are located in Appendix B)

1. A pimple is an example of a:
   a. papule
   b. vesicle
   c. pustule
   d. nodule

2. A Stage III pressure ulcer involves:
   a. erythema of skin
   b. partial loss of epidermis and dermis
   c. full thickness loss of skin up to but not through fascia
   d. full thickness loss of skin with extensive destruction and necrosis

3. This type of dermatitis may be exogenous or endogenous and is common in children and infants:
   a. atopic
   b. irritant contact
   c. stasis
   d. seborrheic

4. Psoriasis, pityriasis, and lichen planus are three types of this disorder:
   a. dermatitis
   b. inflammatory
   c. acne
   d. papulosquamous

5. This condition begins with a herald spot:
   a. psoriasis
   b. pityriasis
   c. lichen planus
   d. dermatitis

6. This skin infection is caused by group A beta-hemolytic *Streptococcus*, and the lesions appear as firm red spots with itching, burning, and tenderness:
   a. furuncles
   b. folliculitis
   c. erysipelas
   d. fasciitis

7. This type of herpes produces cold sores:
   a. herpes zoster
   b. shingles
   c. VZV
   d. herpes simplex

8. This condition is caused by human papillomavirus:
   a. mycoses
   b. verrucae
   c. shingles
   d. folliculitis

9. This type of tumor occurs in hair follicles:
   a. keratoses
   b. nevi
   c. Kaposi's sarcoma
   d. keratoacanthoma

10. This type of superficial carcinoma is rarely metastatic:
    a. squamous cell
    b. basal cell
    c. melanoma
    d. Kaposi's sarcoma

CHAPTER 2: MUSCULOSKELETAL SYSTEM

Anatomy and Terminology

■ Skeletal System

Comprises 206 bones, cartilage, and ligaments

Provides organ protection, movement, framework, stores calcium, hematopoiesis (formation of blood cells)

Classification of Bones
Long Bones (Tubular)
Length exceeds width of bone

Broad at ends, such as thigh, lower leg, upper arm, and lower arm

Short Bones (Cuboidal)
Cubelike bones, such as carpals (wrist) and tarsals (ankle)

Flat
Thin—flattened with curved surfaces

Cover body parts, such as skull, scapula, sternum, ribs

Irregular
Varied shapes, such as zygoma of face or vertebrae

Sesamoid
Rounded

Found near joint, such as patella (kneecap)

Patella is largest sesamoid bone in body

■ Structure

Long Bones (Fig. 2-1)
Diaphysis: shaft

Epiphysis: both ends of long bones—bulbular shape with muscle attachments
- Articular cartilage covers epiphyses and serves as a cushion

Epiphyseal line or plate: growth plate that disappears when fully grown

Metaphysis: flared portion of bone near epiphyseal plate

Periosteum: dense, white outer covering (fibrous)

Cortical or compact bone: hard bone beneath periosteum mainly found in shaft
- Medullary cavity contains yellow marrow (fatty bone marrow)

Cancellous bones: spongy or trabecular
- Contains red bone marrow (blood cell development)

Endosteum is thin epithelial membrane lining medullary cavity of long bone

Two Skeletal Divisions
Axial (trunk)

Appendicular (appendages)

Axial Skeleton, Comprised of 80 Bones
Skull, hyoid bone, vertebral column, sacrum, ribs, and sternum

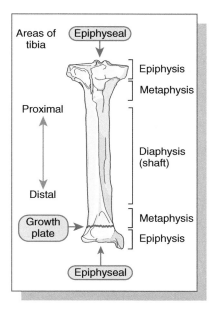

Figure **2-1** Structure of bones.

Skull (Fig. 2-2)
Cranial

Frontal (forehead)

Parietal (sides and top)

Temporal (lower sides)

Occipital (posterior of cranium)

Sphenoid (floor of cranium)

Ethmoid (area between orbits and nasal cavity)

Styloid process (below ear)

Zygomatic process (cheek)

Middle Ear Bones (Fig. 2-3)

Malleus (hammer)

Incus (anvil)

Stapes (stirrup)

Face (Fig. 2-4)

Nasal (bridge of nose)

Maxilla (upper jaw)

Zygomatic (arch of cheekbone)

Mandible (lower jawbone)

Lacrimal (near orbits)

Palate (separates oral and nasal cavities)

Vomer (base, nasal septum)

Nasal conchae (turbinates)

    Interior

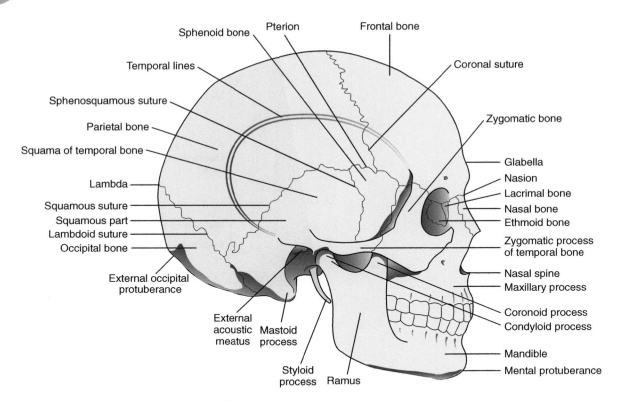

Figure **2-2** Lateral view of skull.

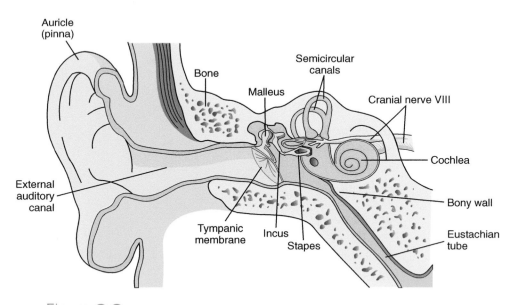

Figure **2-3** Structure of ear and three divisions of external, middle, and inner ear.

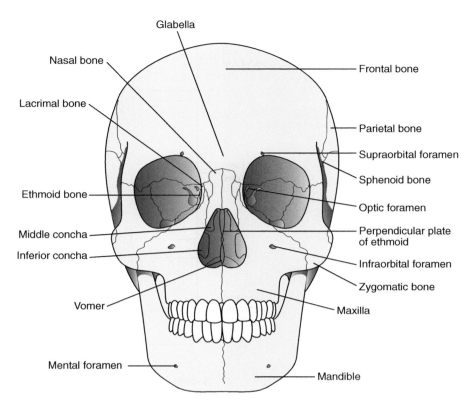

Figure **2-4** Frontal view of skull.

Middle

Superior

Hyoid
Supports tongue

U shaped

Attached by ligaments and muscles to larynx and skull

Spine (33 Vertebrae) (Fig. 2-5)
Cervical vertebrae (7)

- C1-7
- (C1)-atlas
- (C2)-axis

Thoracic vertebrae (12) (T1-12)

Lumbar vertebrae (5) (L1-5)

Sacrum (5)—fused in adults

Coccyx (4)—fused in adults

Thorax (Fig. 2-6)
Ribs, 12 pairs

- True ribs, 1-7
- False ribs, 8-10
- Floating ribs, 11 and 12

Sternum

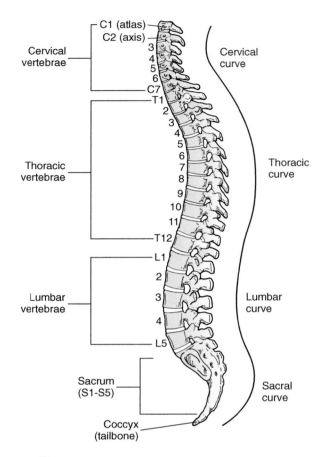

Figure **2-5** Anterior view of vertebral column.

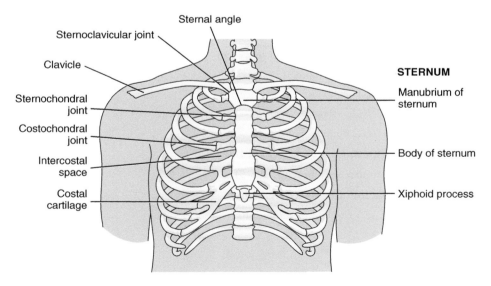

Figure **2-6** The thoracic cage.

Appendicular Skeleton, Comprised of 126 Bones (Fig. 2-7)
Shoulder, Girdle, Pelvic Girdle, and Extremities
Pelvis

Ilium (uppermost part), wing shaped

- Acetabulum, depression on lateral hip surface into which head of femur fits

Ischium (posterior part)

Pubis (anterior part)

Pubis symphysis (cartilage between pubic bones)

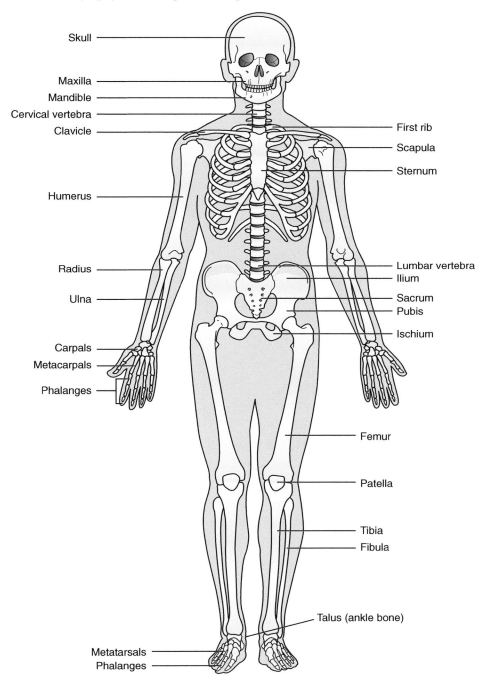

Figure **2-7** Skeletal system.

Lower Extremities
Femur (Thighbone)
Trochanter (processes at neck of femur)

Head fits into acetabulum

Patella (kneecap)

Tibia (shinbone)

Fibula (smaller lateral bone in lower leg)

Talus (ankle bone)

Calcaneus (heel bone)

Metatarsals (foot instep)

Phalanges (toes)

Lateral malleolus (lower part of fibula)

Medial malleolus (lower part of tibia)

Upper Extremities
Clavicle (collarbone)

Scapula (shoulder blade)

Humerus (upper arm)

Radius (forearm, thumb side)

Ulna (forearm, little finger side)

Olecranon (projection of ulna at elbow)

Carpals (wrist)—eight bones bound by ligaments in two rows with 4 bones in each

Metacarpals (hand)—framework or palm of hand (5 bones)

Phalanges (finger)

Olecranon (tip of elbow)

Joints (Articulations)
Condyle, rounded end of bone

Classified by degree of movement
- Synarthrosis (immovable and fibrous)

  Example: joint between cranial bones
- Amphiarthrosis (slightly movable and cartilaginous)

  Example: intervertebral (joint between bodies of vertebra)
- Diarthrosis (considerably movable and synovial)

Types
- Uniaxial—hinge and pivot joints

    Example—elbow (hinge and pivot) and cervical 2 (axis) (pivot)
- Biaxial—saddle and condyloid joints

    Example—thumb and joints between radius and carpal bones
- Multiaxial—ball and socket, gliding

    Example—shoulder and hip joints between articular surfaces of vertebrae

  Example: elbow, hip
- Bursa, sac of synovial fluid located in the tissues to prevent friction

▪ Muscular System

Functions

Heat production

Movement

Posture

Protection

Shape

▪ Muscle Tissue Types

Skeletal—600 Muscles Constituting 40% to 50% of Body Weight

Striated (cross-striped) (Figs. 2-8 and 2-9)

Move body

Voluntary

Attaches to bones

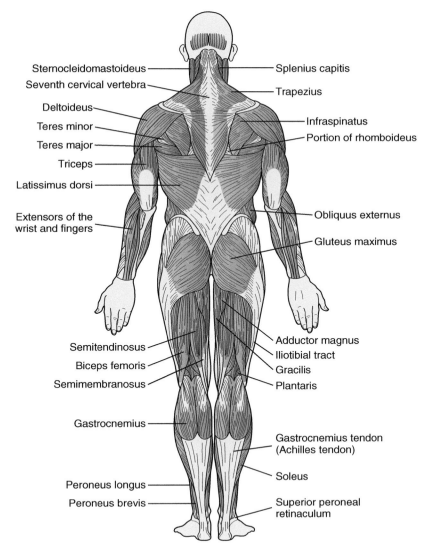

Figure **2-8** Muscular system, posterior view.

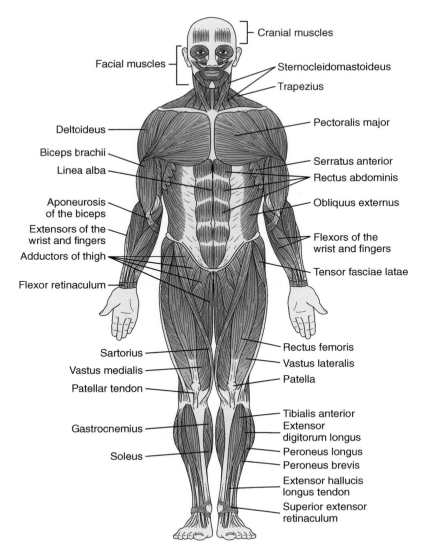

Figure **2-9** Muscular system, anterior view.

- Most attach to two bones with a joint in between
- Origin, point where muscle attaches to stationary bone
- Insertion, where muscle attaches to movable bone
- Body of muscle, main part of muscle

Cardiac/Heart Muscle
Striated and smooth muscle

Specialized cells that interlock so that muscle cells contract together

Involuntary

Moves blood by means of contractions

Smooth/Visceral
Linings such as bowel, urethra, blood vessels

Nonstriated

Involuntary

Tendons Anchor Muscle to Bone
Ligaments Anchor Bones to Bones

■ Muscle Action

Muscle Capabilities

Stretches

Contracts

Receives and responds to stimulus

Returns to original shape and length

Muscle Movement

Prime mover, responsible for movement (agonist)

Synergist, assists prime mover

Antagonist, relaxes as prime mover and synergists contract, resulting in movement

Fixator, acts as joint stabilizer

Terms of Movement—from Midline of Body

Flexion (bend)

Extension (straighten)

Abduction (away)

Adduction (toward)

Rotation (turn on axis)

Circumduction (circular)

Supination (turning palm upward or forward [anteriorly] or lying down with face upward)

Pronation (turning palm downward or backward or act of lying face down)

Hyperextension (overextension)

Inversion (inward)

Eversion (outward)

Names of Muscles

Head and Neck

Facial expression

- Occipitofrontalis (raises eyebrows and wrinkles forehead horizontally)
- Corrugator supercilii (wrinkles forehead vertically)
- Orbicularis oris (opens mouth)
- Zygomaticus (elevates corners of mouth)
- Orbicularis oculi (opens and closes eyelid)
- Buccinator (smiling and blowing)

Mastication (chewing)

- Masseter (used to chew closing jaw)
- Temporalis (closes jaw)
- Pterygoids (grates teeth)

Muscles moving head

- Sternocleidomastoid (flexes head)
- Semispinalis capitis (complexus) (extends head)
- Splenius capitis (extends head, bends and rotates head to side where muscle is contracting)

- Longissimus capitis (trachelomastoid muscle) (extends head, bends and rotates to contracting side)
- Trapezius (extends head)

Upper Extremities

Biceps brachii (flexes elbow)

Triceps brachii and anconeus (extends elbow)

Brachialis (flexes prone forearm)

Brachioradialis (flexes semi-prone/supinated forearm)

Deltoid (abducts upper arm)

Latissimus dorsi (extends upper arm)

Pectoralis major (flexes upper arm)

Trapezius (raises/lowers shoulder)

Trunk

External oblique (compresses abdomen)

Internal oblique (compresses abdomen)

Transversus abdominis (compresses abdomen)

Rectus abdominis (flexes trunk)

Quadratus lumborum (flexes vertebral column laterally)

Respiratory

Diaphragm (enlarges thorax/inspiration)

External intercostals (raise ribs)

Internal intercostal (depress ribs)

Lower Extremities

Thigh

- Gluteus group, maximus, medius, minimus (abducts thigh)
- Tensor fasciae latae (abducts thigh)
- Abductor group, brevis, longus, magnus (adducts thigh)
- Gracilis (adducts thigh)
- Iliopsoas (flexes thigh)
- Rectus femoris (flexes thigh)

Hamstring group, biceps femoris, semitendinosus, semimembranosus (extends thigh)

Quadriceps group, rectus femoris, vastus lateralis, vastus medialis, vastus intermedius (extends lower leg)

Sartorius (flexes, abducts, and rotates leg)

Lower leg

Tibialis anterior (dorsiflexes foot)

Peroneus group, longus, brevis, tertius (everts foot)

Gastrocnemius (calf, with soleus extends foot, also flexes knee)

Soleus (calf, extends foot)

Extensor digitorum longus (extends toes, flexes foot)

Achilles tendon (largest tendon, extending from gastrocnemius to calcaneus)

COMBINING FORMS

1.	acetabul/o	hip socket
2.	ankyl/o	bent, fused
3.	aponeur/o	tendon type
4.	arthr/o	joint
5.	articul/o	joint
6.	burs/o	fluid-filled sac in a joint
7.	calc/o, calci/o	calcium
8.	calcane/o	calcaneus (heel)
9.	carp/o	carpals (wrist bones)
10.	chondr/o	cartilage
11.	clavic/o, clavicul/o	clavicle (collar bone)
12.	cost/o	rib
13.	crani/o	cranium (skull)
14.	disc/o	intervertebral disc
15.	femor/o	thighbone
16.	fibul/o	fibula
17.	humer/o	humerus (upper arm bone)
18.	ili/o	ilium (upper pelvic bone)
19.	ischi/o	ischium (posterior pelvic bone)
20.	kinesi/o	movement
21.	kyph/o	hump
22.	lamin/o	lamina
23.	lord/o	curve
24.	lumb/o	lower back
25.	malleol/o	malleolus (process on lateral ankle)
26.	mandibul/o	mandible (lower jawbone)
27.	maxill/o	maxilla (upper jawbone)
28.	menisc/o	meniscus
29.	menisci/o	meniscus
30.	metacarp/o	metacarpals (hand)

31. metatars/o	metatarsals (foot)
32. myel/o	bone marrow
33. my/o, muscul/o	muscle
34. olecran/o	olecranon (elbow)
35. orth/o	straight
36. oste/o	bone
37. patell/o	patella (kneecap)
38. pelv/i	pelvis (hip)
39. perone/o	fibula
40. petr/o	stone
41. phalang/o	phalanges (finger or toe)
42. plant/o	sole of foot
43. pub/o	pubis
44. rachi/o	spine
45. radi/o	radius (lower arm)
46. rhabdomy/o	skeletal (striated muscle)
47. rheumat/o	watery flow (collection of fluids in joints)
48. sacr/o	sacrum
49. scapul/o	scapula (shoulder)
50. scoli/o	bent
51. spondyl/o	vertebra
52. stern/o	sternum (breast bone)
53. synovi/o	synovial joint membrane
54. tars/o	tarsal (ankle/foot)
55. ten/o	tendon
56. tend/o	tendon (connective tissue)
57. tendin/o	tendon (connective tissue)
58. tibi/o	shin bone
59. uln/o	ulna (lower arm bone)
60. vertebr/o	vertebra

PREFIXES

1.	inter-	between
2.	supra-	above
3.	sym-	together
4.	syn-	together

SUFFIXES

1.	-asthenia	weakness
2.	-blast	embryonic
3.	-clast, -clasia, -clasis	break
4.	-desis	bind together
5.	-listhesia	slipping
6.	-malacia	softening
7.	-physis	to grow
8.	-porosis	passage, cavity formation
9.	-schisis	split
10.	-stenosis	narrowing
11.	-tome	instrument that cuts
12.	-tomy	incision

MEDICAL ABBREVIATIONS

1.	ACL	anterior cruciate ligament
2.	AKA	above-knee amputation
3.	BKA	below-knee amputation
4.	C1-C7	cervical vertebrae
5.	CTS	carpal tunnel syndrome
6.	fx	fracture
7.	L1-L5	lumbar vertebrae
8.	OA	osteoarthritis
9.	RA	rheumatoid arthritis
10.	T1-T12	thoracic vertebrae
11.	TMJ	temporomandibular joint

MEDICAL TERMS

Arthrocentesis	Injection and/or aspiration of joint
Arthrodesis	Surgical immobilization of a joint
Arthrography	Radiography of joint
Arthroplasty	Reshaping or reconstruction of a joint
Arthroscopy	Use of scope to view inside joint
Arthrotomy	Incision into a joint
Articular	Pertains to a joint
Aspiration	Use of a needle and a syringe to withdraw fluid
Atrophy	Wasting away
Bunion	Hallux valgus, abnormal increase in size of metatarsal head that results in displacement of great toe
Bursitis	Inflammation of bursa (joint sac)
Carpal tunnel syndrome	Compression of medial nerve
Chondral	Referring to the cartilage
Closed fracture repair	Not surgically opened with/without manipulation and with/without traction
Closed treatment	Fracture site that is not surgically opened and visualized
Colles' fracture	Fracture at lower end of radius that displaces bone posteriorly
Dislocation	Placement in a location other than original location
Endoscopy	Inspection of body organs or cavities using a lighted scope that may be inserted through an existing opening or through a small incision
Fasciectomy	Removal of band of fibrous tissue
Fissure	Groove
Fracture	Break in a bone
Ganglion	Knot or knotlike mass
Internal/External fixation	Application of pins, wires, screws, placed externally or internally to immobilize a body part
Kyphosis	Humpback
Lamina	Flat plate
Ligament	Fibrous band of tissue that connects cartilage or bone
Lordosis	Anterior curvature of the spine
Lumbodynia	Pain in lumbar area

Lysis	Releasing
Manipulation or reduction	Alignment of a fracture or joint dislocation to normal position
Open fracture repair	Surgical opening (incision) over or remote opening as access to a fracture site
Osteoarthritis	Degenerative condition of articular cartilage
Osteoclast	Absorbs or removes bone
Osteotomy	Cutting into bone
Percutaneous	Through skin
Percutaneous fracture repair	Repair of a fracture by means of pins and wires inserted through the fracture site
Percutaneous skeletal fixation	Considered neither open nor closed; fracture is not visualized, but fixation is placed across fracture site under x-ray imaging
Reduction	Replacement to normal position
Scoliosis	Lateral curvature of the spine
Skeletal traction	Application of pressure to bone by means of pins and/or wires inserted into bone
Skin traction	Application of pressure to bone by means of tape applied to the skin
Spondylitis	Inflammation of vertebrae
Subluxation	Partial dislocation
Supination	Supine position—lying on back, face upward
Synchondrosis	Union between two bones (connected by cartilage)
Tendon	Attaches a muscle to a bone
Tenodesis	Suturing of a tendon to a bone
Tenorrhaphy	Suture repair of tendon
Traction	Application of pressure to maintain normal alignment
Trocar needle	Needle with a cannula that can be removed; used to puncture and withdraw fluid from a cavity

CHAPTER 2: ANATOMY AND TERMINOLOGY QUIZ

(Quiz answers are located in Appendix B)

1. Tubular is another name for these bones:
   a. short
   b. long
   c. flat
   d. irregular

2. These bones are found near joints:
   a. irregular
   b. flat
   c. sesamoid
   d. broad

3. Zygoma is an example of this type of bone:
   a. irregular
   b. flat
   c. sesamoid
   d. broad

4. Diaphysis is this part of bone:
   a. end
   b. surface
   c. shaft
   d. marrow

5. Which is NOT a part of cranium?
   a. condyle
   b. sphenoid
   c. ethmoid
   d. parietal

6. This is NOT an ear bone:
   a. malleus
   b. stapes
   c. incus
   d. styloid

7. This term describes growth plate:
   a. endosteum
   b. epiphyseal
   c. metaphysis
   d. periosteum

8. This is a depression on lateral hip surface into which head of femur fits:
   a. ilium
   b. ischium
   c. patella
   d. acetabulum

9. Tip of elbow is the:
   a. olecranon
   b. trapezium
   c. humerus
   d. tarsal

10. This term describes an immovable joint:
    a. amphiarthrosis
    b. diarthrosis
    c. synarthrosis
    d. ischium

Pathophysiology

■ Injuries

Fractures

Classification of Fractures

Open/Closed

Open (compound): broken bone penetrates skin

Closed (simple): broken bone does not penetrate skin

Complete/Incomplete

Complete: bone is broken all way through

   Example: oblique, linear, spiral, and transverse

Incomplete: bone is not broken all way through

   Example: greenstick, bowing, torus, stress, and transchondral

Treatment

   Closed reduction (realignment of bone fragments by manipulation)

   Reduction (the returning of the bone to normal alignment)

   Immobilization (returns to normal alignment and holds in place)

   Traction (application of pulling force to hold bone in alignment)

- Skeletal traction uses internal devices (pins, screws, wires, etc.) inserted into bone with ends sticking out through skin for attachment of traction device (Fig. 2-10)
- Skin traction is use of strapping, elastic wrap, or tape attached to skin to which weights are attached (Fig. 2-11)

Improper Union

   Nonunion: failure of bone ends to grow together

   Malunion: incorrect alignment of bone ends

   Delayed union: delay of bone union 8 or 9 months

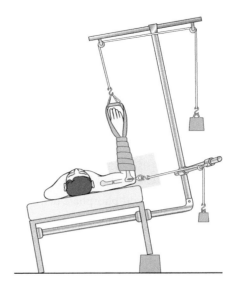

Figure **2-10** Skeletal traction uses patient's bones to secure internal devices to which traction is attached.

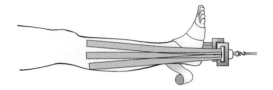

Figure **2-11** Skin traction utilizes strapping, wraps, or tape to which traction is attached.

Dislocations

Bone and soft tissue damage usually caused by trauma

Any part of bone is displaced

Can result in nerve and tissue damage

Treatment

Reduction

Immobilization

Sprains and Strains

Soft tissue damage usually caused by trauma to tendons and ligaments

Strain: partial tear of a tendon

Sprain results from overuse or overextension/tearing or rupture of some part of musculature

■ Bone Disorders

Osteomyelitis

Bone infection

Usually caused by bacteria

- Exogenous osteomyelitis is caused by bacteria that enter from outside body
- Hematogenous osteomyelitis (endogenous) is caused by a bacterial infection within body

Osteoporosis

Common disorder in postmenopausal women and elderly and most common metabolic disease

- Malabsorption of calcium and magnesium; certain trace elements and vitamins C and D contribute to bone loss

Decreased bone mass and density

- Fractures more common due to decrease in strength of bone

Treatment

Increased intake of calcium, magnesium, and vitamin D

Increased weight-bearing activity

Osteomalacia and Rickets

Osteomalacia is softened adult bones, whereas rickets is softened growing bones in children

Caused by vitamin D and phosphate deficiency

Osteitis Deformans (Paget's Disease)

Abnormal bone remodeling and resorption resulting in enlarged, soft bones

Unknown cause but strong genetic considerations

Treatment

Calcitonin and biophosphates

Spinal Curvatures

Lordosis: swayback

- Inward curvature of spine

Kyphosis: humpback

- Outward curvature of spine

Scoliosis

- Lateral curvature of spine

Spina Bifida

Congenital abnormality in which vertebrae do not close correctly around the spinal cord

■ Joint Disorders

Bursitis: inflammation of bursa (joint sac)

Arthritis: inflammation of joints

Osteoarthritis (OA)

This is degenerative or wear/tear arthritis

- DJD, degenerative joint disease

Chronic inflammation of joint

Increased pain on weightbearing or movement

Affects weight-bearing joints

- Loss of articular cartilage
- Sclerosis of bone—eburnation

Turning bone into ivorylike mass—polished

- Osteophytes (bone spurs)

Symptoms

Pain and stiffness

Crepitation (bone on bone creates characteristic grinding sound)

Classifications

Primary (idiopathic)

- No known cause

Secondary

- Associated with joint instability, joint stress, or congenital abnormalities

Treatment

Symptomatic

Arthroplasty

Rheumatoid Arthritis (RA)

Progressive inflammatory connective tissue disease of the joints

Systemic autoimmune disease

- Can invade arteries, lungs, skin, and other organs with inflammation or nodules

Affects small joints

- Destroys synovial membrane, articular cartilage, and surrounding tissues

Leads to loss of function due to fixation and deformity

Treatment

Pharmaceuticals to modify autoimmune and inflammatory processes

Gene therapy and stem cell transplantation are being researched

Symptomatic

Arthroplasty

Infectious and Septic Arthritis

Infectious process

Usually affects single joint

Without antimicrobial intervention, permanent joint damage results

Example: Lyme disease

Treatment

Antibiotics—early intervention

Gout (Gouty Arthritis)

Inflammatory arthritis

Often affects the joint of the great toe

Caused by excessive amounts of uric acid that crystallizes in connective tissue of joints

Leads to inflammation and destruction of joint

Treatment

Pharmaceuticals—nonsteroidal anti-inflammatory drugs

Ankylosing Spondylitis (AS)

Inflammatory disease that is progressive

Affects vertebral joints and insertion points of ligaments, tendons, and joint capsules

Leads to rigid spinal column and sacroiliac joints

Treatment

Nonsteroidal anti-inflammatory drugs relieve symptoms

Analgesics for pain

■ Tendon, Muscle, and Ligament Disorders

Muscular Dystrophy—Familial Disorder

Progressive degenerative muscle disorder

Multiple types of muscular dystrophy

Most often affects boys

- Genetic predisposition—Duchenne muscular dystrophy

Primary Fibromyalgia Syndrome
Symptoms

Generalized aching and pain

Tender points

Fatigue

Depression

Usually Appears in

Middle-aged women

Polymyositis
General muscle inflammation causing weakness

- With skin rash = dermatomyositis

Tumors

Bone Tumors
Origin of Bone Tumors
Osteogenic (bone cells)

Chondrogenic (cartilage cell)

Collagenic (fibrous tissue cell)

Myelogenic (marrow cell)

Osteoma
Benign

Abnormal outgrowth of bone

Chondroblastoma
Rare

Usually benign

Osteosarcoma
Malignant tumor of long bones

Usually in young adults

Typically causes bone pain

Multiple Myeloma
Malignant plasma cells in skeletal system and soft tissue

Progressive and generally fatal

Usually in those over 40

Chondrosarcoma
Malignant cartilage tumor

Usually in middle-aged and older individuals

In late stages, symptoms include local swelling and pain

- Worsens with time

Surgical excision is usually treatment of choice

If diagnosed in early stages, it is treatable with long-term survival possible

Muscle Tumors
Rare

Rhabdomyosarcoma

Aggressive, invasive carcinoma with widespread metastasis

CHAPTER 2: PATHOPHYSIOLOGY QUIZ

(Quiz answers are located in Appendix B)

1. A compound fracture is also known as:
   a. complete
   b. incomplete
   c. closed
   d. open

2. This is a common bone disorder in postmenopausal women resulting from lower levels of calcium and potassium:
   a. Paget's disease
   b. lordosis
   c. osteoporosis
   d. rheumatoid arthritis

3. This inflammatory disease is progressive and leads to a rigid spinal column:
   a. polymyositis
   b. ankylosing spondylitis
   c. primary fibromyalgia syndrome
   d. septic arthritis of spine

4. This type of tumor arises from bone cells:
   a. osteogenic
   b. chondrogenic
   c. collagenic
   d. myelogenic

5. This type of tumor is the most common type of malignant bone tumor that occurs in those over 40 and is progressive and generally fatal:
   a. rhabdomyosarcoma
   b. chondrosarcoma
   c. osteosarcoma
   d. multiple myeloma

6. A general muscle inflammation with an accompanying skin rash is:
   a. muscular dystrophy
   b. dermatologic arthritis
   c. ankylosing spondylitis
   d. dermatomyositis

7. A cartilage tumor that usually occurs in middle-aged and older individuals:
   a. chondrosarcoma
   b. osteosarcoma
   c. chondroblastoma
   d. rhabdomyosarcoma

8. Returning of bone to normal alignment is:
   a. immobilization
   b. traction
   c. reduction
   d. manipulation

9. Result of overuse or overextension of a ligament is:
   a. strain
   b. sprain
   c. fracture
   d. displacement

10. Primary osteoarthritis is also known as:
    a. secondary
    b. functional
    c. congenital
    d. idiopathic

CHAPTER 3: RESPIRATORY SYSTEM

Anatomy and Terminology

Supplies oxygen to body and helps clean body of waste (carbon dioxide)

Two tracts (Fig. 3-1A)

- Upper respiratory tract (nose, pharynx, and larynx)
- Lower respiratory tract (trachea, bronchial tree, and lungs)

Lined with ciliated mucosa

- Purifies air by trapping irritants

Warms and humidifies air

■ Upper Respiratory Tract (URT)

Nose

Sense of smell (olfactory)

Moistens and warms air

Nasal septum divides interior

Sinuses (Paranasal or Accessory Sinuses) (4 Pair)

Frontal

Ethmoid

Maxillary

Sphenoid

Turbinates (Conchae)

Bones on inside of nose

Divided into inferior, middle, and superior (Fig. 3-1B)

Warms and humidifies air

Pharynx (Throat)

Passageway for both food and air

Nasopharynx contains adenoids

Oropharynx contains tonsils

Laryngopharynx leads to larynx

Larynx (Voice Box) (Opening to Trachea)

Contains vocal cords

- Cartilages of larynx, thyroid, epiglottis, and arytenoid

■ Lower Respiratory Tract (LRT)

Trachea (Windpipe)—Air-Conducting Structure

Mucus-lined tube with C-shaped cartilage rings to hold windpipe open

Segmental Bronchi

Trachea divides into right and left main bronchus, which further divide into lobar bronchii—3 on right, 2 on left

Bronchioles

Branches divide into secondary bronchi, then smaller bronchioles

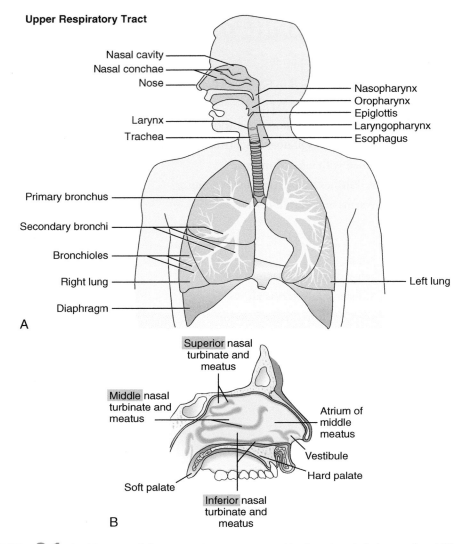

Figure 3-1 A. Upper and lower respiratory system. B. Superior, inferior, and middle nasal turbinates.

Alveolar Ducts (Minute Branches of Bronchial Tree)

End in alveoli (sacs) of simple squamous cells

- Primary gas-exchange units

    Surrounded by capillaries and where exchange of oxygen and carbon dioxide takes place

Lungs

Covered by pleura

Cone-shaped organs filling thoracic cavity

Base rests on diaphragm and apex (top of lungs) extends to above clavicles

Hilum is medial surface of lung where pulmonary artery, pulmonary veins, nerves, lymphatics, and bronchial tubes enter and exit

Left lung contains two lobes divided by fissures

Right lung contains three lobes

Respiration

Inspiration—oxygen moves in, downward movement of lungs enlarging thoracic cavity

Expiration—carbon dioxide moves out, upward movement of diaphragm decreasing lung space

COMBINING FORMS

1.	adenoid/o	adenoid
2.	alveol/o	alveolus
3.	atel/o	incomplete
4.	bronch/o	bronchus
5.	bronchi/o	bronchus
6.	bronchiol/o	bronchiole
7.	capn/o	carbon dioxide
8.	coni/o	dust
9.	cyan/o	blue
10.	diaphragmat/o	diaphragm
11.	epiglott/o	epiglottis
12.	laryng/o	larynx
13.	lob/o	lobe
14.	mediastin/o	mediastinum
15.	muc/o	mucus
16.	nas/o	nose
17.	orth/o	straight
18.	ox/o	oxygen
19.	oxy/o	oxygen
20.	pector/o	chest
21.	pharyng/o	pharynx
22.	phon/o	voice
23.	phren/o	diaphragm
24.	pleur/o	pleura
25.	pneum/o	lung/air
26.	pneumat/o	air
27.	pneumon/o	lung/air
28.	pulmon/o	lung

29. py/o	pus
30. rhin/o	nose
31. sept/o	septum
32. sinus/o	sinus
33. spir/o	breath
34. tel/o	complete
35. thorac/o	thorax
36. tonsill/o	tonsil
37. trache/o	trachea

PREFIXES

1. a-	not
2. an-	not
3. endo-	within
4. eu-	good
5. dys-	difficult
6. pan-	all
7. poly-	many

SUFFIXES

1. -algia	pain
2. -ar	pertaining to
3. -ary	pertaining to
4. -capnia	carbon dioxide
5. -centesis	puncture to remove (drain)
6. -dynia	pain
7. -eal	pertaining to
8. -ectasis	stretching
9. -emia	blood
10. -gram	record
11. -graph	recording instrument
12. -graphy	recording process

13. -itis	inflammation
14. -meter	measurement or instrument that measures
15. -metry	measurement of
16. -osmia	smell
17. -oxia	oxygen
18. -pexy	fixation
19. -phonia	sound
20. -pnea	breathing
21. -ptysis	spitting
22. -rrhage, -rrhagia	abnormal, excessive flow
23. -scopy	to examine
24. -spasm	contraction of muscle
25. -sphyxia	pulse
26. -stenosis	blockage, narrowing
27. -stomy	opening
28. -thorax	chest
29. -tomy	cutting, incision

MEDICAL ABBREVIATIONS

1. ABG	arterial blood gas
2. AFB	acid-fast bacillus
3. ARDS	adult respiratory distress syndrome
4. BiPAP	bi-level positive airway pressure
5. COPD	chronic obstructive pulmonary disease
6. CPAP	continuous positive airway pressure
7. DLCO	diffuse capacity of lungs for carbon monoxide
8. FEF	forced expiratory flow
9. FEV_1	forced expiratory volume in 1 second
10. $FEV_1:FVC$	maximum amount of forced expiratory volume in 1 second
11. FRC	functional residual capacity
12. FVC	forced vital capacity

13.	HHN	hand-held nebulizer
14.	IPAP	inspiratory positive airway pressure
15.	IRDS	infant respiratory distress syndrome
16.	MDI	metered-dose inhaler
17.	MVV	maximum voluntary ventilation
18.	PAWP	pulmonary artery wedge pressure
19.	PCWP	pulmonary capillary wedge pressure
20.	PEAP	positive end-airway pressure
21.	PEEP	positive end-expiratory pressure
22.	PFT	pulmonary function test
23.	PND	paroxysmal nocturnal dyspnea
24.	RDS	respiratory distress syndrome
25.	RSV	respiratory syncytial virus
26.	RV	respiratory volume
27.	RV:TLC	ratio of respiratory volume to total lung capacity
28.	TLC	total lung capacity
29.	TLV	total lung volume
30.	URI	upper respiratory infection
31.	V/Q	ventilation/perfusion scan

MEDICAL TERMS

Ablation	Removal or destruction by cutting, chemicals, or electrocautery
Adenoidectomy	Removal of adenoids
Apnea	Cessation of breathing
Asphyxia	Lack of oxygen
Asthma	Shortage of breath caused by contraction of bronchi
Atelectasis	Incomplete expansion of lung, collapse
Auscultation	Listening to sounds, such as to lung sounds
Bacilli	Plural of bacillus, a rod-shaped bacteria
Bilobectomy	Surgical removal of two lobes of a lung
Bronchiole	Smaller division of bronchial tree

Bronchoplasty	Surgical repair of bronchi
Bronchoscopy	Inspection of bronchial tree using a bronchoscope
Catheter	Tube placed into body to put fluid in or take fluid out
Cauterization	Destruction of tissue by use of cautery
Cordectomy	Surgical removal of vocal cord(s)
Crackle	Abnormal sound when breathing (heard on auscultation)
Croup	Acute viral infection (obstruction of larynx), stridor
Cyanosis	Bluish discoloration
Drainage	Free flow or withdrawal of fluids from a wound or cavity
Dysphonia	Speech impairment
Dyspnea	Shortage of breath, difficult breathing
Emphysema	Air accumulated in organ or tissue
Epiglottidectomy	Excision of covering of larynx
Epistaxis	Nose bleed
Glottis	True vocal cords
Hemoptysis	Bloody sputum
Intramural	Within organ wall
Intubation	Insertion of a tube
Laryngeal web	Congenital abnormality of connective tissue between vocal cords
Laryngectomy	Surgical removal of larynx
Laryngoplasty	Surgical repair of larynx
Laryngoscope	Fiberoptic scope used to view inside of larynx
Laryngoscopy	Direct visualization and examination of interior of larynx with a laryngoscope
Laryngotomy	Incision into larynx
Lavage	Washing out
Lobectomy	Surgical excision of a lobe of lung
Nasal button	Synthetic circular disc used to cover a hole in the nasal septum
Orthopnea	Difficulty in breathing, relieved by assuming upright position
Percussion	Tapping with sharp blows as a diagnostic technique
Pertussis	Whooping cough—highly contagious bacterial infection of pharynx, larynx, and trachea

Pharyngolaryngectomy	Surgical removal of pharynx and larynx
Pleura	Covers lungs and lines thoracic cavity
Pleurectomy	Surgical excision of pleura
Pleuritis	Inflammation of pleura
Pneumocentesis/ pneumonocentesis	Surgical puncturing of a lung to withdraw fluid
Pneumonia	Inflammation of lungs with consolidation
Pneumonolysis/pneumolysis	Surgical separation of lung from chest wall to allow lung to collapse
Pneumonotomy/pneumotomy	Incision of lung
Pulmonary edema	Accumulation of fluid in pulmonary tissues and air spaces
Pulmonary embolism	Thrombus or other foreign material lodged in pulmonary artery or one of its branches
Rales	An abnormal respiratory sound heard in auscultation, indicating some pathologic condition
Rhinoplasty	Surgical repair of nose
Rhinorrhea	Free discharge of a thin nasal mucus
Sarcoidosis	Chronic inflammatory disease with nodules developing in lungs, lymph nodes, other organs
Segmentectomy	Surgical removal of the smaller subdivisions (segment) of lobes of a lung
Septoplasty	Surgical repair of nasal septum
Sinusotomy	Surgical incision into a sinus
Spirometry	Measuring breathing capacity
Tachypnea	Quick, shallow breathing
Thoracentesis/thoracocentesis (pleuracentesis/ pleurocentesis)	Surgical puncture of thoracic cavity, usually using a needle, to remove fluids
Thoracoplasty	Surgical procedure that removes rib(s) and thereby allows collapse of a lung
Thoracoscopy	Use of a lighted endoscope to view pleural spaces and thoracic cavity or to perform surgical procedures
Thoracostomy	Surgical incision into chest wall and insertion of a chest tube
Thoracotomy	Surgical incision into chest wall
Total pneumonectomy	Surgical removal of an entire lung
Tracheostomy	Creation of an opening into trachea
Tracheotomy	Incision into trachea
Transtracheal	Across trachea
Tuberculosis	Infection of the lungs caused by bacteria (tubercle bacillus)

CHAPTER 3: ANATOMY AND TERMINOLOGY QUIZ

(Quiz answers are located in Appendix B)

1. This is NOT a part of lower respiratory tract:
   a. trachea
   b. larynx
   c. bronchi
   d. lungs

2. Another name for voice box is:
   a. oropharynx
   b. pharynx
   c. laryngopharynx
   d. larynx

3. This is the windpipe:
   a. pharynx
   b. larynx
   c. trachea
   d. sphenoid

4. Interior of nose is divided by the:
   a. septum
   b. sphenoid
   c. oropharynx
   d. apical

5. This combining form means "incomplete":
   a. atel/o
   b. alveol/o
   c. ox/i
   d. pneumat/o

6. This combining form means "breath":
   a. py/o
   b. lob/o
   c. spir/o
   d. pleur/o

7. This prefix means "all":
   a. a-
   b. an-
   c. pan-
   d. poly-

8. This abbreviation refers to a syndrome that involves difficulty in breathing:
   a. ABG
   b. ARDS
   c. BiPAP
   d. FEF

9. This abbreviation refers to amount of air patient can expel from the lungs in 1 second:
   a. PFT
   b. PND
   c. RDS
   d. FEV_1

10. This suffix means "breathing":
    a. -stenosis
    b. -spasm
    c. -pexy
    d. -pnea

Pathophysiology

■ Signs and Symptoms of Pulmonary Disorders

Dyspnea
Difficult breathing (sense of air hunger)

Increased respiratory effort

Hypoventilation
Decreased alveolar ventilation

Hyperventilation
Increased alveolar ventilation

Hemoptysis
Bloody sputum

Hypoxia
Reduced oxygenation of tissue cells

Cough
Caused by irritant

Protective reflex

Acute cough is up to 3 weeks

Chronic cough is over 3 weeks

Tachypnea
Rapid breathing

Apnea
Lack of breathing

Orthopnea
Requiring sitting upright to facilitate breathing

■ Pulmonary Diseases and Disorders

Hypercapnia
Increased carbon dioxide in arterial blood

Caused by inadequate ventilation of alveoli

Can result in respiratory acidosis

Hypoxemia
Reduced oxygenation of arterial blood

Acute Respiratory Failure
Inadequate gas exchange

Hypoxemia

Can result from trauma or disease

Adult Respiratory Distress Syndrome (ARDS)
Acute injury to alveolocapillary membrane

Results in edema and atelectasis

In infants, infant respiratory distress syndrome (IRDS)

Pulmonary Edema

Accumulation of fluid in lung tissue

Most common cause is left ventricular failure

Aspiration

Passage of fluid and solid particles into lung

Can cause severe pneumonitis

- Localized inflammation of lung

Atelectasis

Collapse of lung

Three most common types are:

- Adhesive
- Compression
- Obstruction

May be chronic or acute

- Acute, such as compression as a result of an automobile accident
- Chronic from structural defect

Absorption Atelectasis

Results from absence of air in alveoli

Caused by

Foreign body

Tumor

Abnormal external pressure

Bronchiectasis

Chronic, irreversible dilation of bronchi

Common Types that Describe Severity of Condition

- Cylindrical
- Varicose
- Saccular or cystic

Respiratory Acidosis

Decreased level of pH

Due to excess retention of carbon dioxide

Bronchiolitis

Inflammation and obstruction of bronchioles

Usually in children younger than 2 years old—preceded by URI

Viral infection (respiratory syncytial virus, or RSV)

Common Types

- Constrictive
- Proliferative
- Obliterative

Pneumothorax

Air collected in pleural cavity

Leads to lung collapse

Communicating pneumothorax is barometric air pressure in pleural space

Spontaneous pneumothorax is spontaneous rupture of visceral pleura

Secondary pneumothorax is a result of trauma to chest

Pneumoconiosis

Dust particles or other particulate matter in lung

Common Types

- Coal
- Asbestos
- Fiberglass

Pleural Effusion–Fluid in Pleural Space

Common Types

- Hemothorax—hemorrhage into pleural cavity
- Empyema—Infectious materials in pleural space
- Exudate—Fluid remaining after infection, inflammation, malignancy

Empyema

Infectious Pleural Effusion

Pus in pleural space

Complication of respiratory infection

Commonly follows pneumonia and is treated like pneumonia

Pulmonary Embolism

Air, tissue, or clot occlusion

Lodges in pulmonary artery or branch of artery

Risk with congestive heart failure

Most clots originate in leg veins

Cor Pulmonale

Hypertrophy or failure of right ventricle

Result of lung, pulmonary vessels, or chest wall disorders

Acute is secondary to pulmonary embolus

Chronic is secondary to obstructive lung disease

Pleurisy (Pleuritis)

Inflammation of pleura

Often preceded by an upper respiratory infection

Infectious Disease

Upper Respiratory Infection (URI)

Acute inflammatory process of mucous membranes in trachea and above

Common Types

- Common cold
- Croup
- Sinusitis
- Laryngitis

■ Lower Respiratory Infection (LRI)

Pneumonia

Inflammation of lungs with consolidation

Categorized according to causative organism

Can be caused by

  Aspiration

  Bacteria

  Protozoa

  Fungi

  Chlamydia

  Virus

Common Types

  Aspiration pneumonia

  Bacterial

  Chlamydial

  Drug resistant

  Eosinophil

  Fungal

  Hospital acquired (nosocomial)

  Legionnaires' disease

  Mycoplasma

  Pneumococcal

  Viral

Tuberculosis

Communicable lung disease—airborne droplet

Caused by *Mycobacterium tuberculosis* (bacilli)

Chronic Obstructive Pulmonary Disease (COPD)

Irreversible airway obstruction that decreases expiration

Includes

Chronic bronchitis

- Bronchial spasms
- Dyspnea
- Wheezing
- Productive cough
- Cyanosis
- Chronic hypoventilation
- Polycythemia
- Cor pulmonale
- Prolonged expiration

Emphysema

- Loss of elasticity and enlargement of alveoli
- Mimics symptoms of chronic bronchitis but more exaggerated

CHAPTER 3: PATHOPHYSIOLOGY QUIZ

(Quiz answers are located in Appendix B)

1. Acute injury to alveolocapillary membrane that results in edema and atelectasis:
   a. hypoxemia
   b. adult respiratory distress syndrome
   c. bronchiolitis
   d. pneumoconiosis

2. Condition in which pus is in pleural space and is often a complication of pneumonia:
   a. empyema
   b. cor pulmonale
   c. pneumothorax
   d. atelectasis

3. Which of the following is NOT one of the most common types of atelectasis?
   a. adhesive
   b. compression
   c. obstruction
   d. expansion

4. This condition is a result of accumulation of dust particles in lung:
   a. pleurisy
   b. tuberculosis
   c. chronic obstructive pulmonary disease
   d. pneumoconiosis

5. An irreversible airway obstructive disease in which symptoms are bronchial spasm, dyspnea, and wheezing:
   a. pleurisy
   b. empyema
   c. bronchiolitis
   d. COPD

6. Cylindrical, varicose, and secular/cystic are examples of:
   a. bronchiectasis
   b. cor pulmonale
   c. pneumothorax
   d. atelectasis

7. Condition in which there is a loss of elasticity and enlargement of alveoli:
   a. chronic bronchitis
   b. asthma
   c. emphysema
   d. empyema

8. Definition of a chronic cough is one that lasts for more than this number of weeks:
   a. 2
   b. 3
   c. 4
   d. 5

9. A condition marked by an increase in carbon dioxide in arterial blood and decreased ability to breathe that can result in respiratory acidosis:
   a. hypercapnia
   b. hypoxemia
   c. acute respiratory failure
   d. pulmonary edema

10. This condition often follows a viral infection and occurs in children under 2 years of age. Examples of various types of this condition are constrictive, proliferating, and obliterative.
    a. pneumoconiosis
    b. pulmonary edema
    c. bronchiolitis
    d. bronchiectasis

CHAPTER 4: CARDIOVASCULAR SYSTEM

Anatomy and Terminology

Consists of blood, blood vessels, and heart

■ Blood (Function Is to Maintain a Constant Environment)

Composed of cells suspended in plasma (clear, straw-colored liquid)

Carries

Oxygen and nutrients to cells

Waste and carbon dioxide to kidneys, liver, and lungs

Hormones from endocrine system

Regulates

Temperature by circulating blood

Protection

White cells (leukocytes) produce antibodies

Composed of Two Parts

Liquid Part (Extracellular) is Plasma

Water 91%

Protein 1%, albumin, globulins, fibrinogen, ferritin, transferrin

2% ions, nutrients, waste products, gases, regulating substances

Cellular Structures

Leukocytes (WBCs)—granular and agranular—fight infections

- Neutrophils
- Lymphocytes
- Monocytes
- Eosinophils
- Basophils

Erythrocytes (red blood cells)—hemoglobin carries oxygen

Thrombocytes (platelets)—important for hemostasis

Blood types: A, B, AB, and O are genetically endowed

- Blood type O negative is known as universal donor (no Rh and no red cell antigens present)

■ Vessels—Circulatory System

Function

To carry blood delivering nutrients and oxygen (arterial system) and carry away cell waste and carbon dioxide (venous system)

Types

Arteries (Fig. 4-1) Carrying Oxygenated Blood

Inner layer, endothelium

Lead away from heart

Branches are arterioles

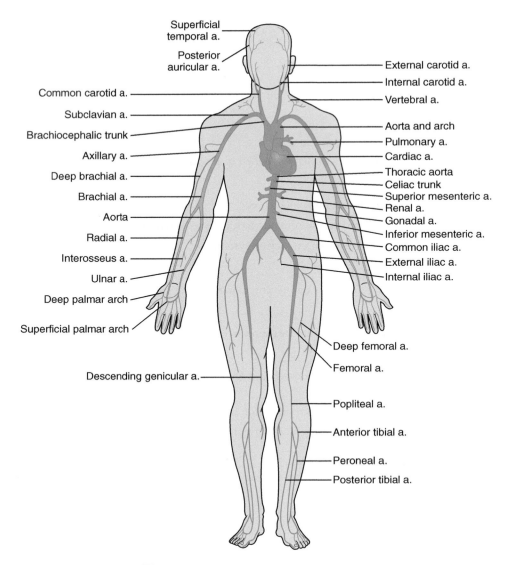

Figure **4-1** Arteries of circulatory system.

Capillaries

Connection between arterioles and venules

Exchange structure (oxygen and carbon dioxide, nutrients, and waste)

Veins (Fig. 4-2) Carrying Deoxygenated Blood

Carry blood to heart

Venules are small branches

■ Heart

Circulates blood

Four Chambers (Fig. 4-3)

Two Upper

Right and left atria (singular: atrium) receive blood

Two Lower

Right and left ventricles discharge blood (pump)

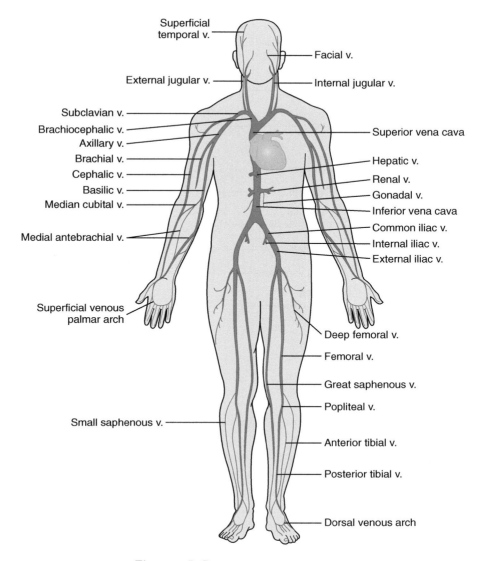

Figure **4-2** Veins of circulatory system.

Chamber Walls
Composed of three layers

- Endocardium: smooth inner layer
- Myocardium: middle muscular layer
- Epicardium: outer layer

Septa (Singular: Septum)
Divide chambers

- Interatrial septum

  Separates two upper chambers
- Interventricular septum

  Separates two lower chambers

Major Blood Vessels
Inferior vena cava—carries deoxygenated blood from lower extremities, pelvic and abdominal viscera to right atrium

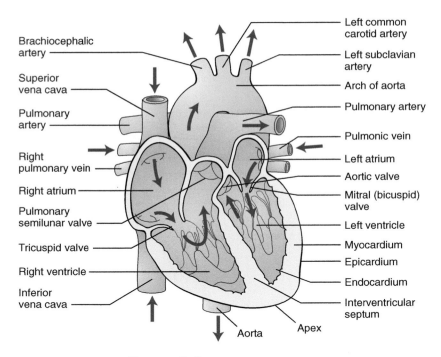

Figure **4-3** Internal view of heart.

Superior vena cava—drains deoxygenated blood from head, neck, upper extremities, and chest to right atrium

Pulmonary artery bifurcates and becomes right and left pulmonary artery—carries deoxygenated blood from right ventricle to lungs

Right and left pulmonary veins (4)—carry oxygenated blood from lungs to left atrium

Aorta—carries oxygenated blood from left side of heart to body

Pericardium
Sac comprised of two layers that covers heart
- Parietal pericardium: outermost covering
- Visceral pericardium: innermost (epicardium)
- Pericardial cavity: contains about 30 cc of fluid

Valves (4 in Heart)
Tricuspid: between right atrium and right ventricle

Pulmonary: at entrance of pulmonary artery leading from right ventricle

Aortic: at entrance of aorta leading from left ventricle

Bicuspid (mitral): between left atrium and left ventricle

Conduction System (Fig. 4-4)
Sinoatrial node: SAN, nature's pacemaker, sends impulses to atrioventricular node

Atrioventricular node (AVN): located on interatrial septum and sends impulses to bundle of His

Bundle of His: divides into right bundle branch (RBB) and left bundle branch (LBB) in septum

Purkinje fibers: merge from bundle branches into specialized cells of myocardium, located in ventricular endocardium

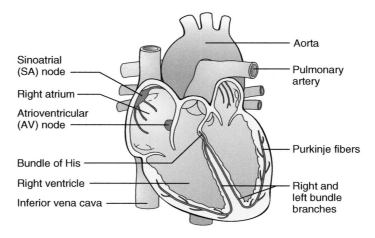

Figure **4-4** Conduction system of heart.

■ Heartbeat

Two Phases—Correspond to Blood Pressure Readouts

Systole: contraction—top number reading

Diastole: relaxation—lower number reading

Trace a drop of blood from trunk of body (deoxygenated) to trunk of body (oxygenated)

　　Inferior vena cava to right atrium

　　Through tricuspid valve to right ventricle

　　From right ventricle to pulmonary artery to lung capillaries

　　From lung capillaries to pulmonary veins

　　To left atrium through mitral (bicuspid) valve to left ventricle

　　Through aortic valve to aorta

COMBINING FORMS

1. angi/o	vessel
2. aort/o	aorta
3. ather/o	yellow plaque (fat)
4. arter/o	artery
5. arteri/o	artery
6. atri/o	atrium
7. brachi/o	arm
8. cardi/o	heart
9. cholesterol/o	cholesterol
10. coron/o	heart
11. cyan/o	blue
12. my/o, muscul/o	muscle

13. myx/o	mucous
14. ox/o	oxygen
15. pericardi/o	pericardium
16. phleb/o	vein
17. sphygm/o	pulse
18. steth/o	chest
19. thromb/o	clot
20. valv/o	valve
21. valvul/o	valve
22. vascul/o	vessel
23. vas/o	vessel
24. ven/o	vein
25. ventricul/o	ventricle

PREFIXES

1. a-	not
2. an-	not
3. bi-	two
4. brady-	slow
5. de-	lack of
6. dys-	bad, difficult, painful
7. endo-	in
8. hyper-	over
9. hypo-	under
10. inter-	between
11. intra-	within
12. meta-	change, after
13. peri-	surrounding
14. tachy-	fast
15. tetra-	four
16. tri-	three

SUFFIXES

1.	-dilation	widening, expanding
2.	-emia	blood
3.	-graphy	recording process
4.	-lysis	separation
5.	-megaly	enlargement
6.	-oma	tumor
7.	-osis	condition
8.	-plasty	repair
9.	-sclerosis	hardening
10.	-stenosis	blockage, narrowing
11.	-tomy	cutting, incision

MEDICAL ABBREVIATIONS

1.	ASCVD	arteriosclerotic cardiovascular disease
2.	ASD	atrial septal defect
3.	ASHD	arteriosclerotic heart disease
4.	AV	atrioventricular
5.	CABG	coronary artery bypass graft
6.	CHF	congestive heart failure
7.	CK	creatine kinase
8.	CPK	creatine phosphokinase
9.	CVI	cerebrovascular insufficiency
10.	DSE	dobutamine stress echocardiography
11.	HCVD	hypertensive cardiovascular disease
12.	LBBB	left bundle branch block
13.	LVH	left ventricular hypertrophy
14.	MAT	multifocal atrial tachycardia
15.	MI	myocardial infarction
16.	NSR	normal sinus rhythm
17.	PAC	premature atrial contraction
18.	PAT	paroxysmal atrial tachycardia

19. PST/PSVT	paroxysmal supraventricular tachycardia
20. PTCA	percutaneous transluminal coronary angioplasty
21. PVC	premature ventricular contraction
22. RBBB	right bundle branch block
23. RSR	regular sinus rhythm
24. RVH	right ventricular hypertrophy
25. SVT	supraventricular tachycardia
26. TEE	transesophageal echocardiography
27. TST	treadmill stress test

MEDICAL TERMS

Acute coronary syndrome (ACS)	An umbrella term used to cover clinical symptoms compatible with acute myocardial ischemia
Anastomosis	Surgical connection of two tubular structures, such as two pieces of the intestine
Aneurysm	Abnormal dilation of vessels, usually an artery
Angina	Spasmotic, choking, or suffocative pain
Angiography	Radiography of blood vessels
Angioplasty	Procedure in a vessel to dilate vessel opening
Atherectomy	Removal of plaque from an artery (can be done by a percutaneous or open procedure)
Auscultation	Listening for sounds within body
Bundle of His	Muscular cardiac fibers that provide heart rhythm to ventricles
Bypass	To go around
Cardiopulmonary	Refers to heart and lungs
Cardiopulmonary bypass	Blood bypasses heart through a heart-lung machine
Circumflex	A coronary artery that circles heart
Cutdown	Incision into a vessel for placement of a catheter
Edema	Swelling due to abnormal fluid collection in tissue spaces
Electrode	Lead attached to a generator that carries electric current from the generator to atria or ventricles
Electrophysiology	Study of electrical system of heart, including study of arrhythmias
Embolectomy	Removal of blockage (embolism) from vessel

Endarterectomy	Incision into an artery to remove inner lining
Epicardial	Over heart
False aneurysm	Sac of clotted blood that has completely destroyed vessel and is being contained by tissue that surrounds vessel
Fistula	Abnormal opening from one area to another area or to outside of the body
Hematoma	Mass of blood that forms outside vessel
Hemolysis	Breakdown of red blood cells
Hypoxemia	Low level of oxygen in blood
Hypoxia	Low level of oxygen in tissue
Implantable defibrillator	Surgically placed or wearable device that directs an electric shock to the heart to restore rhythm
Intracardiac	Inside heart
Invasive	Entering body, breaking skin
Noninvasive	Not entering body, not breaking skin
Nuclear cardiology	Diagnostic specialty that uses radiologic procedures to aid in diagnosis of cardiologic conditions
Order	Shows subordination of one thing to another; family or class
Pericardiocentesis	Procedure in which a surgeon withdraws fluid from pericardial space by means of a needle inserted percutaneously
Pericardium	Membranous sac enclosing heart and ends of great vessels
Swan-Ganz catheter	A catheter that measures pressure in right side of heart and in pulmonary artery
Thoracostomy	Incision into chest wall and insertion of a chest tube
Thromboendarterectomy	Removal of thrombus and atherosclerotic lining from an artery (percutaneous or open procedure)
Transvenous	Through a vein

CHAPTER 4: ANATOMY AND TERMINOLOGY QUIZ

(Quiz answers are located in Appendix B)

1. These carry blood to the heart:
   a. capillaries
   b. arteries
   c. arterioles
   d. veins

2. Relaxation phase of heartbeat:
   a. diastole
   b. systole

3. Nature's pacemaker is this node:
   a. atrioventricular
   b. Bundle of His
   c. sinoatrial
   d. mitral

4. Node located on interatrial septum:
   a. atrioventricular
   b. Bundle of His
   c. sinoatrial
   d. Purkinje

5. Which of the following is NOT one of the three layers of chamber walls of the heart?
   a. endocardium
   b. myocardium
   c. epicardium
   d. parietal

6. Septum that divides upper two chambers of heart:
   a. intraventricular
   b. interatrial
   c. tricuspid
   d. myocardium

7. Valve between right atrium and right ventricle:
   a. pulmonary
   b. aortic
   c. bicuspid
   d. tricuspid

8. Outer two-layer covering of heart:
   a. pericardium
   b. mitral
   c. myocardium
   d. epicardium

9. These are chambers that receive blood:
   a. right and left ventricle
   b. left ventricle and right atrium
   c. right atrium and right ventricle
   d. right and left atria

10. This combining form means "plaque":
    a. atri/o
    b. brachi/o
    c. cyan/o
    d. ather/o

Pathophysiology

■ Vascular Disorders

Coronary Artery Disease (CAD)/Ischemic Heart Disease (IHD)

Thickening and hardening of arterial intima (innermost layer) with lipid and fibrous plaque (atherosclerosis)

- Produces narrowing and stiffening of vessel

Location of lesions leads to various vascular diseases

- Femoral and popliteal arteries = peripheral vascular disease
- Carotid arteries = stroke
- Aorta = aneurysms (dilation/weakening of vessel walls)
- Coronary arteries = ischemic heart disease or myocardial infarction

Resulting in decreased oxygen supply

Risk factors increased by:

- Age
- Family history of CAD
- Hyperlipidemia
- Low HDL-C (good cholesterol)
- Hypertension
- Cigarette smoking
- Diabetes mellitus
- Obesity, particularly abdominal

Ischemia

Deficiency of oxygenated blood

- Often due to constriction or obstruction of blood vessel

Localized Myocardial Ischemia—Most Common Cause: Atherosclerosis of Vessels

Oxygen demand of tissues greater than supply

Presenting symptoms

- Chest pain (angina pectoris)
- Hypotension
- Changes in ECG

Transient Ischemia

Heart muscle begins to perform at a low level due to lack of oxygen (reversible ischemia)

Irreversible Ischemia—is Cause of an MI (Myocardial Infarction)

Heart muscle dies—necrosis (myocardial infarction)

- Prolonged ischemia of 30 minutes or more
- Reestablishment of blood flow reduces residual necrosis
  - Thrombolytic agents to dissolve or split up thrombus
  - Primary percutaneous transluminal coronary angioplasty (PTCA)

Cardiac enzymes are released from damaged cells

- Blood test reveals elevation of enzymes, confirming myocardial infarction

Hypertension (HTN)

Normal is less than 120/80 for adults

- Fig. 4-5 illustrates new hypertension classifications

Leading cause of death in United States due to damage to brain, heart, kidneys, eyes, and arteries of the lower extremities

Cause is unknown in 95% of cases

- Known as
  - Primary hypertension
  - Essential hypertension

5% of cases are secondary to underlying disease

Increased resistance damages heart and blood vessels

- Retinal vascular changes are monitored to assess therapy and disease progression

Chronic hypertension often leads to end-stage renal disease

- Result of progressive sclerosis of renal vessels

Treatment

Medications

- ACE (angiotensin-converting enzyme) inhibitor
- Alpha-adrenergic or beta-adrenergic receptor blocker
- Diuretic
- Calcium channel blocker

Lifestyle changes

Hypotension

Abnormally Low Blood Pressure

Types

Orthostatic (postural) hypotension

- Fall in both systolic and diastolic arterial blood pressure on standing
- Associated with
  - Dizziness

Figure **4-5** Classification of blood pressure.

Classification of blood pressure for adults aged 18 years or older[1]

Category	Systolic (mm Hg)	Diastolic (mm Hg)
Normal	<120	<80
Prehypertension (stays between)	120–139	80–89
Hypertension[2]		
Stage 1 (mild)	140–159	90–99
Stage 2 (moderate)	160–179	100–109
Stage 3 (severe)	≥180	≥110

[1] Not taking antihypertensive drugs and not acutely ill. When systolic and diastolic pressures fall into different categories, the higher category should be selected.

[2] Based on the average of two or more readings taken at each of two or more visits after an initial screening.

- Blurred vision
- Fainting (syncope)
- Caused by insufficient oxygenated blood flow through brain
- Can be acute (temporary) or chronic

Chronic orthostatic hypotension—types

- Primary of unknown cause
- Secondary to certain disease processes
- Such as:
  - Endocrine
  - Metabolic
  - Central nervous system disorders
- Treatment for secondary hypotension is correction of underlying disease

Aneurysm

Dilation of an arterial blood vessel wall or cardiac chamber

- Danger is rupture of aneurysm

Atherosclerosis is common cause

Arteriosclerosis and hypertension also common in persons with aneurysms

True Aneurysm

Involves all three layers of arterial wall

Causes weakening and ballooning of arterial wall

False or Pseudoaneurysm

Usually result of trauma

Also known as saccular

Separation of arterial wall layers (dissecting) in artery wall (crisis situation—a medical emergency)

Bleeds into dissected space and is contained by arterial connective tissue wall

Thrombus

Blood clot that remains attached to vessel wall and occludes vessel

Dislodged thrombus is a thromboembolus

Causes

Trauma

Interior wall lining irritation/roughening

Infection

Inflammation

Low blood pressure/blood stagnation

Obstruction

Atherosclerosis

Risks Related to Thrombus

Dislodges and moves to lungs, brain, heart

Grows to occlude blood flow

Treatment
Pharmacologic, anticoagulants

Heparin

Warfarin derivatives

Noninvasive Intervention
Balloon-tipped catheter to remove or compress thrombus

Thrombophlebitis Caused by Inflammation (Phlebitis)
Causes
Trauma

Infection

Immobility

Commonly Associated With
Endocarditis

Rheumatic heart disease

Embolism
Mass that is present and circulating in blood

Common Types
Air bubble

Fat

Bacterial mass

Cancer cells

Foreign substances

Dislodged thrombus

Amniotic fluid

Obstructs Vessel
Pulmonary emboli travel through venous side or right side of the heart to the pulmonary artery

Systemic or arterial emboli originate in left side of the heart

Associated with

- Myocardial infarction
- Left-sided heart failure
- Endocarditis
- Valvular conditions
- Dysrhythmias

Peripheral Arterial Disease
Thromboangiitis Obliterans (Buerger's Disease)
Occurs most often in young men who are heavy smokers

Inflammatory disease of peripheral arteries creating thombi and vasospasms

Involves small or medium arteries of feet and often hands

- May necessitate amputation

Raynaud's Disease
Vasospasms and constriction of small arterioles of fingers and toes

Affects young women as a secondary condition

Triggered by cold temperatures, emotional stress, cigarette smoking

Fingertips thicken and nails become brittle

Raynaud's phenomenon is secondary to primary disease, such as

- Scleroderma
- Pulmonary hypertension

Treatment of Underlying Condition
No known origin or treatment

Varicose Veins

Blood pools in veins, distending them

Tends to be progressive/vein valve failure

Occurs most commonly in saphenous veins

Hemorrhoids are varicose veins of anus

Leads to
Swelling and discomfort

Fatigue when in legs

Possible ulcerations

Heart Disorders

Congestive Heart Failure (CHF)—Heart Cannot Pump Required Amounts of Blood

Can be left-sided or right-sided heart failure

Left-sided heart failure (systolic); cannot generate adequate output, causing pulmonary edema

Common causes:

Myocardial infarction

Myocarditis

Cardiomyopathies leading to ischemia

Symptoms of left-sided congestive heart failure include:

Shortness of breath

Fatigue

Exercise intolerance

Right-sided heart failure (diastolic) results in right ventricle stasis, inadequate pulmonary circulation, and peripheral edema/hepatosplenomegaly

Abnormal Heart Rhythms (Conduction Irregularities)

Bradycardia and heart block (atrioventricular block)

Inadequate conduction impulses from SA node though AV node to AV bundle

Treatment

Cardiac pacemaker to maintain proper heart rate

Flutter—rapid regular contractions (most commonly of atria)

Symptoms—palpitations

Treatment

Cardioversion (electronic shock to heart)

Ablation (radiofrequency catheter destroying tissue causing arrhythmia)

Fibrillation—rapid, erratic, inefficient contractions of atria and ventricles

    Atrial fibrillation—most common (electrical impulses move randomly in atria)

        Symptoms—palpitation, risk of stroke due to clot formations from poor atrial outputs

    Treatment

        Cardioversion

        Ablation

Ventricular fibrillation—life-threatening, random electrical impulses throughout ventricles

    Symptoms—cardiac death or arrest without immediate treatment

    Treatment

        Cardioversion

        Digoxin—drug used to slow heart rate

        Implantable defibrillator

        Emergency treatment—automatic external defibrillators (AEDs)

        Radiofrequency catheter ablation (RFA) is a minimally invasive technique used to treat cardiac arrhythmias

Infective Endocarditis

Inflammation of interior-most lining of heart

Leads to destruction and permanent damage to heart valves

Caused by

    Bacteria (most commonly streptococci and staphylococci)

    Virus

    Fungi

    Parasites

Patients with heart defects or damage usually take antibiotics prior to invasive procedures

Pericarditis

Inflammation of pericardium of heart

Common Types

- Acute
- Pericardial effusion
- Constrictive

Rheumatic Fever/Rheumatic Heart Disease

Results in formation of scar tissue of the endocardium and heart valves

In 10% of cases leads to rheumatic heart disease

Family tendency to develop

Begins as carditis (inflammation of all layers of heart wall)

Long-term effects:

Mitral and/or aortic valve disease

    Stenosis

    Regurgitation

    Insufficiency

Tricuspid valve

    Affected in about 10% of cases

Pulmonary valve

    Rarely affected

■ Valvular Heart Disease

Valves are extensions of endocardial tissue

Endocardial damage can be congenital or acquired

Damage leads to stenosis and/or incompetent valve

Includes

- Valvular stenosis is narrowing, stiffness, thickening, fusion, or blockage of valve, creating resistance, resulting in increased pressure in cardiac chamber behind valve
- Valvular regurgitation is failure of valve leaflet to close tightly, allowing backflow of blood
  - Result of lesions causing valve leaflets to shrink
  - Functional valvular regurgitation results in increased chamber size (cardiomegaly)

Stenosis

Aortic Valve Stenosis

Caused by

    Congenital malformation

    Degeneration

    Infection

Results in slowing blood circulatory rate

Symptoms

    Bradycardia

    Faint pulse

    May lead to heart murmur and hypertrophy

Mitral Valve Stenosis

Impaired flow from left atrium to left ventricle

Caused by

    Rheumatic fever

    Bacterial infections

Symptom

    Decreased cardiac output

May lead to

- Pulmonary hypertension
- Right ventricular heart failure
- And/or edema

Valvular Regurgitation

Flow in opposite direction from normal

Mitral regurgitation (MR)

    Backflow of blood from left ventricle into left atrium

Aortic regurgitation (AR)

    Backflow of blood from aorta into left ventricle

Pulmonic regurgitation (PR)

    Backflow of blood from pulmonary artery into right ventricle

Tricuspid regurgitation (TR)

Backflow of blood from right ventricle into right atrium

Heart Wall Disorders

Acute Pericarditis

Roughening and inflammation of pericardium (sac around heart)

Treatment

Anti-inflammatory drugs and pain medication

Constrictive Pericarditis (Restrictive Pericarditis)
Forms Fibrous Lesions that Encase Heart

Compresses heart—thickened pericardial sac prevents heart from expanding when blood enters it

Tamponade occurs when fluid builds up in pericardial space

Pressure stops heart from beating—pericardial effusion or bleeding after heart surgery

Reduces output

Pericardial Effusion

Accumulation of fluid in pericardial cavity

Results in pressure on heart

- Sudden development of pressure on heart is tamponade

Cardiomyopathies

Myocardium: muscular wall (middle layer) of heart musculature

Group of diseases that affect myocardium

Cause

Idiopathic (most common)

Underlying condition

Types of Cardiomyopathy

Dilated cardiomyopathy (congestive cardiomyopathy)

- Ventricular distention and impaired systolic function

Hypertrophic cardiomyopathy

- Cause is often hypertensive or valvular heart disease
- Results in thickened interventricular septum (septum between the ventricle chambers)

Restrictive cardiomyopathy

- Myocardium becomes stiffened
- Heart enlarges (cardiomegaly)
- Dysrhythmias common
- Caused by infiltrative diseases such as amyloidosis

Congenital Heart Defects

Coarctation of aorta (CoA)—narrowing of the aorta

- Treatment

Surgical removal of narrow segment/end-to-end anastomosis

Patent ductus arteriosus (PDA)—opening between aorta and pulmonary artery

- Treatment

    Drugs to close/embolize or plug ductus or tying off surgically

Tetralogy of Fallot—malformation of heart includes four defects

1. Pulmonary artery stenosis—
    - Narrowing/obstruction
2. Ventricular septal defect
    - Hole between two bottom chambers (ventricles) of heart
3. Overriding aorta
    - Shift of aorta to right—aorta overrides the interventricular septum
4. Hypertrophy of right ventricle
    - Myocardium enlarges to pump blood through narrowed pulmonary artery

Treatment

- Open-heart technique with heart-lung machine support to relieve right ventricular outflow tract stenosis and repair of ventriculoseptal defect

CHAPTER 4: PATHOPHYSIOLOGY QUIZ

(Quiz answers are located in Appendix B)

1. Lesion of carotid artery may lead to:
   a. heart attack
   b. stroke
   c. peripheral vascular disease
   d. ischemic heart disease

2. This blood pressure is hypertension:
   a. 120/80
   b. 130/70
   c. 140/90
   d. 110/70

3. Infective endocarditis is inflammation of the interior of the lining of the heart, and when caused by streptococci or staphylococci, the infection is:
   a. viral
   b. fungal
   c. bacterial
   d. parasitic

4. Angina pectoris is:
   a. heart block
   b. heart murmur
   c. chest pain
   d. barrel chest

5. In this type of regurgitation, there is a backflow of blood from left ventricle into left atrium:
   a. aortic
   b. pulmonic
   c. tricuspid
   d. mitral

6. In this type of heart wall disorder, fibrous lesions form and encase the heart:
   a. constrictive pericarditis
   b. acute pericarditis
   c. pericardial effusion
   d. cardiomyopathy

7. Which of the following terms means "of unknown cause"?
   a. etiology
   b. manifestation
   c. idiopathic
   d. late effect

8. This condition is also known as congestive cardiomyopathy:
   a. hypertrophic
   b. valvular
   c. dilated
   d. restrictive

9. This peripheral arterial disease most often occurs in young men who are heavy smokers:
   a. Buerger's
   b. Pick's
   c. Addison's
   d. Glasser's

10. This cardiomyopathy results in a thickened interventricular septum:
    a. restrictive
    b. congestive
    c. dilated
    d. hypertrophic

CHAPTER 5: FEMALE GENITAL SYSTEM AND PREGNANCY

Anatomy and Terminology

■ Terminology

Ovaries (Pair)

Produce ova (single female gamete) and hormones; ova: plural; ovum: singular (Fig. 5-1). Each ovum/gamete contains 23 chromosomes.

Fallopian Tubes (Uterine Tubes or Oviducts)

Ducts from ovary to uterus

Uterus (Womb)

Muscular organ that holds embryo

Three layers

- Endometrium: inner mucosa
- Myometrium: middle layer/muscle
- Perimetrium/Uterine serosa: outer layer
  - Cervix: lower narrow portion of uterus
  - Fundus: the upper rounded part of the uterus

Vagina

Tube from uterus to outside of body

Vulva

External genitalia

- Clitoris: erectile tissue
- Labia majora: outer lips of vagina

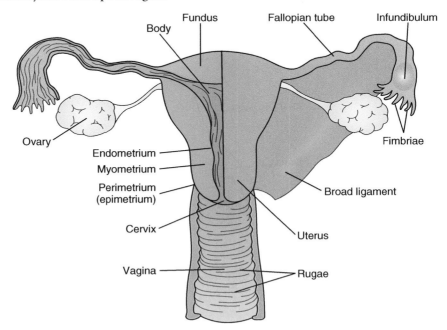

Figure **5-1** Female reproductive system.

- Labia minora: inner lips of vagina
- Urinary meatus: opening to urethra
- Bartholin's gland: glands on either side of vagina
- Hymen: membrane partially or wholly occludes entrance to vagina

Perineum

Area between anus and vaginal orifice

■ Accessory Organs (Fig. 5-2)

Breasts

Mammary glands

Composed of glandular tissue containing milk glands/lactiferous ducts

In response to hormones from pituitary gland, milk is produced in acini (also known as alveoli) (lactation)

Lactiferous ducts transfer milk to nipple

Nipple, surrounded by areola

■ Menstruation and Pregnancy

Proliferation Phase

Menstruation (Days 1-5): discharge of blood fluid containing endometrial cells, blood cells, and glandular secretions from endometrium

Endometrium repair (Days 6-12): maturing follicle in ovary produces estrogen (hormone), which causes endometrium to thicken and ovum (egg) to mature in graafian follicle

Secretory Phase

Ovulation (Days 13-14): occurs when graafian follicle ruptures and ovum travels down fallopian tube

Usually only one graafian follicle develops each month

Premenstruation (Days 15-28): a period of time in which graafian follicle converts to corpus luteum secreting progesterone to stimulate build-up of uterine lining. If after 5 days no fertilization occurs, cycle repeats.

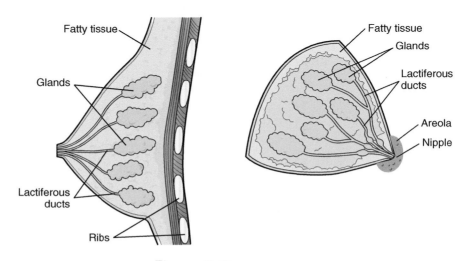

Figure **5-2** Breast structure.

Pregnancy

Prenatal stage of development from fertilization to birth (39 weeks)

Fertilized ovum or zygote develops in a double cavity: yolk sac (produces blood cells) and amniotic cavity (contains amniotic fluid)

Embryo, stage of development from 4th to 8th week

Fetus, unborn offspring, 9 weeks until birth

Placenta Forms Within Uterine Wall and Produces Hormone—Human Chorionic Gonadotropin (HCG)

HCG is hormone tested in urine pregnancy tests

HCG stimulates corpus luteum to produce estrogen and progesterone until the third month of pregnancy

Placenta then produces hormones

Expelled after delivery (afterbirth)

Gestation, Approximately 266 Days

280 days used when calculating estimated date of delivery (EDD) or time from last menstrual period (LMP)

Three trimesters
- First   LMP-12 weeks
- Second   13-27 weeks
- Third   28 weeks-EDD

COMBINING FORMS

1.	amni/o	amnion
2.	arche/o	first
3.	cephal/o	head
4.	cervic/o	cervix
5.	chori/o	chorion
6.	colp/o	vagina
7.	crypt/o	hidden
8.	culd/o	cul-de-sac
9.	episi/o	vulva
10.	fet/o	fetus
11.	galact/o	milk
12.	gynec/o	female
13.	gyn/o	female
14.	hymen/o	hymen
15.	hyster/o	uterus
16.	lact/o	milk

17.	lapar/o	abdominal wall
18.	mamm/o	breast
19.	mast/o	breast
20.	men/o	menstruation, month
21.	metr/o	uterus, measure
22.	metr/i	uterus
23.	my/o, muscul/o	muscle
24.	nat/a	birth
25.	nat/i	birth
26.	obstetr/o	pregnancy/childbirth
27.	olig/o	few
28.	oo/o	egg
29.	oophor/o	ovary
30.	ov/o	egg
31.	ovari/o	ovary
32.	ovul/o	ovulation
33.	perine/o	perineum
34.	peritone/o	peritoneum
35.	phor/o	to bear
36.	salping/o	uterine tube, fallopian tube
37.	top/o	place
38.	uter/o	uterus
39.	vagin/o	vagina
40.	vulv/o	vulva

PREFIXES

1.	ante-	before
2.	dys-	painful
3.	ecto-	outside
4.	endo-	in
5.	extra-	outside
6.	in-	into

7. intra-	within
8. multi-	many
9. neo-	new
10. nulli-	none
11. nulti-	none
12. post-	after
13. primi-	first
14. pseudo-	false
15. retro-	backwards
16. uni-	one

SUFFIXES

1. -arche	beginning
2. -cyesis	pregnancy
3. -gravida	pregnancy
4. -rrhexis	rupture
5. -para	woman who has given birth
6. -parous	to bear
7. -rrhea	discharge
8. -salpinx	uterine tube
9. -tocia	labor
10. -version	turning

MEDICAL ABBREVIATIONS

1. AFI	amniotic fluid index
2. AGA	appropriate for gestational age
3. ARM	artificial rupture of membrane
4. BPD	biparietal diameter
5. BPP	biophysical profile
6. BV	bacterial vaginosis
7. CHL	crown-to-heel length
8. CNM	certified nurse midwife

9.	CPD	cephalopelvic disproportion
10.	CPP	chronic pelvic pain
11.	D&C	dilation and curettage
12.	D&E	dilation and evacuation
13.	DUB	dysfunctional uterine bleeding
14.	ECC	endocervical curettage
15.	EDC	estimated date of confinement
16.	EDD	estimated date of delivery
17.	EFM	electronic fetal monitoring
18.	EFW	estimated fetal weight
19.	EGA	estimated gestational age
20.	EMC	endometrial curettage
21.	ERT	estrogen replacement therapy
22.	FAS	fetal alcohol syndrome
23.	FHR	fetal heart rate
24.	FSH	follicle-stimulating hormone
25.	HPV	human papillomavirus
26.	HSG	hysterosalpingogram
27.	HSV	herpes simplex virus
28.	IVF	in vitro fertilization
29.	LEEP	loop electrosurgical excision procedure
30.	LGA	large for gestational age
31.	PID	pelvic inflammatory disease
32.	PROM	premature rupture of membranes
33.	SHG	sonohysterogram
34.	SROM	spontaneous rupture of membranes
35.	SUI	stress urinary incontinence
36.	TAH	total abdominal hysterectomy
37.	VBAC	vaginal birth after cesarean

MEDICAL TERMS

Abortion	Termination of pregnancy
Amniocentesis	Percutaneous aspiration of amniotic fluid
Amniotic sac	Sac containing fetus and amniotic fluid
Antepartum	Before childbirth
Cesarean	Surgical opening through abdominal wall for delivery
Chorionic villus sampling	CVS, biopsy of outermost part of placenta
Cordocentesis	Procedure to obtain a fetal blood sample; also called a percutaneous umbilical blood sampling
Curettage	Scraping of a cavity using a spoon-shaped instrument
Cystocele	Herniation of bladder into vagina
Delivery	Childbirth
Dilation	Expansion (of cervix)
Ectopic	Pregnancy outside uterus (i.e., in fallopian tube)
Hysterectomy	Surgical removal of uterus
Hysterorrhaphy	Suturing of uterus
Hysteroscopy	Visualization of canal and cavity of uterus using a scope placed through vagina
Introitus	Opening or entrance to vagina
Ligation	Binding or tying off, as in constricting blood flow of a vessel or binding fallopian tubes for sterilization
Multipara	More than one pregnancy
Oophorectomy	Surgical removal of ovary(ies)
Perineum	Area between vulva and anus; also known as pelvic floor
Placenta	A structure that connects fetus and mother during pregnancy
Postpartum	After childbirth
Primigravida	First pregnancy
Primipara	First delivered infant/given birth to only one child
Salpingectomy	Surgical removal of uterine tube
Salpingostomy	Creation of a fistula into uterine tube
Tocolysis	Repression of uterine contractions
Vesicovaginal fistula	Abnormal opening/channel between vagina and bladder

CHAPTER 5: ANATOMY AND TERMINOLOGY QUIZ

(Quiz answers are located in Appendix B)

1. This is NOT one of the three layers of uterus:
   a. perimetrium
   b. endometrium
   c. myometrium
   d. barametrium

2. Located at the lower end of uterus is the:
   a. cervix
   b. vagina
   c. perineum
   d. labia majora

3. Approximate gestation of a human fetus is:
   a. 266 days
   b. 276 days
   c. 290 days
   d. 292 days

4. LMP is the:
   a. later maternity phase
   b. last menstrual period
   c. low metabolic pregnancy
   d. late menstruation phase

5. Name of stage that describes development of fetus from fertilization to birth is:
   a. postpartum
   b. antepartum
   c. prenatal
   d. natal

6. Which of the following correctly identifies three trimesters of gestation?
   a. LMP to less than 14 weeks 0 days, 14 weeks 0 days to less than 28 weeks 0 days, 28 weeks 0 days until deliver
   b. LMP to less than 16 weeks 0 days, 16 weeks 0 days to less than 28 weeks 0 days, 28 weeks 0 days until deliver
   c. LMP to less than 16 weeks 0 days, 16 weeks 0 days to less than 29 weeks 0 days, 29 weeks 0 days until deliver
   d. LMP to less than 13 weeks 0 days, 13 weeks 0 days to less than 27 weeks 0 days, 27 weeks 0 days until deliver

7. Combining form meaning "few":
   a. oopho/o
   b. olig/o
   c. nati/i
   d. top/o

8. Combining form meaning "hidden":
   a. amni/o
   b. crypt/o
   c. chori/o
   d. fet/o

9. Suffix meaning "beginning":
   a. -cyesis
   b. -rrhea
   c. -arche
   d. -orrhexis

10. Prefix meaning "within":
    a. ante-
    b. dys-
    c. ecto-
    d. endo-

Pathophysiology

■ Menstrual and Hormonal Disorders

Dysmenorrhea
Painful menstruation

Common Types
- Primary and secondary

Primary Dysmenorrhea
No underlying condition but begins with commencement of ovulation

Cramping is caused by excess of prostaglandin
- Causes contractions and uterine ischemia
- Develops 24 to 48 hours prior to menstruation

Treatment
- Nonsteroidal anti-inflammatory agents
- Progesterone

Secondary Dysmenorrhea
Caused by an underlying disorder, such as
- Polyps
- Tumors
- Endometriosis
- Pelvic inflammatory disease

Treatment
Directed at underlying disorder

Amenorrhea
Amenorrhea is absence of menstruation

Common Types
- Primary and secondary

Primary Amenorrhea
Menstruation has never occurred

May be genetic disorder
- Turner's syndrome (ovaries do not function)

Secondary Amenorrhea
Cessation of menstruation for 3 cycles or 6 months
- Individual has previously menstruated

Various causes of anovulation/amenorrhea

Examples:
- Tumors
- Stress
- Eating disorders
- Competitive sports participation

Dysfunctional Uterine Bleeding (DUB)

Abnormal bleeding patterns

Occurs when no organic cause can be identified

Abnormal Menstruation Types

Oligomenorrhea: in excess of 6 weeks between periods

Polymenorrhea: less than 3 weeks between periods

Metrorrhagia: bleeding between cycles

Menorrhagia: increase in amount and duration of flow

Hypomenorrhea: light or spotty flow

Menometrorrhagia: irregular cycle with varying amounts and duration of flow

Menorrhea: lengthy menstrual flow

Dysmenorrhea: painful menstruation

Premenstrual Syndrome (PMS)

Also known as premenstrual tension (PMT)

Occurs before onset of menses (luteal phase) and ends at onset of menses

Cluster of Common Symptoms

Weight gain

Breast tenderness

Sleep disturbances

Headache

Irritability

Cause is unknown

Treatment

- Varies depending on individual symptoms

Endometriosis

Endometrial tissue (uterine lining) develops outside the uterus (on ovaries, fallopian tubes, small intestine, etc.)

Responses to Hormone Cycle

Ectopic (out of place) endometrial tissue degenerates, sheds, and bleeds

Causes

- Irritation
- Inflammation
- Pain

Continued cycles produce fibrous tissue

- Adhesions and obstructions can then form
- Interferes with normal bodily function
- For example, fallopian tube endometriosis may lead to obstructed tubes

Primary symptom is dysmenorrhea

- May also cause painful intercourse (dyspareunia)

Risks

Increased risk for cancers

- Breast
- Ovaries
- Non-Hodgkin lymphoma

Treatment Includes

Hormonal suppression

Surgical removal of endometrial tissue

- May require hysterectomy and BSO (bilateral salpingo-oophorectomy)

■ Infection, Inflammation, and Sexually Transmitted Diseases

Pelvic Inflammatory Disease (PID)

Infection and inflammation of reproductive tract

- Primarily ovaries and fallopian tubes
- Usually originates in cervix or vagina
    - Migrates up through reproductive tract

Types

Acute

Chronic

Commonly forms adhesions and strictures

- May lead to infertility

Candidiasis

Yeast infection

- *Candida albicans (Monilia)*

Not sexually transmitted

Opportunistic infection may follow

- Infection treated with antibiotics
- Period of reduced resistance
- Increased glucose or glycogen levels (often associated with diabetes mellitus)

Affects mucous membranes

- Produces a white, thick, curd-like discharge

Result may be dyspareunia and dysuria

Treatment

Antifungal substances such as nystatin

Identification and treatment of underlying condition

Chlamydia

Most common sexually transmitted disease (STD)

Cause

Bacteria, *Chlamydia trachomatis*

Symptoms

Asymptomatic or mild discharge and dysuria

Treatment
Antimicrobial

Genital Herpes
Cause
Virus, herpes simplex 2 (HSV-2)

Symptoms
Ulcers and vesicles

Treatment
Antiviral, manage outbreaks

There is no cure for genital herpes

Genital Warts
Cause
Virus, human papillomavirus

Symptoms
Polyps or grey lesions

Treatment
Excision

Prevention
Vaccine

There is no cure for genital warts

Gonorrhea
Cause
Bacteria, *Neisseria gonorrhoeae*

Symptoms
Dysuria

Discharge

Treatment
Antibacterial drugs

Some strains are drug-resistant

Syphilis
Cause
Bacteria, *Treponema pallidum*

Symptoms
Primary syphilis
- Ulcer or chancre at site of entry

Secondary syphilis
- Headache
- Fever
- Rash
- Tertiary
  - Affects cardiovascular and nervous systems

Treatment

Penicillin

Trichomoniasis

Cause

Protozoan, *Trichomonas vaginalis*

Symptoms

Usually asymptomatic

Treatment

Antimicrobial drugs

■ Benign Lesions

Leiomyomas—Uterine Fibroids

Well-defined, solid uterine tumor

Also known as

- Uterine fibroids
- Fibromyoma
- Fibroma
- Myoma
- Fibroid

Classification is based on location of tumor within uterine wall

Submucous: beneath endometrium

Subserous: beneath serosa

Intramural: in muscle wall

Symptoms

May be asymptomatic

Abnormal uterine bleeding

Pressure on nearby structures, such as bladder and rectum

Constipation

Pain

Sensation of heaviness

Treatment

Surgical excision of lesions

Hysterectomy may be necessary

Adenomyosis

Within uterine myometrium

Symptoms

Usually asymptomatic

Abnormal menstrual bleeding

Enlarged uterus

Commonly develops in late reproductive years

Common in those taking Tamoxifen

Treatment

Symptomatic in mild cases

Surgical in severe cases

- Excision of adenomyosis or hysterectomy

Malignant Lesions

Carcinoma of Breast

Accessory of reproductive system

Most often develops in upper outer quadrant

- Due to location, often spreads to lymph nodes
- May metastasize to lungs, brain, bone, liver, etc.

Majority arise from epithelial cells of ducts and lobules

Second most common cancer of women

Most are adenocarcinoma

- Invasive ductal carcinoma most common type
- Invasive lobular carcinoma second most common type
- Lymph node spread is determined by sentinel node biopsy (SNB)
- Small primary tumors are excised in a lumpectomy (tumor and immediate surrounding tissue only)
- Mastectomy is alternative surgical procedure removing entire breast
- Chemotherapy and radiation may be indicated to prevent recurrence

If neoplasm is responsive to hormone, hormone-blocking agents are administered

Increased Risks

- Heredity
  - Especially history of mother or sister who developed breast cancer
  - Mutated breast cancer gene (BRCA-1)
  - Familial breast cancer syndrome associated with BRCA-2
- Lower socioeconomic status
- Radiation exposure

Carcinoma of Uterus (Endometrial Cancer)

Most frequent pelvic cancer

Usually postmenopausal

Associated with higher levels of estrogen

Increases Risk

Obesity (estrogen produced by fat tissue)

Early menarche

Delayed menopause

Hypertension

Diabetes mellitus

Nulliparity (no viable births)

Some types of colorectal cancer

Oral contraceptives (estrogen)

Estrogen-producing tumors

Symptoms

Abnormal, excessive uterine bleeding

Postmenopausal bleeding

No simple screening test available

- Uterine cells may be aspirated for evaluation

Staging of Endometrial, Cervical, and Ovarian Malignancies

I—Confined to corpus

II—Involves corpus and cervix

III—Extends outside uterus but not outside true pelvis

IV—Extends outside true pelvis or involves rectum or bladder

Treatment

Pharmaceutical

Surgical

Irradiation

Chemotherapy

Combination of above

Carcinoma of Cervix

Routinely found on Papanicolaou (Pap) smear

Dysplasia is an early change in cervical epithelium

Increases Risks

Herpes simplex virus type 2 (HSV-2)

Human papillomavirus (HPV)

Young age of sexual activity

Smoking

Lower socioeconomic status

Stages of cervical cancer

Stage 1—Carcinoma of cervix

Stage 2—Carcinoma spread from cervix to upper vagina

Stage 3—Carcinoma spread to lower portion of vagina/pelvic wall

Stage 4—Most invasive stage spreading to other body parts

Symptoms

Early stages asymptomatic

Later stages

- Bleeding
- Discharge

Biopsy is used to confirm

Treatment

Pharmaceutical

Surgical

Irradiation

Chemotherapy

Combination of above

Carcinoma of Ovary

Cause is unknown—considered silent killer

Increased Risks

Genetic factors (BRCA-1)

Endocrine

- Nulliparous
- Early menarche
- Late menopause
- Non–breast feeding
- Late first pregnancy
- Postmenopausal estrogen replacement therapy (ERT)

Tumor Categories

Germ cell tumors

Arise from primitive germ cells, usually the testis and ovum

Types

- Germinoma
- Yolk sac
- Endodermal sinus tumor
- Teratoma
- Embryonal carcinoma
- Polyembryoma
- Gonadoblastoma
- Some types of choriocarcinoma

Categories

- Dermoid cysts (benign)
- Malignant tumors
- Primitive malignant
  - Embryonic
  - Extraembryonic cells

Epithelial Tumors

Most common gynecologic cancer

Gonadal Stromal Tumors

Symptoms

Pelvic heaviness

Dysuria

Increased urinary frequency

Sometimes vaginal bleeding

Treatment

Excision

Hysterectomy, including bilateral salpingo-oophorectomy with omentectomy (fold of peritoneum)

Chemotherapy

Radiation therapy

Combination of above

Carcinoma of Fallopian Tubes

Primary Fallopian Tube Tumors

Rare

Must be located within tube to be considered primary

- Adenocarcinoma most common primary tumor

Most tumors are secondary

Symptoms

Often asymptomatic

Bleeding or discharge

Irregular menstruation

Pain

Treatment

Hysterectomy, including bilateral salpingo-oophorectomy with any necessary omentectomy (fold of peritoneum)

Chemotherapy

Radiation therapy

Combination of above

Carcinoma of Vulva

Usually squamous cell carcinoma (90%)

Increased risk with STDs

Symptoms

Can be asymptomatic

Pruritic vulvular lesion

Treatment

Radical vulvectomy with node dissection

Wide local excision

Carcinoma of Vagina

Usually squamous cell carcinoma

Increased Risk

Human papillomavirus (HPV)

Postmenopausal hysterectomy

History of abnormal Pap

History of other carcinomas

Symptoms

Often asymptomatic

Vaginal pain, discharge, or bleeding

Treatment

Squamous cell—radiation

Early tumors may be excised

Vaginectomy

Hysterectomy

Lymph node dissection

■ Pregnancy

Placenta Previa

Opening of cervix is obstructed by displaced placenta

Types (Fig. 5-3)

Marginal

Partial

Total

Abruptio Placentae (Fig. 5-4)

Premature separation of placenta from uterine wall

Eclampsia

Serious condition of pregnancy characterized by

- Hypertension
- Edema
- Proteinuria

Ectopic Pregnancy (Extrauterine) (Fig. 5-5)

Implantation of fertilized ovum outside uterus

- Often fallopian tubes (tubal pregnancy)

Hydatidiform Mole

Benign tumor of placenta

Secretes hormone (chorionic gonadotropic hormone, CGH)

Indicates positive pregnancy test

Malpositions and Malpresentations (Fig. 5-6) Vaginal Delivery

Breech

Vertex

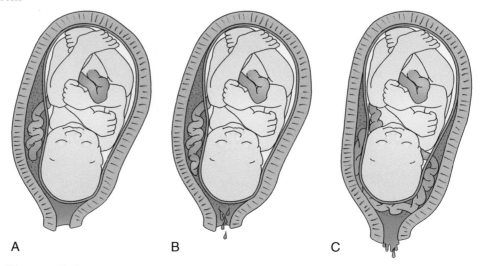

A   B   C

Figure **5-3** **A.** Marginal placenta previa. **B.** Partial placenta previa. **C.** Total placenta previa.

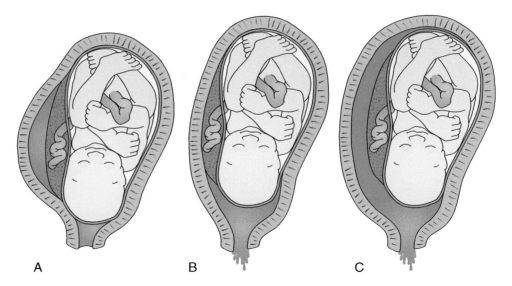

Figure **5-4** Abruptio placentae is classified according to the grade of separation of the placenta from uterine wall. **A.** Mild separation in which hemorrhage is internal. **B.** Moderate separation in which there is external hemorrhage. **C.** Severe separation in which there is external hemorrhage and extreme separation.

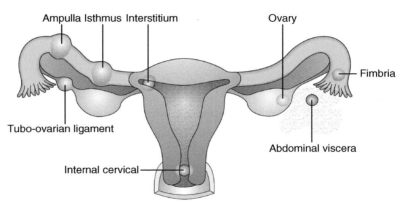

Figure **5-5** Ectopic pregnancy most often occurs in fallopian tube. Pregnancy outside the uterus may end in life-threatening rupture.

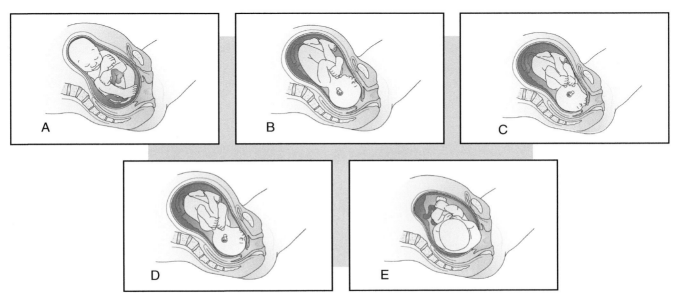

Figure **5-6** Five types of malposition and malpresentation of fetus: **A.** Breech. **B.** Vertex. **C.** Face. **D.** Brow. **E.** Shoulder.

Face

Brow

Shoulder

Abortion
Types
Spontaneous

- Miscarriage
- Happens naturally
- Uterus completely empties

Incomplete

- Uterus does not completely empty
- Requires intervention to remove remaining fetal material

Missed

- Fetus dies naturally
- Requires intervention to remove fetal material

Septic

- Similar to missed
- Has added complication of infection
- Requires intervention to remove fetal material
- Vigorous treatment of infection

Methods
D&C

- Dilation and curettage (scraping)

Evacuation (suction)

Intra-amniotic injections

- Saline (salt) solution

Vaginal suppositories

- Such as prostaglandin

CHAPTER 5: PATHOPHYSIOLOGY QUIZ

(Quiz answers are located in Appendix B)

1. Most common solution used for intra-amniotic injections is:
   a. prostaglandin
   b. saline
   c. estrogen
   d. chorionic gonadotropic hormone

2. This type of dysmenorrhea is treated with nonsteroidal anti-inflammatory agents and progesterone:
   a. secondary
   b. constrictive
   c. periodic
   d. primary

3. In this type of amenorrhea there is a cessation of menstruation:
   a. secondary
   b. constrictive
   c. periodic
   d. primary

For questions 4-6, match the abnormal menstruation type with correct definition from items a-c below.
   a. increased amount and duration of flow
   b. bleeding between cycles
   c. in excess of 6 weeks

4. oligomenorrhea

5. metrorrhagia

6. menorrhagia

7. Increased risks of breast cancer, ovarian cancer, and non-Hodgkin lymphoma exist with this condition:
   a. endometriosis
   b. pelvic inflammatory disease
   c. sexually transmitted disease
   d. dysfunctional uterine bleeding

8. This benign lesion is also known as uterine fibroids:
   a. adenomyosis
   b. squamous cell
   c. leiomyoma
   d. extraembryonic cell primitive

9. Marginal, partial, and total are types of this condition:
   a. abruptio placentae
   b. placenta previa
   c. ectopic pregnancy
   d. hydatidiform mole

10. Which of the following is NOT a malposition of fetus?
   a. breech
   b. shoulder
   c. back
   d. brow

CHAPTER 6: MALE GENITAL SYSTEM

Anatomy and Terminology

Function, reproduction

Structure, essential organs, and accessory organs (Fig. 6-1)

■ Essential Organs

Testes (Gonads)

Produce sperm (male gamete with 23 chromosomes) in seminiferous tubules

Covered by tunica albuginea, located in scrotum

Produce testosterone in Leydig cells

Vas Deferens

Is a tube

End of epididymis

■ Accessory Organs

Ducts (carry sperm from testes to exterior), sex glands (produce solutions that mix with sperm), and external genitalia

Seminal vesicles produce most seminal fluid

Prostate gland produces some seminal fluid and activates sperm

Bulbourethral gland (Cowper's gland) secretes a very small amount of seminal fluid

External genitalia: penis and scrotum

- Penis contains three columns of erectile tissue: two corpora cavernosa and one spongiosum
- Urethra passes through corpora spongiosum
- Scrotum encloses testes

    Passage of sperm from production to exterior

Sperm are produced in seminiferous tubules (testes) and pass into

Epididymis then to vas deferens (within seminal vesicles) to

Ejaculatory duct then through urethra (prostate gland and Cowper's [bulbourethral] gland)

Pass though penis to outside of body

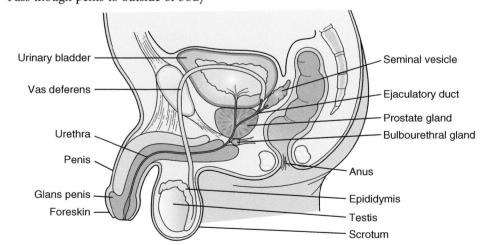

Figure **6-1** Male reproductive system.

COMBINING FORMS

1.	andr/o	male
2.	balan/o	glans penis
3.	cry/o	cold
4.	crypt/o	hidden
5.	epididym/o	epididymis
6.	gon/o	seed
7.	hydr/o	water, fluid
8.	orch/i	testicle
9.	orch/o	testicle
10.	orchi/o	testicle
11.	orchid/o	testicle
12.	prostat/o	prostate gland
13.	semin/i	semen
14.	sperm/o	sperm
15.	spermat/o	sperm
16.	test/o	testicle
17.	varic/o	varicose veins
18.	vas/o	vessel, vas deferens
19.	vesicul/o	seminal vesicles

SUFFIXES

1.	-one	hormone
2.	-pexy	fixation
3.	-ectomy	removal
4.	-stomy	new opening

MEDICAL ABBREVIATIONS

1.	BPH	benign prostatic hypertrophy
2.	PSA	prostate-specific antigen
3.	TURBT	transurethral resection of bladder tumor
4.	TURP	transurethral resection of prostate

MEDICAL TERMS

Cavernosa	Connection between cavity of penis and a vein
Cavernosography	Radiographic recording of a cavity, e.g., pulmonary cavity or main part of penis
Cavernosometry	Measurement of pressure in a cavity, e.g., penis
Chordee	Condition resulting in penis being bent downward
Corpora cavernosa	The two cavities of penis
Epididymectomy	Surgical removal of epididymis
Epididymis	Tube located at the top of testes that stores sperm
Epididymovasostomy	Creation of a new connection between vas deferens and epididymis
Meatotomy	Surgical enlargement of opening of urinary meatus
Orchiectomy	Castration, removal of testes
Orchiopexy	Surgical procedure to release undescended testis and fixate within scrotum
Penoscrotal	Referring to penis and scrotum
Plethysmography	Determining changes in volume of an organ part or body
Priapism	Painful condition in which penis is constantly erect
Prostatotomy	Incision into prostate
Transurethral resection, prostate	Procedure performed through urethra by means of a cystoscopy to remove part or all of prostate
Tumescence	State of being swollen
Tunica vaginalis	Covering of testes
Varicocele	Swelling of a scrotal vein
Vas deferens	Tube that carries sperm from epididymis to ejaculatory duct and seminal vesicles
Vasectomy	Removal of segment of vas deferens
Vasogram	Recording of the flow in vas deferens
Vasotomy	Incision in vas deferens
Vasorrhaphy	Suturing of vas deferens
Vasovasostomy	Reversal of a vasectomy
Vesiculectomy	Excision of seminal vesicle
Vesiculotomy	Incision into seminal vesicle

CHAPTER 6: ANATOMY AND TERMINOLOGY QUIZ

(Quiz answers are located in Appendix B)

1. This gland activates sperm and produces some seminal fluid:
   a. seminal vesicle
   b. bulbourethral gland
   c. prostate gland
   d. scrotum

2. Carries sperm from testes to ejaculatory duct:
   a. vas deferens
   b. sex gland
   c. tunica
   d. seminal

3. Penis contains these erectile tissues:
   a. one corpora cavernosa and two spongiosa
   b. two corpora cavernosa and two spongiosa
   c. one corpora cavernosa and one spongiosum
   d. two corpora cavernosa and one spongiosum

4. Also known as Cowper's gland:
   a. seminal vesicles
   b. bulbourethral gland
   c. prostate gland
   d. scrotum

5. Which of the following is NOT an accessory organ?
   a. gonads
   b. seminal vesicles
   c. prostate
   d. penis

6. Combining form meaning "male":
   a. andr/o
   b. balan/o
   c. orchi/o
   d. test/o

7. Combining form meaning "glans penis":
   a. balan/o
   b. vas/o
   c. vesicul/o
   d. orch/o

8. Testes are covered by the:
   a. seminal vesicles
   b. androgen
   c. chancre
   d. tunica albuginea

9. This abbreviation describes a surgical resection of prostate that is accomplished by means of an endoscope inserted into the urethra:
   a. TURBT
   b. BPH
   c. UPJ
   d. TURP

10. This abbreviation describes a condition of prostate in which there is an enlargement that is benign:
    a. TURBT
    b. BPH
    c. UPJ
    d. TURP

Pathophysiology

■ Male Genital System Disorders

Disorders of Scrotum, Testes, and Epididymis

Cryptorchidism
Undescended testes—condition at birth

- Unilateral or bilateral
- Primarily result from obstruction
- Risk neoplastic processes

Treatment
- May descend spontaneously
- Administration of hormone to stimulate testosterone production
- Surgical intervention (orchiopexy) near age 1 to avoid risk of infertility

Orchitis
Inflammation of testes

Most common cause is virus

- Such as mumps orchitis
- Atrophy with irreversible loss of sperm production at risk

May be associated with

- Mumps or epidemic parotitis
- Gonorrhea
- Syphilis
- Tuberculosis

Symptoms

- Mild to severe pain in testes
- Mild to severe edema
- Feeling of weight in testicular area

Treatment

- Depends on presence of underlying condition

Epididymitis
Inflammation of epididymis

Inflammatory response to trauma or infection

Abscess may form

Types
Sexually transmitted epididymitis

- Gonorrhea
- *T. pallidum*
- *T. vaginalis*

Nonspecific bacterial epididymitis

- *E. coli*
- Streptococci
- Staphylococci
- Associated with underlying urological disorder

Symptoms
Scrotal pain

Swelling

Erythema

Perhaps hydrocele formation

Treatment
Antibiotic

Bed rest

Ice packs

Scrotal support

Analgesics

Hydrocele (Fig. 6-2)
Collection of fluid in membranes of tunica vaginalis

May be congenital or acquired (response to infection or tumors)

Congenital hydrocele may reabsorb due to a communication between the scrotal sac and peritoneal cavity and require no intervention

Symptoms
Scrotal enlargement

Usually painless

- Unless infection is present

Varicocele
Abnormal dilation of plexus of veins

Decreases sperm production and motility

Symptoms
Usually painless

In elderly, may signal renal tumor

Treatment
Surgical intervention

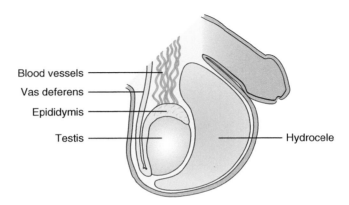

Figure **6-2** Hydrocele.

Torsion of Testes (Fig. 6-3)

Twisting of testes

Congenital abnormal development of tunica vaginalis and spermatic cord

Trauma may precipitate

Symptoms

Sudden onset of severe pain

Nausea

Vomiting

Scrotal edema and tenderness

Fever

Treatment

Immediate surgical intervention

Cancer of Testes

Rare form of cancer

Cure rate high (95%)

Cause unknown

Usually occurs in younger men

Two main groups

- Germ cell tumors (GCT)—90% of testicular tumors
- Sex cord–stromal tumors

Cancer of Scrotum

Rare form of cancer

- Squamous cell carcinoma

Symptoms

Asymptomatic in early stages

Ulcerations in later stages

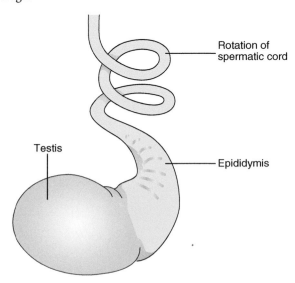

Figure **6-3** Torsion of testis.

Treatment

Wide local excision

Mohs micrographic surgery

- Precise removal of tumor
- Layers are removed until no further microscopic evidence of abnormal cells is seen

Laser therapy

Lymph nodes are examined for metastasis

Disorders of Urethra

Epispadias

Congenital anomaly

Urethral meatus is located on dorsal side of penis

Usually occurs in conjunction with other abnormalities

Treatment

Surgical reconstruction

Hypospadias

Most common abnormality of penis

Urethral opening on ventral side of penis

Results in curvature of penis

- Due to chordee

Treatment

Surgical reconstruction

Urethritis

Inflammation of urethra

Infectious urethritis can be gonococcal or nongonococcal

Nongonococcal organisms

- C. trachomatis
- U. urealyticum

Symptoms

Discharge

Inflammation of meatus

Burning

Itching

Urgent and frequent urination

In nongonococcal, symptoms are fewer

Treatment

Antibiotics based on organism

Disorders of Penis

Balanitis

Inflammation of glans

Causes

Syphilis

Trichomoniasis

Gonorrhea

Candida albicans

Tinea

Underlying disease—diabetes mellitus and candidiasis

No circumcision

Symptoms
Irritation

Tenderness

Discharge

Edema

Ulceration

Swelling of lymph nodes

Treatment
Culture of discharge

Saline irrigation

Antibiotics

Phimosis and Paraphimosis
Phimosis
Condition in which prepuce (foreskin) is constricted

- Prepuce cannot be retracted over glans penis

Can occur at any age

Associated with poor hygiene and chronic infection in uncircumcised males

Symptoms
Erythema

Edema

Tenderness

Purulent discharge

Treatment
Surgical circumcision

Paraphimosis
Condition in which prepuce (foreskin) is constricted

Prepuce is retracted over glans penis and cannot be moved forward

Symptom
Edema

Treatment
Surgical

Peyronie's Disease
Also known as bent nail syndrome

Fibrotic condition

- Results in lateral curvature of penis during erection

Occurs most often in middle-aged men

Cause is unknown but associated with

- Diabetes
- Keloid development
- Dupuytren's contracture (flexion deformity of toes and fingers)

Treatment
Sometimes spontaneous remission

Pharmacologic, oxygen-increasing therapies

Surgical resection of fibrous bands

Cancer of Penis
Rare form of cancer

Occurs most often in men over age 60

Squamous cell carcinoma

Increased risks

- More common in uncircumcised men
- Sexual partner with cervical carcinoma
- Human papillomavirus

Usually begins with small lesion beneath prepuce

Intraepithelial neoplasia is also known as

- Bowen's disease
- Erythroplasia of Queyrat
- Begins as noninvasive

Progresses to invasive if untreated

Metastasis to lymph nodes

Treatment
Excision

Mohs micrographic surgery

Radiation therapy

Laser therapy

Cryosurgery

Advanced tumors are treated with partial or total penectomy and chemotherapy

Disorders of Prostate Gland
Benign Prostatic Hyperplasia/Hypertrophy (BPH)
Multiple fibroadenomatous nodules; usually located on outside of gland, so easily palpable on digital exam

- Related to aging; common in men over 60 years of age
- Enlarging prostate obstructs bladder neck and urethra
- Decreases urine flow

It is thought that increased levels of estrogen/androgen cause BPH

Symptoms
Increased frequency and urgency of urination

Nocturia

Incontinence

Hesitancy

Diminished force

Postvoiding dribble

Screening
Prostate-specific antigen (PSA)

Digital rectal examination (DRE)

Treatment
Partial prostatectomy

Transurethral resection of prostate (TURP)

Excision of nodules

Hormone therapy

Placement of urethral stents

Pharmaceuticals—those that inhibit production of testosterone and those that relax smooth muscle of gland and neck of bladder

Prostatitis
Inflammation of prostate

- Acute or chronic bacterial prostatitis

Bacterial Causes
Escherichia coli

Enterococci

Staphylococci

Streptococci

Chlamydia trachomatis

Ureaplasma urealyticum

Neisseria gonorrhea

Nonbacterial Causes
Spontaneous

Prostatodynia

Symptoms
Acute Prostatitis
Fever and chills

Lower back pain

Perineal pain

Dysuria

Tenderness, suprapubic

Urinary tract infection

Chronic Prostatitis
Recurring

Same as acute only with no infection in urinary tract

Treatment

Acute

Antibiotic based on culture

Chronic

No treatment available

Cancer of Prostate

Most common malignancy diagnosed in men, occurring in men over age 60

Indications are that the cause is related to androgens

Predominately adenocarcinoma (95%)

No relationship between BPH and cancer of prostate

Symptoms

Asymptomatic in early stages

Later symptoms include

- Dysuria
- Back pain
- Hematuria
- Frequent urination
- Urinary retention
- Increased incidence of uremia

Stages

Two systems used to stage prostate cancer

- Whitmore-Jewett stages as indicated in Fig. 6-4
- Tumor-node-metastasis (TNM) as indicated in Fig. 6-5

Treatment

Dependent on stage

WHITMORE-JEWETT STAGES:

Stage A is clinically undetectable tumor confined to the gland and is an incidental finding at prostate surgery.
A1: well-differentiated with focal involvement
A2: moderately or poorly differentiated or involves multiple foci in the gland
Stage B is tumor confined to the prostate gland.
B0: nonpalpable, PSA-detected
B1: single nodule in one lobe of the prostate
B2: more extensive involvement of one lobe or involvement of both lobes
Stage C is a tumor clinically localized to the periprostatic area but extending through the prostatic capsule; seminal vesicles may be involved.
C1: clinical extracapsular extension
C2: extracapsular tumor producing bladder outlet or ureteral obstruction
Stage D is metastatic disease.
D0: clinically localized disease (prostate only) but persistently elevated enzymatic serum acid phosphatase
D1: regional lymph nodes only
D2: distant lymph nodes, metastases to bone or visceral organs
D3: D2 prostate cancer patients who relapse after adequate endocrine therapy

Figure **6-4** Whitmore-Jewett stages.

TNM STAGES:

Primary Tumor (T)

TX: Primary tumor cannot be assessed

T0: No evidence of primary tumor

T1: Clinically inapparent tumor not palpable or visible by imaging

    T1a: Tumor incidental histologic finding in 5% or less of tissue resected

    T1b: Tumor incidental histologic finding in more than 5% of tissue resected

    T1c: Tumor identified by needle biopsy (e.g., because of elevated PSA)

T2: Tumor confined within the prostate

    T2a: Tumor involves half a lobe or less

    T2b: Tumor involves more than half of a lobe, but not both lobes

    T2c: Tumor involves both lobes; extends through the prostatic capsule

T3a: Unilateral extracapsular extension

T3b: Bilateral extracapsular extension

T3c: Tumor invades the seminal vesicle(s)

T4: Tumor is fixed or invades adjacent structures other than the seminal vesicle(s)

    T4a: Tumor invades any of bladder neck, external sphincter, or rectum

    T4b: Tumor invades levator muscles and/or is fixed to the pelvic wall

Regional lymph nodes (N)

NX: Regional lymph nodes cannot be assessed

N0: No regional lymph node metastasis

N1: Metastasis in a single lymph node, 2 cm or less in greatest dimension

N2: Metastasis in a single lymph node, more than 2 cm but not more than 5 cm in greatest dimension; or multiple lymph node metastases, none more than 5 cm in greatest dimension

N3: Metastasis in a single lymph node more than 5 cm in greatest dimension

Distant metastases (M)

MX: Presence of distant metastasis cannot be assessed

M0: No distant metastasis

M1: Distant metastasis

    M1a: Nonregional lymph node(s)

    M1b: Bone(s)

    M1c: Other site(s)

Figure **6-5** TNM stages.

CHAPTER 6: PATHOPHYSIOLOGY QUIZ

(Quiz answers are located in Appendix B)

1. What is the condition in which testes do not descend?
   a. cryptorchidism
   b. Bowen's disease
   c. torsion
   d. hypospadias

2. Orchitis is most often caused by a:
   a. bacteria
   b. virus
   c. parasite
   d. fungus

3. A condition that can be either congenital or acquired through trauma and that involves twisting of testes is:
   a. hydrocele
   b. hypospadias
   c. cryptorchidism
   d. torsion

4. Cancer of the _____ is divided into two main groups of germ cell tumors and sex stromal cord tumors.
   a. testes
   b. penis
   c. scrotum
   d. prostate

5. This type of surgical technique involves excision of a lesion in layers until no further evidence of abnormality is seen:
   a. Bowen's
   b. Addison's
   c. Mohs
   d. laser

6. Epispadias is a disorder of the urethra in which urethral meatus is located on the _____ side of penis:
   a. ventral
   b. dorsal
   c. lateral
   d. medial

7. Inflammation of glans is:
   a. phimosis
   b. paraphimosis
   c. urethritis
   d. balanitis

8. This disease is also known as bent nail syndrome:
   a. Bowen's
   b. Peyronie's
   c. Addison's
   d. Whitmore-Jewett

9. Condition in which multiple fibroadenomatous nodules form and lead to decreased urine flow. Condition is thought to be related to increased levels of estrogen/androgen.
   a. BPH
   b. DRE
   c. GCT
   d. TNM

10. Cancer of prostate is predominately this type of cancer:
    a. sex cord
    b. adenocarcinoma
    c. squamous cell
    d. seminoma

CHAPTER 7: URINARY SYSTEM

Anatomy and Terminology

Removes metabolic waste materials (nitrogenous waste: urea, creatinine, and uric acid)

Conserves nutrients and water

Balances: electrolytes (acids/bases balance)

    Electrolytes are electrically charged molecules required for nerve and muscle function

Assists liver in detoxification

■ Organs (Fig. 7-1)

Kidneys

Ureters

Urinary bladder

Urethra

Kidneys (Fig. 7-2)

Electrolytes and fluid balance

Control pH balance (acid/base)

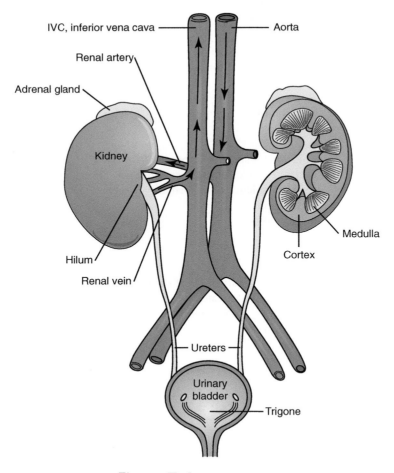

Figure **7-1** Urinary system.

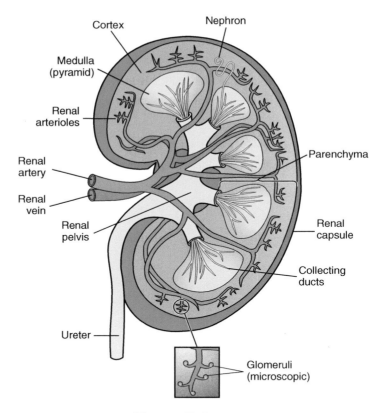

Figure **7-2** Kidney.

Secrete renin (which affects blood pressure) and erythropoietin (which stimulates red blood cell production in bone marrow)

Secrete active vitamin D required for calcium absorption from intestines

Two organs located behind peritoneum (retroperitoneal space)

Kidney Structure

Cortex (outer layer)

Medulla (inner portion)

Hilum (depression on medial border through which blood vessels and nerves pass)

Pyramids (divisions of medulla)

Papilla (inner part of pyramids)

Pelvis (receptacle for urine within kidney)

Calyces surround top of renal pelvis

Nephrons (3 types) are operational units of kidney

Ureters

Narrow tubes transporting urine from kidneys to bladder

Urinary Bladder

Reservoir for urine

Shaped like an upside-down pear with three surfaces

- Posterior (base)

- Anterior (neck)
- Superior (peritoneum)

Trigone

- Smooth triangular area inside bladder—size never changes
- Formed by openings of ureters and urethra

Urethra

Canal from bladder to exterior of body

Urinary meatus, outside opening of urethra

COMBINING FORMS

1.	albumin/o	albumin
2.	azot/o	urea
3.	bacteri/o	bacteria
4.	cali/o	calyx
5.	cyst/o	urinary
6.	dips/o	thirst
7.	glomerul/o	glomerulus
8.	glyc/o	sugar
9.	glycos/o	sugar
10.	hydr/o	water
11.	ket/o	ketone bodies/ketoacidosis
12.	lith/o	stone
13.	meat/o	meatus
14.	nephr/o	kidney
15.	noct/i	night
16.	olig/o	scant, few
17.	pyel/o	renal pelvis
18.	ren/o	kidney
19.	son/o	sound
20.	tripsy	to crush
21.	tryg/o	trigone region/kidney
22.	ur/o	urine
23.	ureter/o	ureter
24.	urethr/o	urethra

25. uria	urination/urinary condition
26. urin/o	urine
27. vesic/o	bladder

PREFIXES

1. dys-	painful
2. peri-	surrounding
3. poly-	many
4. retro-	behind

SUFFIXES

1. -eal	pertaining to
2. -lithiasis	condition of stones
3. -lysis	separation
4. -plasty	repair
5. -rrhaphy	suture
6. -tripsy	crush

MEDICAL ABBREVIATIONS

1. ARF	acute renal failure
2. BUN	blood urea nitrogen
3. ESRD	end-stage renal disease
4. HD	hemodialysis
5. IVP	intravenous pyelogram
6. KUB	kidney, ureter, bladder
7. pH	symbol for acid/base level
8. PKU	phenylketonuria
9. sp gr	specific gravity
10. UA	urinalysis
11. UPJ	ureteropelvic junction
12. UTI	urinary tract infection

MEDICAL TERMS

Bulbocavernosus	Muscle that constricts vagina in a female and urethra in a male
Bulbourethral	Gland with duct leading to urethra
Calculus	Concretion of mineral salts, also called a stone
Calycoplasty	Surgical reconstruction of recess of renal pelvis
Calyx	Recess of renal pelvis
Cystolithectomy	Removal of a calculus (stone) from urinary bladder
Cystometrogram	CMG, measurement of pressures and capacity of urinary bladder
Cystoplasty	Surgical reconstruction of bladder
Cystorrhaphy	Suture of bladder
Cystoscopy	Use of a scope to view bladder
Cystostomy	Surgical creation of an opening into bladder
Cystotomy	Incision into bladder
Cystourethroplasty	Surgical reconstruction of bladder and urethra
Cystourethroscopy	Use of a scope to view bladder and urethra
Dilation	Stretching or expansion
Dysuria	Painful urination
Endopyelotomy	Procedure involving bladder and ureters, including insertion of a stent into renal pelvis
Extracorporeal	Occurring outside of body
Fundoplasty	Repair of the bottom of bladder
Hydrocele	Sac of fluid
Kock pouch	Surgical creation of a urinary bladder from a segment of the ileum
Nephrocutaneous fistula	An abnormal channel from kidney to skin
Nephrolithotomy	Removal of a kidney stone through an incision made into the kidney
Nephrorrhaphy	Suturing of kidney
Nephrostomy	Creation of a channel into renal pelvis of kidney
Transureteroureterostomy	Surgical connection of one ureter to other ureter
Transvesical ureterolithotomy	Removal of a ureter stone (calculus) through bladder
Ureterectomy	Surgical removal of a ureter, either totally or partially
Ureterocutaneous fistula	Channel from ureter to exterior skin
Ureteroenterostomy	Creation of a connection between intestine and ureter

Ureterolithotomy	Removal of a stone from ureter
Ureterolysis	Freeing of adhesions of ureter
Ureteroneocystostomy	Surgical connection of ureter to a new site on bladder
Ureteropyelography	Ureter and renal pelvis radiography
Ureterotomy	Incision into ureter
Urethrocystography	Radiography of bladder and urethra
Urethromeatoplasty	Surgical repair of urethra and meatus
Urethropexy	Fixation of urethra by means of surgery
Urethroplasty	Surgical repair of urethra
Urethrorrhaphy	Suturing of urethra
Urethroscopy	Use of a scope to view urethra
Vesicostomy	Surgical creation of a connection of viscera of bladder to skin

CHAPTER 7: ANATOMY AND TERMINOLOGY QUIZ

(Quiz answers are located in Appendix B)

1. The outer covering of kidney:
   a. medulla
   b. pyramids
   c. cortex
   d. papilla

2. Which is not a division of kidneys?
   a. pelvis
   b. pyramids
   c. cortex
   d. trigone

3. The inner portion of kidneys:
   a. medulla
   b. pyramids
   c. cortex
   d. papilla

4. The smooth area inside bladder:
   a. pyramids
   b. calyces
   c. trigone
   d. cystocele

5. The narrow tube connecting kidney and bladder:
   a. urethra
   b. ureter
   c. meatus
   d. trigone

6. Which of the following is NOT a surface of urinary bladder?
   a. posterior
   b. anterior
   c. superior
   d. inferior

7. Combining form that means "stone":
   a. azot/o
   b. cyst/o
   c. lith/o
   d. olig/o

8. Term meaning "painful urination":
   a. pyuria
   b. dysuria
   c. diuresis
   d. hyperemia

9. Combining form meaning "scant":
   a. glyc/o
   b. hydr/o
   c. meat/o
   d. olig/o

10. Term that describes renal failure that is acute:
    a. ARF
    b. ESRD
    c. HD
    d. BPH

Pathophysiology

Renal Failure

Acute Renal Failure
Sudden onset of renal failure

Causes
Extreme hypotension

Trauma

Infection

Inflammation

Toxicity

Obstructed vascular supply

Symptoms
Uremia

Oliguria (decreased output) or anuria (no output)

Hyperkalemia (high potassium in blood)

Pulmonary edema

Types
Prerenal

- Associated with poor systemic perfusion
- Decreased renal blood flow
  - Such as with congestive heart failure

Intrarenal

- Associated with renal parenchyma disease (functional tissue of kidney)
  - Such as acute interstitial nephritis, glomerulopathies, and malignant hypertension

Postrenal

- Resulting from urine flow obstruction outside kidney (ureters or bladder neck)

Treatment
Underlying condition

Dialysis

Monitoring of fluid and electrolyte balance

Chronic Renal Failure
Gradual loss of function

- Progressively more severe renal insufficiency until end stage of
  - Renal disease
  - Irreversible kidney failure

Stages—Based on Level of Creatinine Clearance
Stage 1: Blood flow through kidney increases, kidney enlarges

Stage 2 (mild): Small amounts of blood protein (albumin) leak into urine (microalbuminuria)

Stage 3 (moderate): Albumin and other protein losses increase; patient may develop high blood pressure and kidney loses ability to filter waste

Stage 4 (severe): Large amounts of urine pass through kidney; blood pressure increases

Stage 5: End-stage renal failure. Ability to filter waste nearly stops; dialysis or transplant only option

Causes

Long-term exposure to nephrotoxins

Diabetes

Hypertension

Symptoms

No symptoms until well advanced

Polyuria

Nausea or anorexia

Dehydration

Neurologic manifestations

Stages of Nephron Loss

Decreased reserve

- 60% loss

Renal insufficiency

- 75% loss

End-stage renal failure

- 90% loss

Treatment

No cure

Dialysis

Kidney transplant

■ Urinary Tract Infections (UTI)

Cystitis—Bacterial

Cause

Bacteria, usually *E. coli*

Symptoms

Lower abdominal pain

Dysuria

Lower back pain

Urinary frequency and urgency

Cloudy, foul-smelling urine

Systemic Signs

Fever

Malaise

Nausea

Treatment

Antibiotics

Increased fluid intake

Cystitis—Noninfectious, Nonbacterial

Cause

Radiation, chemotherapy, autoimmune disorder, etc.

May later produce bacterial infection

Symptoms

Urinary frequency and urgency

Dysuria

Negative urine culture

Treatment

No known treatment

Acute Pyelonephritis (Fig. 7-3)

Bacterial infection with multiple abscesses of renal pelvis and medullary tissue

- May involve one or both kidneys

Causes

E. coli

Proteus

Pseudomonas

Obstruction and reflux of urine from bladder

Symptoms

Fever

Chills

Groin or flank pain

Dysuria

Pyuria

Nocturia

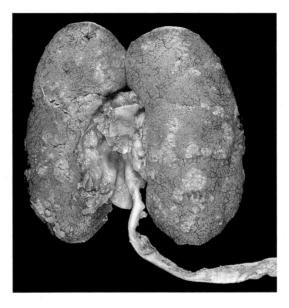

Figure **7-3** Acute pyelonephritis. Cortical surface exhibits grayish white areas of inflammation and abscess formation.

Treatment
Antibiotics

Surgical correction of obstruction

Chronic Pyelonephritis
Recurrent infection that causes scarring of kidney

Cause is difficult to determine

- Repeated infections
- Obstructive conditions

Symptoms
Hypertension

Dysuria

Flank pain

Increased frequency of urination

Treatment
Antibiotics for extended periods when reoccurring

Surgical reduction of obstruction

■ Glomerular Disorders

May be acute or chronic

Function of glomerulus is blood filtration

Glomerulonephritis
Inflammation of glomerulus

Causes
Drugs or toxins

Systemic disorder affecting many organs or idiopathic

May follow acute infections—most commonly streptococcal infections

Vascular pathology

Immune disorders

Treatment
Follows cause

Nephrotic Syndrome (Nephrosis)
Disease of kidneys that includes damage to membrane of the glomerulus causing excessive protein loss to urine

Accompanied by

- Hypoalbuminemia
- Hypercholesterolemia
- Hypercoagulability (excessive clotting)
- Prone to infections
- Edema
- Protein loss of >3.5 g

Damage to glomerulus results from

- Infection
- Immune response
  - Most predominant cause of dysfunction is exposure to toxins

May be a manifestation of an underlying condition, such as diabetes

Symptoms

Edema

Weight gain

Pallor

Proteinuria

Lipiduria

Treatment

Glucocorticoids, such as prednisone

- Reduces inflammation

Sodium- and fat-reduced diet

Protein supplements

Careful monitoring for continued inflammation

Acute Poststreptococcal Glomerulonephritis (APSGN)

Cause

Streptococcus infection

- With certain types of group A beta-hemolytic *Streptococcus*

Creates an antigen-antibody complex

- Infiltrates glomerular capillaries
- Results in inflammation in kidneys
- Inflammation interferes with normal kidney function
- Fluid and waste build-up
- Can lead to acute renal failure and scarring

Usually occurs in children 3 to 7 years of age

- Most often in boys

Symptoms

Back and flank pain

Cloudy, dark urine

Oliguria (decreased output)

Edema

Elevated blood pressure

Fatigue

Malaise

Headache

Nausea

Treatment

Sodium reduction

Antibiotics

Careful monitoring for continued inflammation

■ Urinary Tract Obstructions

Interference with urine flow

Causes urine backup behind obstruction of urinary system

Damage occurs to structures behind blockages

Increased urinary tract infection

Obstruction can be

- Functional
- Anatomic
    - Also known as obstructive uropathy

Kidney Stones (nephrolithiasis—renal calculi)

Formed of mineral salts (uric and calcium)

Develop anywhere in urinary tract

Tend to form in presence of excess salt and decreased fluid intake

- Most stones are formed of calcium salts
- Staghorn calculus forms in renal pelvis

Symptoms

Asymptomatic until obstruction occurs

Obstruction results in renal colic

- Extremely intense pain in flank
- Nausea
- Vomiting
- Cold, clammy skin
- Increased pulse rate

Treatment

Stone usually passes spontaneously

May use extracorporeal ultrasound or laser lithotripsy to break up stone (also known as extracorporeal shock wave lithotripsy, or ESWL)

Drugs may be used to dissolve stone

Preventative treatment to adjust pH level

- Increased fluid intake

Bladder Carcinoma

Malignant Tumor

Most common site of malignancy in urinary system

Tumors originate in transitional epithelial lining

Tends to recur

Often metastatic to liver and bone

Tumor Staging for Renal Cancer

Stage 1—Tumor of kidney capsule only

Stage 2—Tumor invading renal capsule/vein but within fascia

Stage 3—Tumor extending to regional lymph nodes/vena cava

Stage 4—Other organ metastasis

Symptoms

Often asymptomatic in early stage

Hematuria

Dysuria

Frequent urination

Infections common

Increased Risks

Cigarette smoking

Males age 50+

Working with industrial chemicals

Analgesics used in large amounts

Recurrent bladder infections

Treatment

Immunotherapy (Bacillus Calmette-Guérin [BCG] vaccine)

Excision

Chemotherapy

Radiation therapy

Hydronephrosis

Distention of kidney with urine

- Due to an obstruction
- Usually as a result of a kidney stone
- May also be due to scarring, tumor, edema from infection, or other obstruction

Symptoms

Usually asymptomatic

Mild flank pain

Infection may develop

May lead to chronic renal failure

Treatment

Treat underlying condition, such as removal of stone or antibiotics for infection

Dilation of stricture

■ Vascular Disorders

Nephrosclerosis

Excessive hardening and thickening of vascular structure of kidney

- Reduces blood supply
  - Increases blood pressure
  - Results in atrophy and ischemia of structures
  - May lead to chronic renal failure

Symptoms

Asymptomatic in early stages

Treatment

Diuretics

ACE (angiotensin-converting enzyme) inhibitors

Beta blockers that block release of resin

Antihypertensive drugs

Sodium intake reduction

Congenital Disorders

Polycystic Kidney Disease (PKD)

Numerous kidney cysts

Genetic disease

Symptoms

Asymptomatic until 40s

Cysts progressive in development (both kidneys)

Nephromegaly, hematuria, UTI, hypertension, uremia

Develops chronic renal failure

Cysts may spread to other organs, such as liver

Treatment

As for chronic renal failure

Wilms' Tumor—Nephroblastoma

Usually unilateral kidney tumors

Most common tumor in children

Usually advanced at time of diagnosis

- Metastasis to lungs at time of diagnosis is common

Symptoms

Asymptomatic until abdominal mass becomes apparent at age 1 to 5

Treatment

Excision

Radiation therapy

Chemotherapy

Usually a combination of above

CHAPTER 7: PATHOPHYSIOLOGY QUIZ

(Quiz answers are located in Appendix B)

1. Which of the following is NOT a type of acute renal failure?
   a. prerenal
   b. intrarenal
   c. interrenal
   d. postrenal

2. The loss of nephron function in end-stage renal disease is:
   a. 60%
   b. 70%
   c. 80%
   d. 90%

3. The cause of bacterial cystitis is usually:
   a. *Proteus*
   b. *Pseudomonas*
   c. *Staphylococcus*
   d. *E. coli*

4. The primary treatment for acute pyelonephritis would be:
   a. prednisone
   b. sodium reduction
   c. antibiotics
   d. BCG

5. APSGN stands for:
   a. advanced poststaphylococcal glomerulonephritis
   b. acute poststreptococcal glomerulonephritis
   c. acute poststaphylococcal glomerulonephritis
   d. advanced poststreptococcal glomerulonephritis

6. Obstructive uropathy is also known as:
   a. pyelonephritis
   b. renal failure
   c. urinary tract obstruction
   d. nephrotic syndrome

7. A treatment for kidney stone may be:
   a. ESWL
   b. prednisone
   c. open surgical procedure
   d. diuretics

8. The treatment for hydronephrosis involves:
   a. an open surgical procedure
   b. use of diuretics
   c. treatment of the underlying condition
   d. BCG

9. This is a congenital condition in which numerous cysts form in the kidney:
   a. Wilms' tumor
   b. polycystic kidney
   c. nephrosclerosis
   d. nephrotic syndrome

10. The treatment of Wilms' tumor would NOT include which of the following?
    a. excision
    b. chemotherapy
    c. diuretic
    d. radiation therapy

CHAPTER 8: DIGESTIVE SYSTEM

Anatomy and Terminology

Function: digestion, absorption, and elimination

Includes gastrointestinal tract (alimentary canal) and accessory organs

■ Mouth (Fig. 8-1)

Roof: hard palate, soft palate, uvula (projection at back of mouth)

Floor: contains tongue (Fig. 8-2), muscles, taste buds, and lingual frenulum, which anchors tongue to floor of mouth

■ Teeth

Thirty-two teeth (permanent)

Names of teeth: incisor, cuspid, bicuspid, and tricuspid

Tooth has crown (outer portion), neck (narrow part below gum line), root (end section), and pulp cavity (core)

■ Salivary Glands (Fig. 8-3)

Surround mouth and produce saliva—1.5 liters daily

Parotid

Submandibular

Sublingual

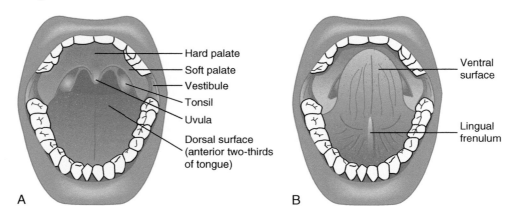

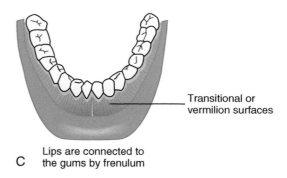

Figure **8-1** Anatomic structures of the mouth.

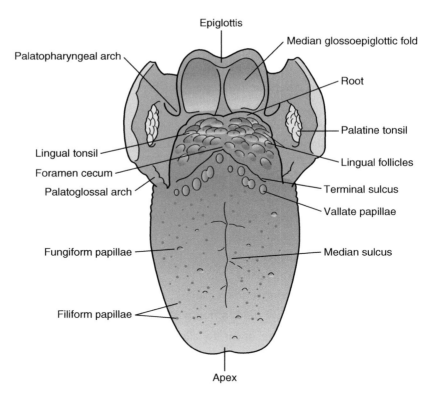

Figure **8-2** Dorsum of the tongue.

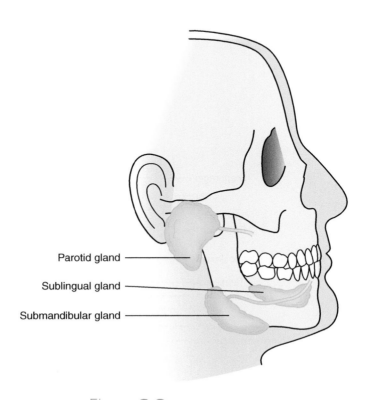

Figure **8-3** Major salivary glands.

■ Pharynx or Throat (Fig. 8-4)

Muscular tube (5 inches long) lined with mucous membrane through which air and food/water travel

Epiglottis covers larynx/esophagus when swallowing

■ Esophagus

Muscular tube (9-10 inches long) that carries food from pharynx to stomach by means of peristalsis (rhythmic contractions)

■ Stomach

Sphincter (ring of muscles) at entry into stomach (gastroesophageal or cardiac)

Three parts of stomach:

Fundus (upper part)

Body (middle part)

Antrum/pylorus (lower part)

Lined with rugae (folds of mucosal membrane)

Pyloric sphincter opens to allow chyme (thick liquid) to leave stomach and enter small intestine

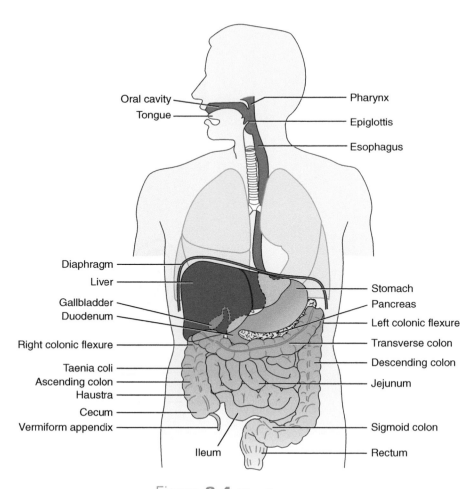

Figure **8-4** Digestive system.

■ Small Intestine

Duodenum (2 inches long): first portion beyond stomach—bile and pancreatic juice delivered here

Jejunum (96 inches long): connects duodenum to ileum

Ileum (132 inches long): attaches to large intestine

■ Large Intestine

Extends from ileum to anus

Cecum, from which appendix extends, connects ileum and colon

Colon (60 inches long), divided into:

    Ascending

    Transverse

    Descending

    Sigmoid

Sigmoid colon connected to rectum, which terminates at anus

■ Accessory Organs

Liver produces bile, sent to gallbladder via hepatic duct and cystic duct

Gallbladder stores bile, sent to duodenum from cystic duct into common bile duct

Bile emulsifies fat (breaks up large globules)

Pancreas produces enzymes sent through pancreatic duct to hepatopancreatic ampulla (ampulla of Vater) then to duodenum

Pancreatic cells—islets of Langerhans produce insulin and glucagon

■ Peritoneum

Serous membrane lines abdominal cavity and maintains organs in correct anatomic position

Food passes through digestive tract via:

    Mouth—including salivary glands

    Pharynx

    Esophagus

    Stomach

    Duodenum—pancreatic enzymes and bile produced in liver and stored in gallbladder enter

    Jejunum

    Ileum

    Cecum

    Ascending colon

    Transverse colon

    Descending colon

    Sigmoid colon

    Rectum

    Anus

COMBINING FORMS

1.	abdomin/o	abdomen
2.	an/o	anus
3.	appendic/o	appendix
4.	bil/i	bile
5.	bilirubin/o	bile pigment
6.	bucc/o	cheek
7.	cec/o	cecum
8.	celi/o	abdomen
9.	cheil/o	lip
10.	chol/e	gall/bile
11.	cholangio/o	bile duct
12.	cholecyst/o	gallbladder
13.	choledoch/o	common bile duct
14.	col/o	colon
15.	dent/i	tooth
16.	diverticul/o	diverticulum
17.	duoden/o	duodenum
18.	enter/o	small intestine
19.	esophag/o	esophagus
20.	faci/o	face
21.	gastr/o	stomach
22.	gingiv/o	gum
23.	gloss/o	tongue
24.	hepat/o	liver
25.	herni/o	hernia
26.	ile/o	ileum
27.	jejun/o	jejunum
28.	labi/o	lip
29.	lapar/o	abdomen
30.	lingu/o	tongue

31.	lip/o	fat
32.	lith/o	stone
33.	or/o	mouth
34.	ordont/o	tooth
35.	palat/o	palate
36.	pancreat/o	pancreas
37.	peritone/o	peritoneum
38.	pharyng/o	throat
39.	polyp/o	polyp
40.	proct/o	rectum
41.	pylor/o	pylorus
42.	rect/o	rectum
43.	sial/o	saliva
44.	sialaden/o	salivary gland
45.	sigmoid/o	sigmoid colon
46.	steat/o	fat
47.	stomat/o	mouth
48.	uvul/o	uvula

SUFFIXES

1.	-ase	enzyme
2.	-cele	hernia
3.	-chezia	defecation
4.	-iasis	abnormal condition
5.	-phagia	eating
6.	-prandial	meal

MEDICAL ABBREVIATIONS

1.	EGD	esophagogastroduodenoscopy
2.	EGJ	esophagogastric junction
3.	ERCP	endoscopic retrograde cholangiopancreatography
4.	GERD	gastroesophageal reflux disease

5.	GI	gastrointestinal
6.	HJR	hepatojugular reflux
7.	LLQ	left lower quadrant
8.	LUQ	left upper quadrant
9.	PEG	percutaneous endoscopic gastrostomy
10.	RLQ	right lower quadrant
11.	RUQ	right upper quadrant

MEDICAL TERMS

Anastomosis	Surgical connection of two tubular structures, such as two pieces of intestine
Biliary	Refers to gallbladder, bile, or bile duct
Cholangiography	Radiographic recording of bile ducts
Cholecystectomy	Surgical removal of gallbladder
Cholecystoenterostomy	Creation of a connection between gallbladder and intestine
Colonoscopy	Fiberscopic examination of entire colon that may include part of terminal ileum
Colostomy	Artificial opening between colon and abdominal wall
Diverticulum	Protrusion in wall of an organ
Dysphagia	Difficulty swallowing
Enterolysis	Releasing of adhesions of intestine
Eventration	Protrusion of bowel through an opening in abdomen
Evisceration	Pulling viscera outside of the body through an incision
Exstrophy	Condition in which an organ is turned inside out
Fulguration	Use of electric current to destroy tissue
Gastrointestinal	Pertaining to stomach and intestine
Gastroplasty	Operation on stomach for repair or reconfiguration
Gastrostomy	Artificial opening between stomach and abdominal wall
Hernia	Organ or tissue protruding through wall or cavity that usually contains it
Ileostomy	Artificial opening between ileum and abdominal wall
Imbrication	Overlapping
Incarcerated	Regarding hernias, a constricted, irreducible hernia that may cause obstruction of an intestine
Intussusception	Slipping of one part of intestine into another part

Jejunostomy	Artificial opening between jejunum and abdominal wall
Laparoscopy	Exploration of the abdomen and pelvic cavities using a scope placed through a small incision in abdominal wall
Lithotomy	Incision into an organ or a duct for the purpose of removing a stone
Lithotripsy	Crushing of a stone by sound wave or force
Paraesophageal or hiatal hernia	Protrusion of any structure through esophageal hiatus of diaphragm
Proctosigmoidoscopy	Fiberscopic examination of sigmoid colon and rectum
Sialolithotomy	Surgical removal of a stone of salivary gland or duct
Varices	Varicose veins
Volvulus	Twisted section of intestine

CHAPTER 8: ANATOMY AND TERMINOLOGY QUIZ

(Quiz answers are located in Appendix B)

1. This is NOT a part of the small intestine:
   a. ileum
   b. cecum
   c. duodenum
   d. jejunum

2. Term meaning "ring of muscles":
   a. pyloric
   b. parotid
   c. epiglottis
   d. sphincter

3. The throat is also known as the:
   a. larynx
   b. epiglottis
   c. esophagus
   d. pharynx

4. The three parts of the stomach:
   a. pyloric, rugae, fundus
   b. fundus, body, antrum
   c. antrum, pyloric, rugae
   d. ilium, fundus, pyloric

5. The projection at the back of the mouth:
   a. palate
   b. sublingual
   c. uvula
   d. parotid

6. Mucosal membrane that lines the stomach:
   a. cecum
   b. rugae
   c. frenulum
   d. fundus

7. The parts of the colon are:
   a. ascending, transverse, descending, sigmoid
   b. ascending, descending, sigmoid
   c. transverse, descending, sigmoid
   d. descending, sigmoid

8. Combining form meaning "abdomen":
   a. an/o
   b. cec/o
   c. celi/o
   d. col/o

9. Term that means connecting two ends of a tube:
   a. anastomosis
   b. amylase
   c. aphthous stomatitis
   d. atresia

10. Abbreviation that means a scope placed through the esophagus, into the stomach, and to the duodenum:
    a. ERCP
    b. EGD
    c. GERD
    d. PEG

Pathophysiology

■ Disorders of Oral Cavity

Cleft Lip and Cleft Palate (Orofacial Cleft) (Fig. 8-5)

Congenital defect

Cleft lip and palate

> Lip and palate do not properly join together

Causes feeding problems

- Infants cannot create sufficient suction for feeding
- Danger of aspirating food
- Results in speech defects

Treatment

> Surgical repair of defects

Ulceration

Canker sore—caused by herpes simplex virus

- Ulceration of oral mucosa

Also known as

- Aphthous ulcer (aphtha: small ulcer)
- Aphthous stomatitis

Heals spontaneously

Infections

Candidiasis

Candida albicans is naturally found in mouth

Thrush (oral candidiasis) is overarching infection

Causes

Antibiotic regimen

Chemotherapy

Glucocorticoids

Common in patients with diabetes and AIDS patients

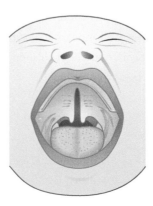

Figure **8-5** Cleft palate.

Treatment

Nystatin (topical fungal agent)

Herpes Simplex Type 1

Herpetic stomatitis

- Viral cold sores and blisters
- Associated with herpes simplex virus type 1 (HSV-1)

Treatment

No cure

May be alleviated somewhat by antiviral medications

Cancer of Oral Cavity

Most common type is squamous cell carcinoma

Kaposi's sarcoma is type seen in AIDS patients

Increased in smokers

  Lip cancer also increased in smokers, particularly pipe smokers

Poor prognosis

Usually asymptomatic until later stages

Metastasis through lymph nodes

■ Esophageal Disorders

Scleroderma

Also known as progressive systemic sclerosis

Atrophy of smooth muscles of lower esophagus

Lower esophageal sphincter (LES) does not close properly

- Leads to esophageal reflux
- Strictures form

Symptom

Predominantly dysphagia

Esophagitis

Inflammation of esophagus

Types

  Acute

Most common type is that caused by hiatal hernia

Infectious esophagitis is common in patients with AIDS

Ingestion of strong alkaline or acid substances

- Such as those in household cleaners

Inflammation leads to scarring

  Chronic

Most common type is that caused by LES reflux

Cancer of Esophagus

Most common type is squamous cell or secondary adenocarcinoma

Usually caused by continued irritation

- Smoking
- Alcohol

- Hiatal hernia
- Chronic esophagitis/GERD

Poor prognosis

Hiatal Hernia (Diaphragmatic hernia)
Diaphragm goes over stomach

- Esophagus passes through diaphragm at natural opening (hiatus)
- Part of the stomach protrudes (herniates) through opening in diaphragm into thorax

Types (Fig. 8-6)
Sliding

- Stomach and gastroesophageal junction protrude through the hiatus

Paraesophageal/rolling hiatal

- Part of fundus protrudes

Symptoms
Heartburn

Reflux

Belching

Lying down causes discomfort

Dysphagia

Substernal pain after eating

Gastroesophageal Reflux Disease (GERD)
Associated with hiatal hernias

- Reflux of gastric contents

Lower esophageal sphincter does not constrict properly

Treatment
Reduce irritants, such as

- Smoking
- Spicy foods
- Alcohol

Antacids

Elevate head of bed

Avoid tight clothing

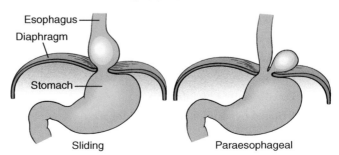

HIATAL HERNIAS

Esophagus

Diaphragm

Stomach

Sliding   Paraesophageal

Figure **8-6** Sliding and paraesophageal hernias (hiatal hernias).

■ Stomach and Duodenum Disorders

Gastritis
Inflammation of stomach mucosa

Acute Superficial Gastritis
Mild, transient irritation

Causes
Excessive alcohol

Infection

Food allergies

Spicy foods

Aspirin

H. pylori (Helicobacter pylori)

Symptoms
Nausea

Vomiting

Anorexia

Bleeding in more severe cases

Epigastric pain

Treatment
Usually spontaneous remission in 2 to 3 days

Removal of underlying irritation

Antibiotics for infection

Chronic Atrophic Gastritis
Progressive atrophy of epithelium

Types
Type A, atrophic or fundal
- Involves fundus of stomach
- Autoimmune disease
  - Decreases acid secretion
  - Results in high gastrin levels

Type B, antral
- Involves antrum region of stomach
- Often associated with elderly
  - May be associated with pernicious anemia
- Low gastrin levels
- Usually caused by infection
- Irritated by alcohol, drugs, and tobacco

Symptom abatement
- Bland diet
- Alcohol avoidance

- ASA avoidance
- Antibiotics for *H. pylori*

Peptic Ulcers

Erosive area on mucosa

- Extends below epithelium
- Chronic ulcers have scar tissue at base of erosive area

Ulcers can occur anywhere on gastrointestinal tract but typically are found on the

- Lower esophagus
- Stomach
- Proximal duodenum

Some Causes

Alcohol

Smoking

Aspirin

Severe stress

Bacterial infection caused by *Helicobacter pylori (H. pylori)*, 90% of the time

Genetic factor

Constant use of anti-inflammatory drugs

Symptoms

Epigastric pain when stomach is empty

- Relieved by food or antacid

Burning

May include

- Vomiting blood
- Nausea
- Weight loss
- Anorexia

Severe cases may include

- Obstruction
- Hemorrhage
- Perforation

Treatment

Surgical intervention

Antacids

Dietary restrictions

Rest

Antibiotics

Gastric Cancer (Malignant Tumor of Stomach)

Most often occurs in men over 40

Cause is unknown, but often associated with *Helicobacter pylori* (bacterial infection)

Predisposing Factors

Atrophic gastritis

Pernicious anemia

History of nonhealing gastric ulcer

Blood type A

Geographic factors

Environmental factors

Carcinogenic foods

- Smoked meats
- Nitrates
- Pickled foods

Symptoms

Usually asymptomatic in early stages

Treatment

Excision

Chemotherapy

Radiation (poor response)

Prognosis is poor

Pyloric Stenosis

Narrowing of the pyloric sphincter

Signs appear soon after birth

- Failure to thrive
- Projectile vomiting

Treatment

Surgery to relieve stenosis (pyloromyotomy)

■ Intestinal Disorders

Small Intestine

Malabsorption Conditions
Celiac Disease

Most important malabsorption condition

Villi atrophy in response to food containing gluten and lose ability to absorb

- Gluten is a protein found in wheat, rye, oats, and barley

Symptoms

Malnutrition

Muscle wasting

Distended abdomen

Diarrhea

Fatigue

Weakness

Steatorrhea (excess fat in feces)

Treatment

Gluten-free diet

Steroids when necessary

Lactase Deficiency

Enzyme deficiency

- Secondary to gastrointestinal damage, such as
  - Regional enteritis
  - Infection
- Common in African Americans, occurring in adulthood

Symptoms

Intolerance to milk

Intestinal cramping

Diarrhea

Flatulence

Treatment

Elimination of milk products

Crohn's Disease (Regional Enteritis)

Inflammatory Bowel Disease (IBD)—Affects Terminal Ileum and Colon

Cause

Unknown

Symptoms

Vary greatly

Inflammatory disease of GI tract

Diarrhea

Gas

Fever

Abdominal pain

Malaise

Anorexia

Weight loss

Treatment

No specific treatment

Palliative medications to control symptoms

Resection of affected section of intestine with anastomosis

Diet modifications

Duodenal Ulcers

Most common ulcer

Develop in younger population

Common in type O blood types

Appendicitis

Inflammation of vermiform appendix that projects from cecum

Obstruction of lumen leads to infection

- Appendix becomes hypoxic (decreased oxygen levels)
- May cause gangrene
- May rupture, causing peritonitis

Symptoms

Periumbilical (around umbilicus) pain, initially

Right lower quadrant (RLQ) pain as inflammation progresses

Nausea

Vomiting

Possible diarrhea

Treatment

Appendectomy

Management of any perforation or abscess

Meckel's Diverticulum

- Appendage of ileum near cecum derived from an unobliterated yolk stalk in fetal development
- Symptoms can mimic appendicitis

Peritonitis

Inflammation of peritoneum (membrane that lines abdominal cavity)

Usually a result of

- Spread of infection from abdominal organ
- Puncture wound to abdomen
- Rupture of gastrointestinal tract—appendicitis or Meckel's diverticulum

Abscesses form, resulting in adhesions

- May result in obstruction

Types

Acute, chronic

Symptoms

Abdominal pain

Vomiting

Rigid abdomen

Fever

Leukocytosis (increased white cells in blood)

Treatment

Antibiotics

Suction of stomach and intestines

If possible, surgical removal of origin of infection, such as appendix

Fluid replacement

Bed rest

Obstruction

Any interference with passage of intestinal contents

May be

- Acute
- Chronic
- Partial
- Total

Types

Nonmechanical

- Paralytic ileus
- Result of trauma or toxin

Mechanical

- Result of tumors, adhesions, hernias
- Simple mechanical obstruction
  - One point of obstruction
- Closed-loop obstruction
  - At least two points of obstruction
- Diverticulosis
- Twisted bowel (volvulus)
- Telescoping bowel (intussusception)

Symptoms

Abdominal distention

Pain

Vomiting

Total constipation

Treatment

Surgical intervention

Symptomatic treatment

Large Intestine

Diverticulosis

Herniation of intestinal mucosa

- Forms sacs in lining, called diverticula

Diverticulitis

Sacs fill and become inflamed

- Common in aged persons

Symptoms

Diarrhea or constipation

Gas

Abdominal discomfort

Complications

Perforation

Bleeding

Peritonitis

Abscess

Obstruction

Treatment

Antimicrobials as necessary

High-fiber diet (greater than 20 g daily)

Stool softeners

Dietary restrictions of solid foods

Surgical intervention if necessary

Ulcerative Colitis (Fig. 8-7)

Inflammation of rectum that progresses to sigmoid colon

Intermittent exacerbations and remissions

May develop into toxic megacolon

- Leads to obstruction and dilation of colon

Increased risk for colorectal cancer

Symptoms

Diarrhea

- Blood and mucus may be present

Cramping

Fever

Weight loss

Treatment

Remove physical or emotional stressors

Anti-inflammatory medications

Antimotility agents

Nutritional supplementation

Surgical intervention, if necessary

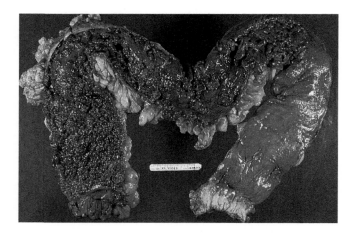

Figure **8-7** Ulcerative colitis.

Colorectal Cancer

Usually develop from polyp

- In those 55 and older

Increased Risks

Genetic factors

40 years of age and older

Diets high in

- Fat
- Sugar
- Red meat

Low-fiber diets

Symptoms

Asymptomatic until advanced

Some may experience

- Cramping
- Ribbon stools
- Feeling of incomplete evacuation
- Fatigue
- Weight loss
- Change in bowel habits
- Blood in stool

Treatment

Surgical excision

Radiation

Chemotherapy

Combination of above

■ Disorders of Liver, Gallbladder, and Pancreas

Disorders of Liver

Jaundice (Hyperbilirubinemia)

A sign of biliary disease, not a disease itself

- Results in yellow eyes (sclera) and skin

Types

Prehepatic

- Excess destruction of red blood cells
- Result of hemolytic anemia or reaction to transfusion

Intrahepatic

- Impaired uptake of bilirubin and decreased blending of bilirubin by hepatic cells
- Result of liver disease, such as cirrhosis or hepatitis

Posthepatic

- Excess bile flows into blood
- Result of obstruction
  - Due to conditions such as inflammation of liver, tumors, cholelithiasis

Treatment
Removal of cause

Cancer of Liver
Most commonly a metastasis; primary CA rare

Risk for primary liver CA

- Hepatitis B, C, and D
- Cirrhosis
- Myotoxins
- Heavy smoking/alcohol use

Treatment
Surgical resection if localized

Survival typically 3 or 4 months

Viral Hepatitis
Liver cells are damaged

Results in inflammation and necrosis

Damage can be mild or severe

Scar tissue forms in liver

- Leads to ischemia

Hepatitis A (HAV)
Infectious hepatitis—caused by hepatitis A virus

Transmission

- Most commonly fecal-oral route—contaminated food or water

Does not have a chronic state

Slow onset—complete recovery characteristic

Vaccine available for those who are traveling

Gamma globulin may be administered to those just exposed

Hepatitis B (HBV)
Serum hepatitis

Carrier state is common

Caused by hepatitis B virus

- Asymptomatic but contagious

Long incubation period

Transmission

- Intravenous drug users
- Transfusion
- Exposure to blood and bodily fluids
- Sexual transmission
- Mother-to-fetus transmission
- Immune globulin is temporary prophylactic
- Vaccine is now routine for children and is given to those at risk

Severe forms cause liver cell destruction, cirrhosis, death

Hepatitis C (HCV)

Transmission of virus

- Most commonly by transfusion
- IV drug users

Half of cases develop into chronic hepatitis

Increases risk of hepatocellular cancer

Carrier state may develop

Hepatitis D (HDV)

Transmission of hepatitis D virus

- Blood
- Intravenous drug users

Hepatitis B is present for this type to develop

Hepatitis E (HEV)

Transmission of hepatitis E virus

- Fecal-oral route

Does not develop into chronic or carrier

Hepatitis G

Transmission of hepatitis G virus

- IV drug use
- Sexual transmission

Symptoms of Hepatitis

Stages

Preicteric

- Anorexia
- Nausea and vomiting

Liver enzymes may be elevated—indication of liver cell damage

- Fatigue
- Malaise
- Generalized pain with low-grade fever
- Cough

Icteric

- Jaundice
- Hepatomegaly (enlarged liver)
- Biliary obstruction
- Light-colored stools and dark urine
- Pruritus
- Abdominal pain

Posticteric (recovery)

- Reduction of symptoms

Treatment

None

In early stages gamma globulins may be used

Interferon may be used for cases of chronic hepatitis B and C

Nonviral Hepatitis

Hepatitis that results from hepatotoxins

Symptoms

- Similar to viral hepatitis

Treatment

- Removal of hepatotoxin

Cirrhosis

Profuse liver damage

- Extensive fibrosis
  - Results in inflammation

Progressive disorder

Leads to liver failure

Types

Alcoholic liver

- Known as Laënnec's cirrhosis or portal cirrhosis
- Largest group

Biliary

- Associated with immune disorders
- Obstructions (intrahepatic or extrahepatic blood vessels) occur and disrupt normal function

Postnecrotic

- Associated with chronic hepatitis (A or C) and exposure to toxins

Symptoms

Asymptomatic in early stages

Nausea

Vomiting

Fatigue

Weight loss

Pruritus

Jaundice

Edema

Treatment

Symptomatic

Dietary restrictions

- Reduced protein and sodium
- Increased vitamins and carbohydrates

Diuretics

Antibiotics

Liver transplant

Disorders of Gallbladder

Cholecystitis

Inflammation of gallbladder and cystic duct

Cholangitis
Inflammation of bile duct

Cholelithiasis
Formation of gallstones (Fig. 8-8)

- Consists of cholesterol or bilirubin
- Occurs most often in those with high levels of cholesterol, calcium, or bile salts

Stones cause irritation and inflammation

- May lead to infection
- Obstruction
  - May result in pancreatitis
  - Rupture is possible

Symptoms
Often asymptomatic

Dietary intolerance particularly to fat

Right upper quadrant (RUQ) pain

Pain in back and/or shoulder

Epigastric discomfort

Bloating heartburn, flatulence

Treatment
Surgical intervention (laparoscopic cholecystectomy)

Lithotripsy

Medical management by use of drugs that break down stone

Disorders of Pancreas

Pancreatitis
Inflammation of pancreas resulting from digestive enzyme attack to pancreas

Acute and chronic forms

Commonly associated with alcoholism, biliary tract obstruction, drug toxicity, gallstone obstruction of common bile duct, and viral infections

Symptoms
Severe pain

Fever

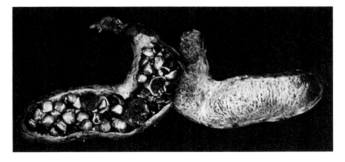

Figure **8-8** Resected gallbladder containing mixed gallstones.

Acute form is a medical emergency

Neurogenic shock

Septicemia

General sepsis

Complications
Adult respiratory distress syndrome (ARDS)

Renal failure

Treatment
No oral intake

- IV fluids given and carefully monitored

Analgesics

Stop process of autodigestion

Prevent systemic shutdown

Pancreatic Cancer
Increased Risk
Cigarette smoking

Diet high in fat and protein

Symptoms
Weight loss

Jaundice

Anorexia

Most types of pancreatic cancer are asymptomatic until well advanced

Treatment
Surgery

Chemotherapy and radiation therapy

CHAPTER 8: PATHOPHYSIOLOGY QUIZ

(Quiz answers are located in Appendix B)

1. This type of hyperbilirubinemia is characterized by excess bile flow into the blood:
   a. intrahepatic
   b. prehepatic
   c. posthepatic
   d. jaundice

2. This type of hepatitis is transmitted by the fecal-oral route:
   a. A
   b. B
   c. C
   d. D

3. Which of the following is the recovery stage of hepatitis?
   a. prehepatic
   b. posthepatic
   c. preicteric
   d. posticteric

4. This type of cirrhosis is also known as portal cirrhosis:
   a. biliary
   b. alcoholic liver
   c. postnecrotic
   d. traumatic

5. This condition is the inflammation of the bile ducts:
   a. cholangitis
   b. cholecystitis
   c. cholelithiasis
   d. cholangioma

6. Formation of gallstones most often occurs with high levels of the following:
   a. bile salts and toxins
   b. cholesterol and toxins
   c. cholesterol and bile salts
   d. toxins

7. The primary factor that increases the risk of pancreatic cancer is:
   a. smoking
   b. alcohol
   c. intravenous drug use
   d. hepatitis

8. A potential complication of this condition is ARDS:
   a. hyperbilirubinemia
   b. hepatitis
   c. pancreatitis
   d. pancreatic cancer

9. The primary treatment for jaundice is:
   a. removal of cause
   b. antibiotics
   c. dialysis
   d. vaccine

10. This condition has the largest group of those who abuse alcohol:
    a. cirrhosis
    b. hepatitis
    c. pancreatitis
    d. pancreatic cancer

CHAPTER 9: MEDIASTINUM AND DIAPHRAGM

Anatomy and Terminology

Not an organ system

Mediastinum

That area between lungs that a median (partition) divides (Fig. 9-1) into

- Superior
- Anterior
- Posterior
- Middle

Space that houses heart, thymus gland, trachea, esophagus, nerves, lymph and blood vessels, and major blood vessels

- Aorta
- Inferior vena cava

Diaphragm

A dome-shaped muscular partition that separates abdominal cavity from thoracic cavity

- Assists in breathing
  - Expands to assist lungs in exhalation/relaxation of diaphragm
  - Flattens out during inspiration/contraction of diaphragm
- Diaphragmatic hernia: esophageal hernia

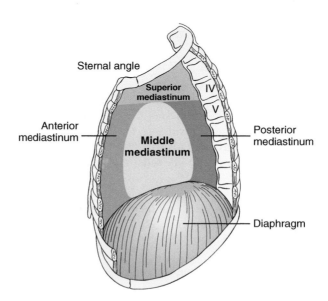

Figure **9-1** Mediastinum and diaphragm.

CHAPTER 9: ANATOMY AND TERMINOLOGY QUIZ

(Quiz answers are located in Appendix B)

1. The mediastinum is NOT an organ system.
   a. true
   b. false

2. The mediastinum is divided into:
   a. superior, anterior, posterior
   b. superior, anterior, posterior, middle
   c. anterior, posterior, middle
   d. middle, anterior, superior

3. During inspiration, the diaphragm:
   a. expands
   b. moves upward
   c. collapses
   d. flattens out

4. Term meaning "partition":
   a. middle
   b. aspect
   c. median
   d. diaphragm

5. The diaphragm is said to be this shape:
   a. square
   b. flat
   c. dome
   d. round

6. This separates the abdominal cavity from the thoracic cavity:
   a. mediastinum
   b. diaphragm
   c. superior
   d. inferior

7. This is the area between the lungs:
   a. mediastinum
   b. diaphragm
   c. superior
   d. inferior

8. This is an esophageal hernia:
   a. mediastinal
   b. diaphragmatic
   c. paraesophageal
   d. hiatal

9. A diaphragmatic hernia is also known as:
   a. esophageal
   b. epiglottis
   c. partitional
   d. medial

10. The diaphragm assists in:
    a. percussion
    b. auscultation
    c. contraction
    d. breathing

CHAPTER 10: HEMIC AND LYMPHATIC SYSTEM

Anatomy and Terminology

Hemic refers to blood

Lymphatic system removes excess tissue fluid

- Lymph tissue is scattered throughout body
- Composed of lymph nodes, vessels, and organs

■ Lymph

Colorless fluid containing lymphocytes and monocytes

Originates from blood and after filtering, returns to blood

Transports interstitial fluids and proteins that have leaked from blood system into venous system

Absorbs and transports fats from villi of small intestine to venous system

Assists in immune function

■ Lymph Vessels

Similar to veins

Organized circulatory system throughout body

■ Lymph Organs

Lymph nodes, spleen, bone marrow, thymus, tonsils, and Peyer's patches (lymphoid tissue on mucosa of small intestine)

Lymph nodes, areas of concentrated tissue (Fig. 10-1)

Spleen, located in left upper quadrant (LUQ) of abdomen

- Composed of lymph tissue
  - Function is to filter blood; activates lymphocytes and B cells to filter antigens
  - Stores blood

Thymus secretes thymosin, causing T cells to mature

- Larger in infants and shrinks with age

Tonsils

- Palatine tonsils
- Pharyngeal tonsils/adenoids

■ Hematopoietic Organ

Bone marrow, contains tissue that produces RBCs, WBCs, and platelets

- Produces stem cells

COMBINING FORMS

1. aden/o	gland
2. adenoid/o	adenoids

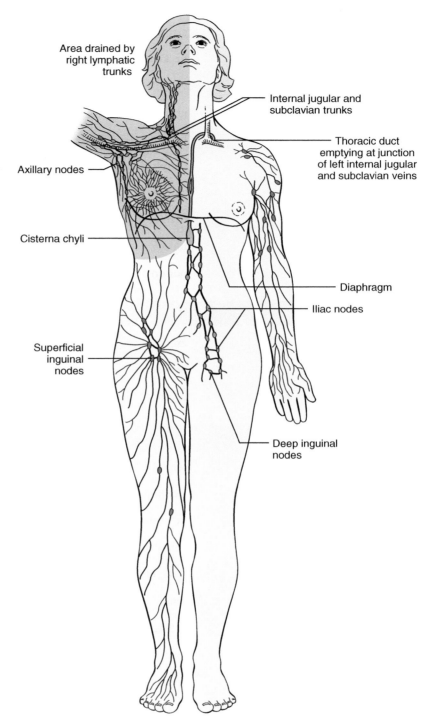

Area drained by right lymphatic trunks

Internal jugular and subclavian trunks

Thoracic duct emptying at junction of left internal jugular and subclavian veins

Axillary nodes

Cisterna chyli

Diaphragm

Iliac nodes

Superficial inguinal nodes

Deep inguinal nodes

Figure **10-1** Lymphatic system.

3. axill/o	armpit
4. cervic/o	neck/cervix
5. immune/o	immune
6. inguin/o	groin
7. lymph/o	lymph
8. lymphaden/o	lymph gland
9. splen/o	spleen
10. thym/o	thymus gland
11. tonsill/o	tonsil
12. tox/o	poison

PREFIXES

1. hyper-	excess
2. inter-	between
3. retro-	behind

SUFFIXES

1. -ectomy	removal
2. -edema	swelling
3. -itis	inflammation
4. -megaly	enlargement
5. -oid	resembling
6. -oma	tumor
7. -penia	deficient
8. -pexy	fixation
9. -phylaxis	protection
10. -poiesis	production

MEDICAL TERMS

Axillary nodes	Lymph nodes located in armpit
Cloquet's node	Also called a gland; it is highest of deep groin lymph nodes
Inguinofemoral	Referring to groin and thigh
Jugular nodes	Lymph nodes located next to large vein in neck

Lymph node	Station along lymphatic system
Lymphadenectomy	Excision of a lymph node or nodes
Lymphadenitis	Inflammation of a lymph node
Lymphangiography	Radiographic recording of lymphatic vessels and nodes
Lymphangiotomy	Incision into a lymphatic vessel
Lymphangitis	Inflammation of lymphatic vessel or vessels
Parathyroid	Produces a hormone to mobilize calcium from bones to blood
Splenectomy	Excision of spleen
Splenography	Radiographic recording of spleen
Splenoportography	Radiographic procedure to allow visualization of splenic and portal veins of spleen
Stem cell	Immature blood cell
Thoracic duct	Largest lymph vessel; it collects lymph from portions of body below diaphragm and from left side of body above diaphragm
Transplantation	Grafting of tissue from one source to another

CHAPTER 10: ANATOMY AND TERMINOLOGY QUIZ

(Quiz answers are located in Appendix B)

1. The spleen is located in this quadrant of the abdomen:
   a. RUQ
   b. LUQ
   c. LLQ
   d. LRQ

2. Produces RBCs and platelets:
   a. thymus
   b. tonsils
   c. lymph node
   d. bone marrow

3. Which of the following is NOT a lymph organ?
   a. adrenal
   b. spleen
   c. thymus
   d. tonsil

4. Lymph transports fluids and _____ that have leaked from the blood system back to veins.
   a. stem cells
   b. lymphocytes
   c. B cells
   d. proteins

5. This is largest in infants and shrinks with age:
   a. tonsils
   b. spleen
   c. thymus
   d. bone marrow

6. Combining form meaning "gland":
   a. axill/o
   b. thym/o
   c. aden/o
   d. tox/o

7. Prefix meaning "excess":
   a. hyper-
   b. hypo-
   c. inter-
   d. retro-

8. Suffix meaning "enlargement":
   a. -edema
   b. -poiesis
   c. -penia
   d. -megaly

9. Lymph node located on neck:
   a. thoracic
   b. jugular
   c. Cloquet's
   d. axillary

10. These cells originate in the bone marrow:
    a. B cells
    b. antigens
    c. erythrocytes
    d. stem cells

Pathophysiology

■ Anemia

Reduction in number of erythrocytes or decrease in quality of hemoglobin

- Less oxygen is transported in the blood

Aplastic Anemia

Diverse group of anemias

Characterized by bone marrow failure with reduced numbers of red and white blood cells and platelets

Causes

Genetic or acquired (primary or secondary)

Toxins/chemical agents

- Benzene and antibiotics such as chloramphenicol

Irradiation

Immunologic

Idiopathic (unknown)

Treatment

Blood transfusion

Bone marrow transplant

Iron Deficiency Anemia

Characterized by small erythrocytes and a reduced amount of hemoglobin

Caused by low or absent iron stores or serum iron concentrations

- Blood loss
- Decreased intake of iron
- Malabsorption of iron

Symptoms

Pallor

Headache

Stomatitis

Oral lesions

Gastrointestinal complaints

Retinal hemorrhages

Thinning, brittle nails and hair

Treatment

Iron supplement

Pernicious Anemia

Megaloblastic anemia (large stem cells)

Inability to absorb vitamin B_{12} due to a lack of intrinsic factor (found in gastric juices)

Usually in older adults

Caused by impaired intestinal absorption of vitamin B_{12}

Symptoms

Pallor

Weakness

Neurologic manifestations

Gastric discomfort

Treatment

Injections of vitamin B_{12}

Transfusions

Hemolytic Anemia

May be acute or chronic

Shortened survival of mature erythrocytes—excessive destruction of RBCs

- Inability of bone marrow to compensate for decreased survival of erythrocytes

Treatment

Treat cause

Sickle Cell Anemia

Occurs primarily in those of West African descent

Abnormal sickle-shaped erythrocytes (sickle cell) caused by an abnormal type of hemoglobin (Hemoglobin S)

Symptoms

Abdominal pain

Arthralgia

Ulceration of lower extremities

Fatigue

Dyspnea

Increased heart rate

Treatment

Symptomatic

■ Granulocytosis

Increase in granulocytes

- Neutrophils
- Eosinophils
- Basophils

■ Eosinophilia

Increase in number of eosinophilic granulocytes

Cause

Allergic disorders

Dermatologic disorders

Parasitic invasion

Drugs

Malignancies

■ Basophilia

Increase in basophilic granulocytes seen in leukemia

■ Monocytosis

Increased number of monocytes

Cause
Infection

Hematologic factors

■ Leukocytosis

Increased number of leukocytes

Cause
Acute viral infections, such as hepatitis

Chronic infections, such as syphilis

■ Leukocytopenia

Decreased number of leukocytes

Cause
Neoplasias

Immune deficiencies

Drugs

Virus

Radiation

■ Infectious Mononucleosis

Acute Infection of B Cells
Epstein-Barr virus most common cause

Symptoms
Fatigue

Fever

Weakness (asthenia)

Pharyngitis

Atypical lymphocytes in blood

Lymph node enlargement

Splenomegaly

Hepatomegaly

Transmission
Saliva

- Known as kissing disease

Treatment
Rest

Treatment of symptoms

■ Leukemia

Malignant disorder of blood and blood-forming organs

Leads to dysfunction of cells

- Primarily leads to proliferation of abnormal leukocytes—filling bone marrow and bloodstream

Acute Myelogenous Leukemia (AML)

Rapid onset

Short survival time

Symptoms

Abrupt onset

Fatigue

Lymphadenopathy

Bone pain and tenderness

Anemia

Bleeding

Fever

Infection

Anorexia

Splenomegaly

Hepatomegaly

Headache, vomiting, paralysis

Treatment

Chemotherapy

Bone marrow transplant following high-dose chemotherapy to eradicate leukemic cells

Acute Lymphocytic Leukemia (ALL)

Immature lymphocytes (lymphoblasts)

Most cases occur in children and adolescents

Sudden onset

Treatment

Chemotherapy with drugs that suppress cell division and destroy rapidly dividing cells

Remission

Relapse—leukemia cells in bone marrow and blood requiring treatment

Chronic Myelogenous Leukemia (CML)

Mature and immature granulocytes in bone marrow and blood

Slow, progressive disease (those over 55 years live many years without life threat)

Cells are more differentiated

Gradual onset with milder symptoms

- Majority of cases are in adults

Symptoms

Extreme fatigue

Weight loss

Splenomegaly

Night sweats

Fever

Infections

Treatment

Chemotherapy—target abnormal proteins

Bone marrow transplant following high-dose chemotherapy

Chronic Lymphocytic Leukemia (CLL)

Increased numbers of mature lymphocytes in marrow, lymph nodes, spleen

Most common form seen in elderly

Slowly progressive

Treatment

Chemotherapy

Lymphadenopathy

Lymphadenopathy

Any abnormality of lymph node

Enlargement of lymph node

Lymphangitis

Inflammation of lymphatic vessel

Lymphadenitis

Inflammation of lymph node

Localized inflammation associated with inflamed lesion

Generalized inflammation associated with disease

Inflammation can occur as result of

- Trauma
- Infection
- Drug reaction
- Autoimmune disease
- Immunologic disease

Malignant Lymphoma

Hodgkin Disease

Initial sign is a painless mass commonly located on neck

Giant Reed-Sternberg cells are present in lymphatic tissue

Presentation

Enlarged spleen (splenomegaly)

Abdominal mass

Mediastinal mass

Localized node involvement

- Orderly spreading of node involvement
- Cervical, axillary, inguinal, and retroperitoneal lymph node involvement

Symptoms

Night sweats

Fever

Weight loss

Itching (pruritus)

Anorexia

Weakness

Treatment

If localized: radiation therapy and chemotherapy

If systemic: chemotherapy alone

High probability of cure with new treatments

Non-Hodgkin Lymphoma

No giant Reed-Sternberg cells present

Involves multiple nodes scattered throughout body (follicular lymphoma)

Large cell lymphoma (large lymphocytes in diffuse nodes and lymph tissue)

- Noncontiguous spread of node involvement
- Not localized

Usually begins as a painless enlargement of node

Symptoms

Presents similar to Hodgkin disease

Treatment

Chemotherapy cures or stops disease progression

Burkitt's Lymphoma

Type of non-Hodgkin lymphoma

Usually found in Africa and New Guinea

Characterized by lesions in jaw and face

Epstein-Barr (herpes virus) has been found in Burkitt's lymphoma

Treatment

Radiation and chemotherapy for African type

■ Myeloma

Multiple Myeloma

B-cell cancer—lymphocytes that produce antibodies destroying bone tissue

- Also known as plasma cell myeloma

Increased plasma cells replace bone marrow

Overproduction of immunoglobulins—Bence Jones protein (found in urine)

Multiple tumor sites cause bone destruction

Results in weakened bone

Hypercalcemia

Anemia

Renal damage

Increased susceptibility to infections

Cause

Unknown

Treatment

Chemotherapy

Radiotherapy

Autologous bone marrow transplant (ABMT) prolongs remission—may be a cure

Palliative treatments

CHAPTER 10: PATHOPHYSIOLOGY QUIZ

(Quiz answers are located in Appendix B)

1. This condition involves a reduced number of erythrocytes and decreased quality of hemoglobin:
   a. monocytosis
   b. eosinophilia
   c. anemia
   d. leukocytosis

2. This condition is characterized by a shortened survival of mature erythrocytes and inability of bone marrow to compensate for decreased survival:
   a. hemolytic anemia
   b. granulocytosis
   c. eosinophilia
   d. monocytosis

3. The most common cause of this disease is Epstein-Barr virus:
   a. leukocytopenia
   b. infectious mononucleosis
   c. leukocytosis
   d. hemolytic anemia

4. Inflammation of the lymphatic vessels is:
   a. lymphadenitis
   b. lymphoma
   c. lymphadenopathy
   d. lymphangitis

5. What giant cell is present in Hodgkin disease?
   a. B cell
   b. Reed-Sternberg
   c. T cell
   d. C cell

6. This condition increases plasma cells, which replace bone marrow:
   a. Burkitt's lymphoma
   b. Multiple myeloma
   c. Hodgkin disease
   d. leukemia

7. Injection of vitamin B may be prescribed for this type of anemia:
   a. pernicious
   b. aplastic
   c. sideroblastic
   d. sickle cell

8. These are large stem cells:
   a. megaloblasts
   b. leukocytes
   c. erythrocytes
   d. granulocytes

9. This is known as the kissing disease:
   a. monocytosis
   b. leukocytopenia
   c. infectious mononucleosis
   d. granulocytosis

10. This lymphoma is usually found in Africa:
    a. multiple
    b. Burkitt's
    c. B-cell
    d. T-cell

CHAPTER 11: ENDOCRINE SYSTEM

Anatomy and Terminology

Regulates body through hormones (chemical messengers)

Ductless endocrine glands secrete hormones directly to bloodstream

Affects growth, development, and metabolism

■ Endocrine Glands (Fig. 11-1)

Pituitary (Hypophysis): Master Gland

Located at base of brain in a depression in skull (sella turcica)

Anterior pituitary (adenohypophysis)

- Adrenocorticotropic hormone (ACTH)—stimulates adrenal cortex and increases production of cortisol
- Follicle-stimulating hormone (FSH)—males, stimulates sperm and testosterone production; females, with luteinizing hormone (LH) stimulates secretion of estrogen and follicle development and ovulation

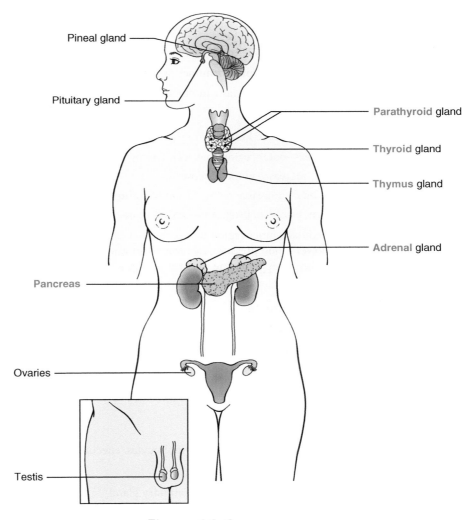

Figure **11-1** Endocrine system.

- Growth hormone (GH or somatotropin STH)—stimulates protein processing resulting in growth of bones, muscle, and fat metabolism, and maintains blood glucose levels
- Luteinizing hormone (LH)—males, stimulates testosterone production; females, stimulates secretion of progesterone and estrogen
- Melanocyte-stimulating hormone (MSH)—increases skin pigmentation
- Prolactin (PRL)—secreted by anterior pituitary, stimulates milk production and breast development
- Thyroid-stimulating hormone (TSH or thyrotropin)—stimulates thyroid gland

Posterior pituitary (neurohypophysis)—stores and releases hormones

- Antidiuretic hormone (ADH) or vasopressin—stimulates reabsorption of water by kidney tubules and increases blood pressure by constricting arterioles
- Oxytocin (OT)—stimulates contractions during childbirth, production and release of milk

Thyroid

Two lobes overlying trachea

Secretes two hormones that increase cell metabolism—thyroxine (T_4) and triiodothyronine (T_3)—synthesized from iodine

Secretes one hormone that decreases blood calcium—thyrocalcitonin (nasal spray used to treat osteoporosis)

Parathyroid Glands (4)

Located on posterior side of thyroid

Secretes PTH (parathyroid hormone) or parathormone

Promotes calcium homeostasis in bloodstream

Adrenal Gland (Pair)

Located on top of each kidney

Adrenal cortex—outer region that secretes corticosteroids

- Cortisol—increases blood glucose
- Aldosterone—increases reabsorption of sodium (salt)
- Androgen, estrogen, progestin—sexual characteristics

Adrenal medulla—inner region that secretes catecholamines (epinephrine to dilate blood vessels to lower blood pressure, increase heart rate, dilate bronchial tubes, and release glycogen for energy and norepinephrine to constrict blood vessels to raise blood pressure)

Pancreas

Located behind stomach

Contains specialized cells (islets of Langerhans) that produce insulin and glycogen hormones

Insulin (decreases blood glucose), glucagon (converts glycogen to glucose, raising blood sugar), and somatostatin (regulates other cells of pancreas)

Thymus

Located behind sternum

Atrophies during adolescence

Produces thymosin—stimulates T-lymphocytes, effecting a positive immune response

Hypothalamus (Part of Brain)

Located below thalamus and above pituitary gland

Stimulates anterior pituitary to release hormones and posterior hypothalamus to store and release hormones

Pineal

Located between two cerebral hemispheres and above third ventricle

Secretes melatonin—more so at night, which affects sleep cycle

Also responsible for delaying sexual maturation in children

Also has neurotransmitters such as somatostatin, norepinephrine, serotonin, and histamine

Ovaries (Pair, Females)

Estrogen production stimulates ova production and secondary female sex characteristics

Progesterone—prepares the uterus for and maintains pregnancy

Placenta

Produces HCG (human chorionic gonadotropin) to sustain a pregnancy

Testes (Pair, Males)

Testosterone—male sex characteristics

COMBINING FORMS

1.	aden/o	in relationship to a gland
2.	adren/o	adrenal gland
3.	adrenal/o	adrenal gland
4.	andr/o	male
5.	calc/o, calc/i	calcium
6.	cortic/o	cortex
7.	crin/o	secrete
8.	dips/o	thirst
9.	estr/o	female
10.	gluc/o	sugar
11.	glyc/o	sugar
12.	gonad/o	ovaries and testes
13.	home/o	same
14.	hormon/o	hormone
15.	kal/i	potassium
16.	lact/o	milk
17.	myx/o	mucus
18.	natr/o	sodium
19.	pancreat/o	pancreas
20.	parathyroid/o	parathyroid gland

21. phys/o	growing
22. pituitar/o	pituitary gland
23. somat/o	body
24. ster/o, stere/o	solid, having three dimensions
25. thry/o	thyroid gland
26. thyroid/o	thyroid gland
27. toc/o	childbirth
28. toxic/o	poison
29. ur/o	urine

PREFIXES

1. eu-	good/normal
2. oxy-	sharp, oxygen
3. pan-	all
4. tetra-	four
5. tri-	three
6. tropin-	act upon

SUFFIXES

1. -agon	assemble
2. -drome	run, relationship to conducting, to speed
3. -emia	blood condition
4. -in	a substance
5. -ine	a substance
6. -tropin	act upon
7. -uria	urine

MEDICAL TERMS

Adrenals	Glands, located at top of kidneys, that produce steroid hormones (cortex) and catecholamines (medulla)
Contralateral	Opposite side
Hormone	Chemical substance produced by body's endocrine glands
Isthmus	Connection of two regions or structures

Isthmus, thyroid	Tissue connection between right and left thyroid lobes
Isthmusectomy	Surgical removal of isthmus
Lobectomy	Removal of a lobe
Thymectomy	Surgical removal of thymus
Thymus	Gland that produces hormones important to immune response
Thyroglossal duct	A duct in embryo between thyroid and posterior tongue that occasionally persists into adult life and causes cysts, fistulas, or sinuses
Thyroid	Part of endocrine system that produces hormones that regulate metabolism
Thyroidectomy	Surgical removal of thyroid

CHAPTER 11: ANATOMY AND TERMINOLOGY QUIZ

(Quiz answers are located in Appendix B)

1. Which of the following is NOT affected by the endocrine system?
   a. digestion
   b. development
   c. progesterone
   d. metabolism

2. Gland that overlies the trachea:
   a. parathyroid
   b. adrenal
   c. pancreas
   d. thyroid

3. Gland that is located on the top of each kidney:
   a. parathyroid
   b. adrenal
   c. pancreas
   d. thyroid

4. The outer region of the adrenal gland that secretes corticosteroids:
   a. cortex
   b. medulla
   c. sternum
   d. medullary

5. Located on the thyroid:
   a. hypophysis
   b. thymus
   c. pineal
   d. parathyroid

6. Located at the base of the brain in a depression in the skull:
   a. pituitary
   b. thymus
   c. adrenal
   d. pineal

7. Stimulates contractions during childbirth:
   a. cortisol
   b. PTH
   c. ADH
   d. oxytocin

8. Produced only during pregnancy by the placenta:
   a. estrogen and progesterone
   b. melatonin
   c. thymosin
   d. adrenocorticotropic hormone

9. Combining form meaning "secrete":
   a. dips/o
   b. crin/o
   c. gluc/o
   d. kal/i

10. Prefix meaning "good":
    a. tri-
    b. tropin-
    c. pan-
    d. eu-

Pathophysiology

■ Diabetes Mellitus

Caused by a deficiency in insulin production or poor use of insulin by body cells

Islets of Langerhans (pancreatic cells) secrete glucagon and insulin to regulate fat, carbohydrate, and protein metabolism

Types of Diabetes Mellitus

Type 1, IDDM (Insulin-Dependent Diabetes Mellitus), Immune Mediated

Onset before age 30—peak onset age 12

Includes beta islet cell destruction, insulin deficiency

Acute onset

Positive family history

Requires insulin

Ketoacidosis (fats improperly burned leads to ketones and acids circulating)

Type 2, NIDDM (Non–Insulin-Dependent Diabetes Mellitus)

Adult onset, after age 30, but it is now occurring earlier

Insidious onset/asymptomatic

Positive in immediate family

Dietary management and/or oral hypoglycemics and/or insulin

Most common type—85% are obese at onset

Insulin is present

Ketoacidosis does not occur

Symptoms

Polyuria

Polydipsia

Glycosuria

Hyperglycemia

Polyphagia

Unexplained weight loss

Acute Complications

Hypoglycemia

Hyperglycemia with coma

Diabetic ketoacidosis

Chronic Complications

Diabetic neuropathy (Fig. 11-2)

Retinopathy

Coronary artery disease (atherosclerosis)

Stroke

Peripheral vascular disease

Infection

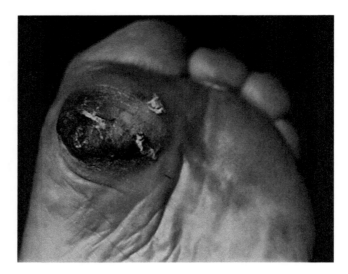

Figure **11-2** Patient with diabetes mellitus and neuropathy had severe claw toes, and shear forces across plantar surface of first metatarsal head caused recurrent ulceration.

Gestational Diabetes Mellitus—Predisposition to Diabetes

Most often recognized in second trimester

Glucose intolerance may be temporary, occurring only during pregnancy

Many will develop diabetes mellitus within 15 years

■ Pituitary Disorders

Tumors

    Most common cause of pituitary disorders

    May secrete hormone

        Such as prolactin or ACTH

Anterior Pituitary
Dwarfism (Hypopituitarism)

Can be caused by deficiency of somatotropin (growth hormone)

Gigantism (Fig. 11-3) (Hyperpituitarism)

Can be caused by excess of somatotrophin (growth hormone) in childhood

Treatment

Resection of tumor or irradiation of pituitary

Acromegaly (Hyperpituitarism)

Increased GH in adulthood

Enlargement of facial bones, feet, and hands

Treatment

Pituitary adenoma is irradiated or removed

Posterior Pituitary
Diabetes Insipidus

Insufficient antidiuretic hormone—kidney tubules fail to retain needed water and salts

Causes polyuria, polydipsia, and dehydration

ADH or SIADH—syndrome of inadequate antidiuretic hormone

Excessive secretion of antidiuretic hormone

Causes excessive water retention

Treatment

Some types have no treatment

Others can be controlled with vasopressin (drug)

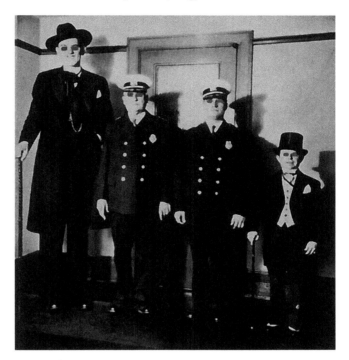

Figure **11-3** Gigantism. A pituitary giant and dwarf contrasted with normal-size men.

▪ Thyroid Disorders

Goiter (Fig. 11-4)
Enlargement of thyroid gland in the neck

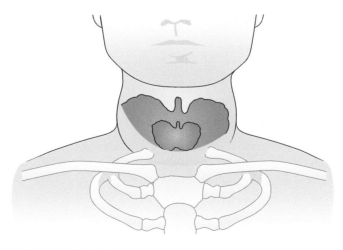

Figure **11-4** Goiter is an enlargement of thyroid gland.

Cause

Hypothyroid disorders

Hyperthyroid disorders

Hyperthyroidism—Thyrotoxicosis

Excessive thyroid hormone production

Most common form: Graves' disease (familial)—results of autoimmune process

Characterized by

Goiter

Tachycardia

Atrial fibrillation

Dyspnea

Palpitations

Fatigue

Tremor

Nervousness

Weight loss

Exophthalmos (protruding eyes)

- Decreased blinking

Treatment

Medication (antithyroid drugs)

Radioactive iodine

Surgical excision

Thyrotoxicosis Storm/Crisis

Thyroid storm/crisis is an acute, life-threatening hypermetabolic state induced by excessive release of thyroid hormones

- Most extreme state of thyrotoxicosis

Hypothyroidism

Primary: inadequate thyroid hormone production

Resulting in increasing levels of thyroid-stimulating hormone (TSH) production

Secondary: inadequate amounts of thyroid-stimulating hormone synthesized

Types

Cretinism

- Congenital
- Occurs in children
- If not treated, it will cause a severe delay in physical and mental development

Myxedema

- Severe form
- Occurs in adults
  - Atherosclerosis
- Symptoms
  - Cold intolerance
  - Weight gain

- Mental sluggishness
- Fatigue

Hashimoto's thyroiditis

- Autoimmune disorder

Treatment
Medication (levothyroxine synthetic hormone replacement)

■ Parathyroid Disorders

Hyperparathyroidism—Excessive Parathyroid Hormone (PTH)
Leads to hypercalcemia

- Affects heart and bones and damages kidneys

Symptoms
Brittle bones

Kidney stones

Cardiac disturbances

Treatment
Surgical excision

Hypoparathyroidism—Abnormally Low PTH
Leads to hypocalcemia

Symptoms
Nerve irritability—twitching or spasms

Muscle cramps

Tingling and burning (paresthesias) of fingertips, toes, and lips

Anxiety, nervousness

Tetany (constant muscle contraction)

Treatment
Calcium and vitamin D

■ Adrenal Gland Disorders

Cushing Syndrome—Hypercortisolism
Excess levels of adrenocorticotropic hormone (ACTH)

Cause
Hyperfunction of adrenal cortex

Long-term use of steroid medications

Symptoms
Weight gain

- Fat deposits on face (moonface) and trunk (buffalo hump)

Glucose intolerance

- Diabetes may develop (20%)

Hypernatremia

Hypokalemia

Virilization

Hypertension

Muscle wasting

Osteoporosis

Change in mental status

Delayed healing

Treatment
Medication

Radiation therapy

Surgical intervention

Addison's Disease—Primary Adrenal Insufficiency
Deficiency of Adrenocortical Hormones Resulting from Destruction of Adrenal Glands
- Glucocorticoids
- Mineralocorticoids

Cause
Tumors

Autoimmune disorders

Viral

Tuberculosis

Infection

Symptoms
Decreased blood glucose levels

Elevated serum ACTH

Fatigue

Lack of ability to handle stress

Weight loss

Infections

Hypotension

Decreased body hair

Hyperpigmentation

Treatment
Hormone (glucocorticoid) replacement

Hyperaldosteronism
Excess aldosterone secreted by adrenal cortex

Types
Primary hyperaldosteronism (Conn's syndrome)
- Caused by an abnormality of adrenal cortex
  - Usually an adrenal adenoma

Secondary hyperaldosteronism
- Caused by other than adrenal stimuli

Symptoms

Hypertension

Hypokalemia

Neuromuscular disorders

Treatment

Treat the underlying condition that caused hyperaldosteronism

- Such as adrenal adenoma

Adrenal Medulla

Hypersecretion

Pheochromocytoma—benign tumor of medulla

Excessive production of epinephrine and norepinephrine

Symptoms

Severe headaches

Sweating

Flushing

Hypertension

Muscle spasms

Treatment

Antihypertensive drugs

Remove tumor

Androgen and Estrogen Hypersecretion

Androgen, male characteristic hormone

- Virilization, development of male characteristics

Hypersecretion of estrogen, female characteristic hormone

- Feminization

Cause

Underlying condition

- Adrenal tumor
- Cushing syndrome
- Adenomas or carcinomas
- Defects in steroid metabolism

Treatment

Surgical intervention for tumor

Underlying condition

CHAPTER 11: PATHOPHYSIOLOGY QUIZ

(Quiz answers are located in Appendix B)

1. This type of diabetes typically occurs before age 30:
   a. type 1
   b. type 2

2. The acronym that indicates that insulin is not required is:
   a. IDDM
   b. NIDDM
   c. PIDDM
   d. NDDMI

3. The most common cause of pituitary disorders is:
   a. hypersecretion
   b. hyposecretion
   c. tumor
   d. infection

4. In excess, this hormone can cause gigantism:
   a. somatotrophin
   b. thyroid
   c. mineralocorticoids
   d. adrenocortical

5. Goiter can be caused by which of the following:
   a. hypothyroidism
   b. parathyroidism
   c. hyperthyroidism
   d. both a and c

6. This type of hypothyroidism is an autoimmune disorder:
   a. myxedema
   b. Hashimoto's
   c. cretinism
   d. hypokalemia

7. Tetany can be caused by:
   a. hypoparathyroidism
   b. hyperthyroidism
   c. hyperparathyroidism
   d. hyperaldosteronism

8. Conn's syndrome is also known as:
   a. primary hypoparathyroidism
   b. primary hyperthyroidism
   c. primary hyperparathyroidism
   d. primary hyperaldosteronism

9. Development of male characteristics is known as:
   a. virilization
   b. feminization
   c. hypertrophy
   d. hyperaldosteronism

10. The treatment for Addison's disease is often:
    a. chemotherapy
    b. radiation
    c. hormone replacement
    d. all of the above

CHAPTER 12: NERVOUS SYSTEM

Anatomy and Terminology

Controlling, regulating, and communicating system

Organization

- Central nervous system (CNS), brain and spinal cord
- Peripheral nervous system (PNS), cranial and spinal nerves
  - Autonomic nervous system—motor and sensory nerves of viscera (involuntary)
  - Somatic nervous system—motor and sensory nerves of skeletal muscles

Cells of the Nervous System (Fig. 12-1)

Neurons—Primary Cells of Nervous System

Classified according to function (afferent [sensory], efferent [motor], interneurons [associational])

- Dendrites (receive signals)
- Cell body (nucleus, within cell body)
- Axon (carries signals from cell body)
- Myelin sheath (insulation around axon)

Glia

Astrocytes

Star shaped—transport water and salts between capillaries and neurons

Microglia

Multiple branching processes—protect neurons from inflammation

Oligodendrocytes

Form myelin sheath

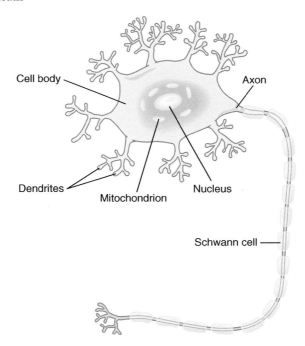

Figure **12-1** Myelinated axon.

Ependymal

Lining membrane of brain and spinal cord where central spinal fluid circulates

■ Divisions of Central Nervous System (CNS) (Fig. 12-2)

Brain—Housed in Cranium (Box Comprised of 8 Bones)—Functioning to Enclose and Protect

Listing from inferior to superior

Brainstem

Medulla oblongata—crossover area left to right and center of respiratory and cardiovascular systems

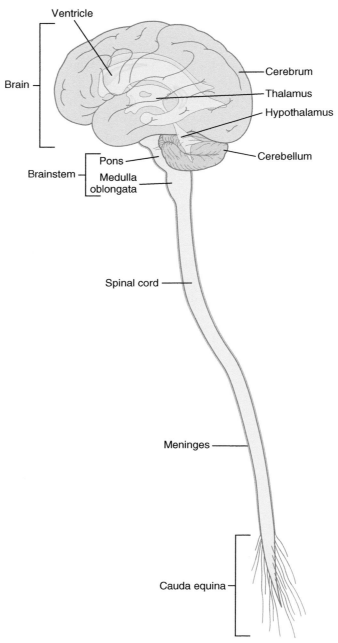

Figure **12-2** Brain and spinal cord.

Pons—connection of nerves (face and eyes)

Midbrain

Diencephalon

Hypothalamus controls autonomic nervous system, body temperature, sleep, appetite, and control of pituitary

Thalamus relays impulses to cerebral cortex for sensory system (pain)

Cerebellum

Controls voluntary movement and balance

Cerebrum

Largest part of brain

Functions

Mental processes, personality, sensory interpretation, movements, and memory

Two Hemispheres

Right controls left side of body

Left controls right side of body

Divided into Five Lobes

- Frontal
- Parietal
- Temporal
- Occipital
- Insula

Vertebral Column—33 Vertebrae

7 cervical

12 thoracic

5 lumbar

5 sacrum (fused)

4 coccygeal (fused)—tailbone

Spinal Cord—Housed Within Vertebrae from Medulla Oblongata to Second Lumbar

Spinal and brain meninges (coverings—dura mater [external], arachnoid, pia mater [internal])

Spine and brain spaces bathed by cerebrospinal fluid (CSF) (subarachnoid space)

Cavities within brain contain cerebrospinal fluid (ventricles)

■ Peripheral Nervous System (PNS)

Cranial nerves, 12 pair

Spinal nerves, 31 pair

■ Autonomic Nervous System (ANS)—Housed Within Both PNS and CNS

Two divisions

- Sympathetic system—functions in fight and flight (stress)
- Parasympathetic system—functions to restore and conserve energy

COMBINING FORMS

1.	cephal/o	head
2.	cerebell/o	cerebellum
3.	cerebr/o	cerebrum
4.	crani/o	cranium
5.	dur/o	dura mater
6.	encephal/o	brain
7.	gangli/o	ganglion
8.	ganglion/o	ganglion
9.	gli/o	glial cells
10.	lept/o	slender
11.	mening/o	meninges
12.	meningi/o	meninges
13.	ment/o	mind
14.	mon/o	one
15.	myel/o	bone marrow, spinal cord
16.	neur/o	nerve
17.	phas/o	speech
18.	phren/o	mind
19.	poli/o	gray matter
20.	pont/o	pons
21.	psych/o	mind
22.	quadr/i	four
23.	radic/o	nerve root
24.	radicul/o	nerve root
25.	rhiz/o	nerve root
26.	vag/o	vagus nerve

PREFIXES

1.	hemi-	half
2.	per-	through
3.	quadri-	four
4.	tetra-	four

SUFFIXES

1.	-algesia	pain sensation
2.	-algia	pain
3.	-cele	hernia
4.	-esthesia	feeling
5.	-iatry	medical treatment
6.	-ictal	pertaining to
7.	-kines/o	movement
8.	-paresis	incomplete paralysis
9.	-plegia	paralysis

MEDICAL ABBREVIATIONS

1.	ANS	autonomic nervous system
2.	CNS	central nervous system
3.	CSF	cerebrospinal fluid
4.	CVA	stroke/cerebrovascular accident
5.	EEG	electroencephalogram
6.	LP	lumbar puncture
7.	PNS	peripheral nervous system
8.	TENS	transcutaneous electrical nerve stimulation
9.	TIA	transient ischemic attack

MEDICAL TERMS

Burr	Drill used to create an entry into the cranium
Central nervous system	Brain and spinal cord
Craniectomy	Permanent, partial removal of skull
Craniotomy	Opening of the skull
Cranium	That part of the skeleton that encloses the brain
Discectomy	Removal of a vertebral disc
Electroencephalography	Recording of the electric currents of the brain by means of electrodes attached to the scalp
Laminectomy	Surgical excision of posterior arch of vertebra—includes spinal process

Peripheral nerves	12 pairs of cranial nerves, 31 pairs of spinal nerves, and autonomic nervous system; connects peripheral receptors to the brain and spinal cord
Shunt	An artificial passage
Skull	Entire skeletal framework of the head
Somatic nerve	Sensory or motor nerve
Stereotaxis	Method of identifying a specific area or point in the brain
Sympathetic nerve	Part of the peripheral nervous system that controls automatic body function and sympathetic nerves activated under stress
Trephination	Surgical removal of a disk of bone
Vertebrectomy	Removal of vertebra

CHAPTER 12: ANATOMY AND TERMINOLOGY QUIZ

(Quiz answers are located in Appendix B)

1. Portion of nervous system that contains cranial and spinal nerves:
   a. central
   b. peripheral
   c. autonomic
   d. parasypathetic

2. Part of neuron that receives signals:
   a. dendrites
   b. cell body
   c. axon
   d. myelin sheath

3. NOT associated with glia:
   a. monocytes
   b. astrocytes
   c. microglia
   d. oligodendrocytes

4. Largest part of brain:
   a. cerebellum
   b. cerebrum
   c. cortex
   d. pons

5. Divided into two hemispheres:
   a. cerebellum
   b. cerebrum
   c. cortex
   d. pons

6. Number of pairs of cranial nerves:
   a. 10
   b. 11
   c. 12
   d. 13

7. Controls right side of body:
   a. left cerebrum
   b. right cerebrum
   c. right cortex
   d. left cortex

8. Combining form that means "brain":
   a. mening/o
   b. mon/o
   c. esthesi/o
   d. encephal/o

9. Prefix that means "four":
   a. per-
   b. tetra-
   c. para-
   d. bi-

10. Combining form that means "speech":
    a. phas/o
    b. rhiz/o
    c. poli/o
    d. myel/o

Pathophysiology

■ Dementias—Classified by Causative Factor

Cognitive deficiencies

Causes
Alzheimer's disease

Vascular disease

Head trauma

Tumors

Infection

Toxins

Substance abuse

AIDS

Alzheimer's Disease
Most common type of dementia

Progressive intellectual impairment

- Results in damage to neurons (neurofibrillary tangles)
- Fatal within 3 to 20 years

Causes
Mostly unknown

Perhaps genetic defect, autoimmune reaction, or virus

Symptoms
Behavior change

Memory loss

Confusion

Disorientation

Restlessness

Speech disturbances

Personality change—anxiety, depression

Irritability

Inability to complete activities of daily living

Treatment
- No cure
- Aricept (drug has modest effect in early stages)
- Symptomatic treatment
- Support for family

Vascular Dementia
Result of brain infarctions (vascular occlusion resulting in loss of brain function)

Nutritional Degenerative Disease
Deficiency

- B vitamins

- Niacin
- Pantothenic acid

Associated with alcoholism

Amyotrophic Lateral Sclerosis (ALS)

Motor neuron disease (MND)

Also known as Lou Gehrig's disease

- Baseball player who died of ALS

Deterioration of neurons of spinal cord and brain

Results in atrophy of muscles and loss of fine motor skills

Difficulty walking, talking, and breathing

Mental functioning remains normal

Survival is 2 to 5 years after diagnosis

Genetic cause—familial chromosome 21 aberration

- Death usually results from respiratory failure

Treatment

Symptomatic only

Emotional support

No cure

Huntington's Disease—Chorea

Inherited progressive atrophy of cerebrum

Symptoms

Restlessness

Rapid, jerky movements in arms and face (uncontrollable jerking and facial grimacing)

Rigidity

Intellectual impairment, bradyphrenia, apathy

Treatment

Genetic defect of chromosome 4

No cure

Symptomatic

Parkinson's Disease (Parkinsonism)

Decreased secretion of dopamine

Typically occurs after age 40

Cause unknown

Symptoms

Muscle rigidity and weakness

Bradykinesia—slow voluntary movements

Postural instability, stooped

Shuffling gait

Tremors at rest

Masklike facial appearance

Depression

Treatment

Medications to reduce symptoms

Dopamine replacement

Multiple Sclerosis (MS)

Common neurologic condition

- Demyelination of central nervous system—replaced by sclerotic tissue

Diagnosed in young adults 20–40 years old

Results in myelin destruction and gliosis of white matter of central nervous system

Speculation that it is an autoimmune condition or result of a virus

Exacerbations and remission patterns

Symptoms

Precipitated by "an event," e.g., infection, pregnancy, stress

Loss of feeling (paresthesias)

Vision problems

Bladder disorder

Mood disorders

Weakness of limbs—unsteady gait and paralysis

Treatment

Symptomatic

Management of relapses

Reducing relapses and disease progression—disease-modifying drugs (DMDs)

Myasthenia Gravis (MG)

Means grave muscle weakness

Autoimmune neuromuscular condition—antibodies block neurotransmission to muscle cells

Most have pathologic changes of thymus

Symptoms

Insidious

Muscle weakness and fatigability

May be localized or generalized

Often affects

- Swallowing
- Breathing
- Compromised swallowing and breathing may lead to crisis

Treatment

Anticholinesterase drugs

- Restores normal muscle strength and recoverability after fatigue

Corticosteroids (prednisone) and immunosuppressive drugs

Thymectomy

Tourette Syndrome

Symptoms

Spasmodic, twitching movements, uncontrollable vocal sounds, inappropriate words

Begins with twitching eyelids and facial muscles (tics)

Verbal outbursts

Causes
Unknown

Excess dopamine or hypersensitivity to dopamine

Treatment
Antipsychotic drugs

Antidepressant drugs

Mood-elevating drugs

Poliomyelitis
Contagious viral disease

Affects motor neurons

Causes paralysis and respiratory failure

Prevent with vaccination

Postpolio Syndrome (PPS)
Also known as postpoliomyelitis neuromuscular atrophy

Progressive muscle weakness

- Past history of paralytic polio

Symptoms
Muscle weakness and fatigability

- May include atrophy and muscle twitching

Treatment
Symptomatic

Maintenance of respiratory function

Guillain-Barré Syndrome
Also known as

- Idiopathic polyneuritis
- Acute inflammatory polyneuropathy
- Landry's ascending paralysis

Demyelination of peripheral nerves—acquired disease

Symptoms
Primary ascending motor paralysis

Variable sensory disturbances

Treatment
Supportive

■ Congenital Neurologic Disorders

Hydrocephalus
Excessive amounts of circulating cerebrospinal fluid in ventricles of brain

Circulation is impaired in brain or spinal cord

Compresses brain

Treatment

Surgical placement of a shunt

Spina Bifida (Fig. 12-3)

Developmental birth defect that causes incomplete development of spinal cord and its coverings

Vertebrae overlying open portions of spinal cord do not fully form and remain unfused and open

- Spina bifida occulta—may not be noticed, no protrusion through defect
- Spina bifida manifesta, which includes:
  - Myelomeningocele (spina bifida cystica)
    - Meninges and spinal cord protrude through defect

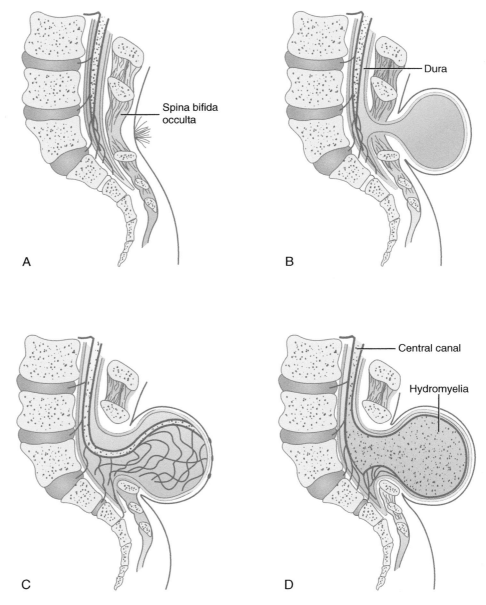

Figure **12-3** **A.** Spina bifida occulta. **B.** Meningocele. **C.** Myelomeningocele. **D.** Myelocystocele or hydromyelia.

- Meningocele
  - Meninges herniated through defect

Results in neurologic deficiencies

Treatment

Surgical repair

■ Mental Disorders

Schizophrenia

Variety of syndromes

Results in changes in brain

Hereditary factors are considered a cause

- Also, fetal brain damage caused by viral infections, complications of pregnancy, nutritional deficiencies

Stress usually precipitates onset

Symptoms

Delusions of persecution and/or grandeur

Disorganized thought

Repetitive behaviors

Behavior issues

Decreased speech

Decreased ability to solve problems

Loss of emotions/flat affect

Hallucinations

Types are based on characteristics

Treatment

Antipsychotic drugs

Drugs have very unpleasant side effects, such as tardive dyskinesia, with symptoms as follows:

- Excessive movement
- Grimacing
- Jerking
- Tremors
- Shuffling gait
- Dry mouth
- Blurred vision

Depression

Mood (sustained emotional state) disorder

Exact cause is unknown

Symptoms

Sadness

Hopelessness

Lethargy

Insomnia

Anorexia

Treatment

Antidepressant drugs

Electroconvulsive therapy

Central Nervous System (CNS) Disorders

Vascular Disorder

Transient Ischemic Attack (TIA)

Temporary reduction of blood flow to brain that produces strokelike symptoms but no lasting damage

Often a warning sign before cerebrovascular accident

Symptoms

Depend on location of ischemia

- Usual recovery within 24 hours

No loss of consciousness

Slurred, indiscernible speech

May display muscle weakness in legs/arms

Paresthesia (numbness) of face

Mental confusion may be present

Repeated attacks common in the presence of atherosclerotic disease

Cerebrovascular Accident (CVA) or Stroke

Infarction of brain due to lack of blood/oxygen flow

Necrosis of tissue with total occlusion of vessel

Causes

Atherosclerotic disease—thrombus formation

Embolus

Hemorrhage—arterial aneurysm

Symptoms

Depend on location of obstruction

- Thrombus
  - Gradual onset
  - Often occurs at rest
  - Intracranial pressure (ICP) minimal
  - Localized damage
- Embolus
  - Sudden onset
  - Occurs anytime
  - ICP minimal
  - Localized damage unless multiple emboli
- Hemorrhage
  - Sudden onset
  - Occurs most often with activity

- ICP high
- Widespread damage
- May be fatal

Treatment

Anticoagulant drugs (clot dissolving) if caused by thrombus or embolus—tissue plasminogen activator (tPA)

Carotid endarterectomy (removes artherosclerotic plaque)

Oxygen treatment

Underlying condition treated, such as

- Hypertension
- Atherosclerosis
- Thrombus

Aneurysm—Cerebral

Dilation of artery

- May be localized or multiple

Rupture possible, often on exertion

- Fatal if rupture is massive

Symptoms

May display visual effects, such as

- Loss of visual fields
- Photophobia
- Diplopia

Headache

Confusion

Slurred speech

Weakness

Stiff neck (nuchal rigidity)

Treatment

Dependent on diagnosis prior to rupture

Surgical intervention

Encephalitis

Infection of parenchymal tissue of brain or spinal cord

- Often viral

Accompanying inflammation

Usually results in some permanent damage

Symptoms

Stiff neck

Headaches

Vomiting

Fever

May have seizure

Lethargy

Some Types of Encephalitis
Herpes simplex

Lyme disease

West Nile fever

Western equine

Treatment
Symptomatic

Supportive

Reye's Syndrome
Associated with viral infection
- Especially when aspirin has been administered

Changes occur in brain and liver
- Leads to increased intracranial pressure

Symptoms
Headaches

Vomiting

Lethargy

Seizures

Treatment
Symptomatic treatment

Brain Abscess
Localized infection

Necrosis of tissue

Usually spread from infection elsewhere, such as ears or sinus

Symptoms
Neurologic deficiencies

Increased intracranial pressure

Treatment
Antibiotics for bacterial infections

Surgical drainage

Epilepsies

Chronic seizure disorder

Types
Partial Seizures (Focal)
State of altered focus but conscious—simple

Impaired consciousness—complex

Specialized epileptic seizures

Aura
- Auditory or visual sign that precedes a seizure

Generalized Seizures
Absence seizures—petit mal

- Brief loss of awareness
- Most common in children (febrile causation)

Tonic-clonic—grand mal or ictal event

- Loss of consciousness
- Alternate contraction and relaxation
- Incontinence
- No memory of seizure

Causes
Tumor

Hemorrhage

Trauma

Edema

Infection

Excessive cerebrospinal fluid

High fever

Treatment
Correct cause

Anticonvulsant drugs

Neurosurgery

Postictal event—after seizure—neurologic symptoms (weakness, etc.)

Trauma

Head Injury—Traumatic Brain Injury (TBI)
Concussion
Mild blow to head

Temporary axonal disturbances

Grade 1: temporary confusion and amnesia (brief)

Grade 2: memory loss for very recent events and confusion

Grade 3: amnesia for recent events and disorientation (longer duration)

Results in reversible interference with brain function

- Recovery within 24 hours with no residual damage

Contusion
Bruising of brain

Force of blow determines outcome

Hematomas—Blood Accumulation (Clot)
Compresses surrounding structures

Classified based on location

- Epidural
  - Develops between dura and skull

- Subdural
  - Develops between dura and arachnoid
    - Development within 24 hours is acute
    - Development within a week is subacute
  - ICP increases with enlargement of hematoma
- Subarachnoid
  - Develops between pia and arachnoid
  - Blood mixes with cerebrospinal fluid
    - No localized hematoma forms
  - Intracerebral
    - As a result of a contusion

Symptoms

Increased ICP

Others dependent on location and severity of injury

Treatment

Identification of the location of hematoma

Medications to decrease edema

Antibiotics

Surgical intervention—burr hole if necessary to decrease the ICP

Spinal Cord Injury

Result of trauma to vertebra, cord, ligaments, intervertebral disc

Vertebral Injuries Classified As

- Simple—affects spinous or transverse process
- Compression—anterior fracture of vertebrae
- Comminuted—vertebral body is shattered
- Dislocation—vertebrae are out of alignment
- Flexion injury in which hyperflexion compresses vertebra

Dislocation

Rotation

Symptoms

Depend on vertebral level and severity

Paralysis

Loss of sensation

Drop in blood pressure

Loss of bladder and rectal control

Decreased venous circulation

Treatment

Identification of area of injury

Immobilization

Corticosteroids to decrease edema

Bladder and bowel management

Rehabilitation

Tumors of Brain and Spinal Cord

Increases ICP

Life threatening

Rarely metastasize outside of central nervous system

Secondary brain tumors are common

Metastasis from lung or breast

Gliomas Common Type

Primary malignant tumor—encapsulated and invasive

Types based on cell from which tumor arises and location of tumor

Glioblastoma

Located in cerebral hemispheres (deep in white matter)

Highly aggressive

Oligodendrocytoma

Usually located in frontal lobes

Oligodendroblastoma, more aggressive form

Ependymoma

Located in ventricles

Most often occurs in children

Ependymoblastoma, more aggressive form

Astrocytoma

Located anywhere in brain and spinal cord

Invasive but slow growing

Pineal Region
Germ Cell Tumors

Usually in adolescents

Rare

Variable growth rate

Several Other Pineal Tumors

Pineocytoma

Teratoma

Germinoma

Blood Vessel
Angioma

Usually located in posterior cerebral hemispheres

Slow growing

Hemangioblastoma

Located in cerebellum

Slow growing

Medulloblastoma

Aggressive tumor

Located in posterior cerebellar vermis (fourth ventricle)

Meningioma

Originates in arachnoid

Slow growing

Pituitary Tumor

Related to aging

Slow growing

- Such as macroadenomas

Cranial Nerve Tumors

Neurilemmomas most common location: cranial nerve VIII

Slow growing

Metastatic

Spinal Cord Tumors

Symptoms are based on location of spinal compression

Intramedullary

- Originates in neural tissue

Extramedullary

- Originates outside the spinal cord

Metastatic tumors of spinal cord are more common

- Myeloma—marrow
- Lymphoma—lymph
- Carcinomas—lung, breast, prostate

Most common type of primary extramedullary tumor

- Meningiomas—anyplace in spine
- Neurofibromas—common in thoracic and lumbar regions

CHAPTER 12: PATHOPHYSIOLOGY QUIZ

(Quiz answers are located in Appendix B)

1. Most common dementia is:
   a. Alzheimer's disease
   b. secondary
   c. nutritional degenerative disease
   d. Lou Gehrig's disease

2. MND stands for:
   a. maximal neuron disorder
   b. migrating niacin disorder
   c. motor neuron disease
   d. motor neuropathic disorder

3. Dopamine replacement is useful in treating:
   a. multiple sclerosis
   b. Parkinson's disease
   c. Huntington's disease
   d. CVA

4. Condition in which primary symptoms are muscle weakness and fatigability:
   a. amyotrophic lateral sclerosis
   b. multiple sclerosis
   c. dyskinesis
   d. myasthenia gravis

5. Another name for idiopathic polyneuritis is:
   a. Guillain-Barré syndrome
   b. multiple sclerosis
   c. amyotrophic lateral sclerosis
   d. postpolio syndrome

6. This condition is thought to be caused by genetic factors and, possibly, fetal brain damage:
   a. Parkinson's
   b. schizophrenia
   c. spina bifida
   d. Guillain-Barré syndrome

7. This condition is associated with viral infection, especially when aspirin has been administered:
   a. Reye's syndrome
   b. Guillain-Barré syndrome
   c. Lou Gehrig's disease
   d. Conn's syndrome

8. Concussion is a mild blow to the head in which recovery is expected within

   _____.
   a. 12 hours
   b. 24 hours
   c. 48 hours
   d. 1 week

9. ICP means:
   a. intercranial pressure
   b. intracranial pressure
   c. interior cranial pressure
   d. intensive cranial pressure

10. In this type of hematoma, blood mixes with cerebrospinal fluid:
    a. epidural
    b. subdural
    c. subarachnoid
    d. intracerebral

CHAPTER 13: SENSES

Anatomy and Terminology

Sight	Eyes
Hearing	Ears
Smell	Nose
Taste	Tongue
Touch	Skin

■ Sight: Three Layers of Eye (Fig. 13-1)

Cornea (Outer Layer)

Fibrous, transparent layer that extends over dome of eye

Refracts (bends) light to focus on receptor cells (posterior eye)

Avascular (nourished by aqueous humor and tears)

Sclera (Extension of Outer Layer)

White of eye

Extends from edge of cornea (anterior surface) to optic nerve (posterior surface)

- Lies over choroid

Choroid (Middle Layer)

Vascular layer between sclera and retina

- Supplies nutrients

Retina (Inner Layer)

Contains rods and cones

- Rods provide night and peripheral vision
- Cones provide day and color vision and are stimulated by primary colors of red, green, and blue

Conjunctiva

Covers anterior sclera and lines eyelid (contiguous layer)

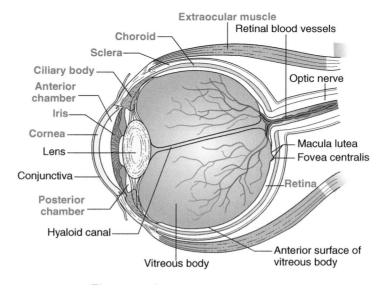

Figure **13-1** Eye and ocular adnexa.

Lens

Behind pupil

Lens is connected by zonules to ciliary body

Ciliary body muscles cause lens to change shape to refract light rays (accommodation)

Fluids

Aqueous humor (front of lens)—watery substance secreted by ciliary body

  Maintains shape of front portion of eye

  Refracts light

  Nourishes cornea

Vitreous humor (behind lens)—gel-like substance (not readily re-formed) filling large space behind lens

  Maintains shape of eyeball

  Refracts light

Optic Nerve

Light rays from rods and cones travel from eye to brain via optic nerve

Optic nerve meets retina in optic disc (no light receptors)—blind spot

Pathway of light ray

  Cornea—refraction site

  Anterior chamber (aqueous humor)—refraction site

  Pupil

  Lens—refraction site

  Posterior chamber (vitreous humor)—refraction site

  Retina (rods and cones)

  Optic nerve fibers—nerve cells act as a cable connecting the eye with the brain

  Optic chiasm

  Thalamus

  Cerebral cortex (occipital lobe)—light is interpreted

■ Hearing, Three Divisions of Ear

External Ear

Auricle (pinna)—sound waves enter ear

External auditory canal—tunnel from auricle to middle ear

Middle Ear

Begins with tympanic membrane (eardrum)

Ossicles—small bones conducting sound waves from middle to inner ear

- Malleus
- Incus
- Stapes

Eustachian tube—leads to pharynx

Inner Ear (Labyrinth)

Vestibule

Semicircular canals/vestibular apparatus

Cochlea contains perilymph and endolymph (liquids through which sound waves are conducted)

- Organ of Corti—auditory receptor area

Auditory nerve—electrical impulse is conducted to cerebral cortex for interpretation (hearing)

Pathway of sound vibration (exterior to brain)

Pinna

External auditory canal

Tympanic membrane

Malleus

Incus

Stapes

Oval window

Cochlea

Auditory fluid/receptors in organ of Corti

Auditory nerve

Cerebral cortex

■ Smell

Olfactory Sense Receptors

Located in nasal cavity

Closely related to sense of taste

Cranial nerve I

■ Taste

Gustatory sense—sweet, salty, and sour differentiated

Taste buds located on anterior portion of tongue

Cranial nerves VII and IX

■ Touch

Mechanoreceptors

Widely distributed throughout body

React to touch and pressure

- Meissner corpuscles (touch)
- Pacinian corpuscles (pressure)

Proprioceptors

Position and orientation

Dysfunctions

- Vestibular nystagmus—involuntary movement of eyes
- Vertigo—sense of spinning/dizziness

Thermoreceptors

Under skin

Sense temperature changes

Nociceptors

Pain sensors

In skin and internal organs

COMBINING FORMS

1.	ambly/o	dim, dullness
2.	aque/o	water
3.	audi/o	hearing
4.	blephar/o	eyelid
5.	conjunctiv/o	conjunctiva
6.	cor/o, core/o	pupil
7.	corne/o	cornea
8.	cycl/o	ciliary body
9.	dacry/o	tear
10.	essi/o, esthesi/o	sensation
11.	glauc/o	gray
12.	ir/o	iris
13.	irid/o	iris
14.	kerat/o	cornea
15.	lacrim/o	tear
16.	mi/o	smaller
17.	myring/o	eardrum
18.	ocul/o	eye
19.	ophthalm/o	eye
20.	opt/o	eye, vision
21.	optic/o	eye
22.	ot/o	ear
23.	palpebr/o	eyelid
24.	papill/o	optic nerve
25.	phac/o	eye lens
26.	phak/o	eye lens
27.	phot/o	light
28.	presby/o	old age
29.	pupill/o	pupil
30.	retin/o	retina

31. scler/o	sclera
32. scot/o	darkness
33. staped/o	stapes
34. tympan/o	eardrum
35. uve/o	uvea
36. vitre/o	glassy
37. xer/o	dry

PREFIXES

1. audi-	hearing
2. eso-	inward
3. exo-	outward

SUFFIXES

1. -opia	vision
2. -omia	smell
3. -tropia	to turn

MEDICAL ABBREVIATIONS

1. AD	right ear
2. AS	left ear
3. AU	both ears
4. H or E	hemorrhage or exudate
5. IO	intraocular
6. IOL	intraocular lens
7. OD	right eye
8. OS	left eye
9. OU	each eye
10. PERL	pupils equal and reactive to light
11. PERRL	pupils equal, round, and reactive to light
12. PERRLA	pupils equal, round, and reactive to light and accommodation
13. REM	rapid eye movement
14. TM	tympanic membrane

MEDICAL TERMS

Anterior segment	Those parts of eye in the front of and including lens (cornea, iris, ciliary body, aqueous humor)
Apicectomy	Excision of a portion of temporal bone
Astigmatism	Condition in which refractive surfaces of eye are unequal
Aural atresia	Congenital absence of external auditory canal
Blepharitis	Inflammation of eyelid
Cataract	Opaque covering on or in lens
Chalazion	Granuloma around sebaceous gland
Cholesteatoma	Tumor that forms in middle ear
Conjunctiva	The lining of eyelids and covering of anterior sclera
Dacryocystitis	Blocked, inflamed infection of nasolacrimal duct
Dacryostenosis	Narrowing of lacrimal duct
Ectropion	Eversion (outward sagging) of eyelid
Entropion	Inversion of eyelid (lashes rubbing cornea)
Enucleation	Removal of an organ or organs from a body cavity
Episclera	Connective covering of sclera
Exenteration	Removal of an organ all in one piece, commonly used to describe radical excision
Exophthalmos	Protrusion of eyeball
Exostosis	Bony growth
Fenestration	Creation of a new opening in inner wall of middle ear
Glaucoma	Eye diseases that are characterized by an increase of intraocular pressure
Hordeolum	Stye—infection of sebaceous gland (nodule on lid margin)
Hyperopia	Farsightedness, eyeball is too short from front to back
Keratomalacia	Softening of cornea associated with a deficiency of vitamin A
Keratoplasty	Surgical repair of the cornea
Labyrinth	Inner connecting cavities, such as internal ear
Labyrinthitis	Inner ear inflammation
Lacrimal	Related to tears
Mastoidectomy	Removal of mastoid bone
Ménière's disease	Condition that causes dizziness, ringing in ears, and deafness
Myopia	Nearsightedness, eyeball too long from front to back

Myringotomy	Incision into tympanic membrane
Ocular adnexa	Orbit, extraocular muscles, and eyelid
Ophthalmoscopy	Examination of the interior of eye by means of a scope, also known as fundoscopy
Otitis media	Noninfectious inflammation of middle ear; serous otitis media produces liquid drainage (not purulent), and suppurative otitis media produces purulent (pus) matter
Otoscope	Instrument used to examine ear
Papilledema	Swelling of optic disc (papilla)
Posterior segment	Those parts of eye behind lens
Ptosis	Drooping of upper eyelid
Sclera	Outer covering of eye
Strabismus	Extraocular muscle deviation resulting in unequal visual axes
Tarsorrhaphy	Suturing together of eyelids
Tinnitus	Ringing in the ears
Transmastoid	Creates an opening in mastoid for drainage antrostomy
Tympanolysis	Freeing of adhesions of the tympanic membrane
Tympanometry	Test of the inner ear using air pressure
Tympanostomy	Insertion of ventilation tube into tympanum
Uveal	Vascular tissue of the choroid, ciliary body, and iris
Vertigo	Dizziness
Xanthelasma	Yellow plaque on eyelid (lipid disorder)

CHAPTER 13: ANATOMY AND TERMINOLOGY QUIZ

(Quiz answers are located in Appendix B)

1. The middle layer of the eye:
   a. sclera
   b. retina
   c. episclera
   d. choroid

2. The covering of the anterior sclera and lining of eyelid:
   a. aqueous humor
   b. ossicles
   c. vitreous
   d. conjunctiva

3. Which of the following is NOT a bone of the middle ear?
   a. cochlea
   b. stapes
   c. malleus
   d. incus

4. This cranial nerve controls the sense of smell:
   a. I
   b. II
   c. III
   d. IV

5. Which of the following is NOT part of the inner ear?
   a. pinna
   b. vestibule
   c. semicircular canals
   d. cochlea

6. These receptors react to touch:
   a. nociceptors
   b. mechanoreceptors
   c. proprioceptors
   d. thermoreceptors

7. These receptors react to position and orientation:
   a. nociceptors
   b. mechanoreceptors
   c. proprioceptors
   d. thermoreceptors

8. Combining form meaning "eyelid":
   a. aque/o
   b. blephar/o
   c. optic/o
   d. uve/o

9. Combining form meaning "eye lens":
   a. cor/o
   b. irid/o
   c. ocul/o
   d. phak/o

10. Abbreviation meaning the pupils are equal, round, and reactive to light and accommodation:
    a. PERRLA
    b. PERRL
    c. PERL
    d. PURL

Pathophysiology

■ Eye

Visual Disturbances

Astigmatism

Irregular curvature of refractive surfaces (cornea or lens) of eye

Can be congenital or acquired (as a result of disease or trauma)

Image is distorted

Treatment

Corrected with cylindrical lens

Diplopia

Double vision

Amblyopia

Dimness of vision—impairment of vision without detectable organic lesion of eye

Hyperopia

Farsightedness

Shortened eyeball

- Can see objects in distance, not close up

Treatment

Corrected with convex lens

Presbyopia

Age-related farsightedness

Treatment

Magnification (reading glasses or bifocals)

Myopia

Nearsightedness

Elongated eyeball

- Can see objects up close, not in distance

Treatment

Corrected with concave lens thicker at periphery

Nystagmus—Unilateral or Bilateral

Rapid, involuntary eye movements

Movements can be

- Vertical
- Horizontal
- Rotational
- Combination of above

Cause

Brain tumor or inner ear disease

Normal in newborns

Due to underlying condition or adverse effect of drug

Various types, such as

- Vestibular nystagmus
- Rhythmic eye movements

Strabismus
Cross-eyed

Due to muscle weakness or neurologic defect

Forms of strabismus

- Hypotropia (downward deviation of one eye)
- Hypertropia (upward deviation of one eye)
- Estropia (one eye turns inward)
- Exotropia (one eye turns outward)

Treatment

- Eye exercises/patching of normal eye
- Surgery to establish muscle balance

Infections
Conjunctivitis (Pink Eye)
Inflammation of conjunctival lining of eyelid or covering of sclera

Due to

- Infection
- Allergy
- Irritation

Treatment

- Varies with cause
- Antibiotic eye drops

Hordeolum (Stye)
Bacterial infection of eyelid hair follicle

- Usually *Staphylococcus*

Results in mass on eyelid

Treatment

- Antibiotics
- Incision and drainage may be necessary

Keratitis
Corneal inflammation

May be caused by herpes simplex virus, contact lens issue, or exposure

Causes tearing and photophobia, pain

Macular Degeneration
Destruction of fovea centralis

- Fovea centralis is small pit in center of retina (fovea centralis retinae)

Usually age related—leading cause of blindness in elderly

Results from exposure to ultraviolet rays or drugs

- Also may have a genetic component

Central vision is lost

Two types of macular degeneration

- Wet—development of new vascularization and leaking blood vessels near macula
- Dry (85% of cases)—atrophy and degeneration of retinal cells and deposits of drusen (clumps of extracellular waste)

Treatment

None for "dry" macular degeneration

Surgical intervention with laser for "net" macular degeneration to coagulate leaking vessels; success is limited

Medications

Detached Retina

Retinal tear—two layers of retina separate from each other

- Vitreous humor then leaks behind retina
- Retina then pulls away from choroid

Results in increasing blind spot in visual field

Condition is painless

Pressure continues to build if left unattended

Final result is blindness

Treatment

Surgical intervention with laser to repair tear (emergency/urgency)—photocoagulation for small tears

Scleral buckle for large retinal detachments

Pneumatic retinopexy for medium to large retinal detachment. Gas bubble is injected into vitreous cavity; pressure to tear resulting in retinal reattachment.

Cataracts

Lens becomes opaque with protein aggregates

Classified by Morphology

Size

Shape

Location

Also may be classified by etiology (cause) or time cataract occurs

Examples of Classification

Congenital cataract

- Bilateral opacity present at birth
- Also known as developmental cataract

Heat cataract

- Also known as glassblowers' cataract
- Caused by exposure to radiation

Traumatic cataract (Fig. 13-2)

- Result of injury to eye

Senile cataract

- Age related
- Usually forms on anterior lens

Symptoms

Blurring of vision

Halos around lights

Treatment

Removal of cataract with intraocular lens implantation

If no intraocular lens implant, then glasses or contact lenses for refraction

Glaucoma

Excess accumulation of intraocular aqueous humor

- High pressure results in decreased blood flow and edema
- Damages retinal cells and optic nerve

Stages of Glaucoma

Mild, moderate, severe

- Based on visual field loss caused by disease

Narrow-Angle Glaucoma

Acute type of glaucoma

Rapid onset is painful

Chronic Glaucoma

Also known as

- Wide-angle glaucoma
- Open-angle glaucoma

Asymptomatic

Diagnosed in eye examination using tonometry to test anterior chamber pressure and visual field exams

Treatment

Medications that decrease output of aqueous humor and decrease intraocular pressure (IOP)

Laser treatment to provide drainage

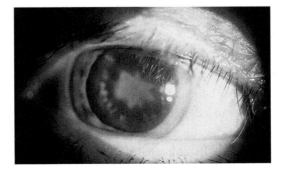

Figure **13-2** A concussive injury that resulted in a traumatic cataract.

◾ Ear

Infections

Otitis Media

Infection or inflammation of middle ear cavity

Chronic infection produces adhesions

Results in loss of hearing

Often occurs in children in combination with URI (upper respiratory infection)

Causes severe ear pain (otalgia)

Treatment

Antibiotics

Surgical intervention with placement of tubes to allow for drainage

- Useful in patients with recurrent infection

Otitis Externa

Also known as swimmer's ear

Infection of external auditory canal and pinna (exterior ear)

Caused by bacteria or fungus

Results in pain and discharge

Treatment

Antibiotic

Encouraged to keep ear dry

Hearing Loss

Conductive Hearing Loss

Due to a defect of sound-conducting apparatus

- Accumulation of wax
- Scar tissue on tympanic membrane

Also known as:

- Transmission hearing loss
- Conduction deafness

Treatment

- Hearing aids

Sensorineural

Due to a lesion of cochlea or central neural pathways

Also known as

- Perceptive deafness

May be divided into

- Cochlear hearing loss
  - Due to a defect in receptor or transducing mechanisms of cochlea
- Retrocochlear hearing loss
  - Due to defect located proximal to cochlea (vestibulocochlear nerve or auditory area of brain)

Presbycusis is age-related sensorineural hearing loss

Treatment

- Medication, implant, surgery

Ototoxic Hearing Loss

Caused by ingestion of toxic substance

Also known as toxic deafness

Ménière's Disease

Inner ear disturbance

Also known as idiopathic endolymphatic hydrops

Cause unknown

Common cause of vertigo (dizziness)

Other symptoms include hearing loss and tinnitus

CHAPTER 13: PATHOPHYSIOLOGY QUIZ

(Quiz answers are located in Appendix B)

1. This condition can be acquired or congenital and results in an irregular curvature of the refractive surfaces of the eye:
   a. diplopia
   b. hyperopia
   c. nystagmus
   d. astigmatism

2. In this condition, the eyeball is shorter than normal and results in being able to see objects in the distance but not close up:
   a. diplopia
   b. hyperopia
   c. nystagmus
   d. astigmatism

3. Rapid, involuntary eye movement is the predominant symptom of this condition:
   a. diplopia
   b. hyperopia
   c. nystagmus
   d. astigmatism

4. Age-related farsightedness is:
   a. presbyopia
   b. hyperopia
   c. diplopia
   d. myopia

5. Another name for a stye is:
   a. keratitis
   b. hordeolum
   c. hyperopia
   d. strabismus

6. An inflammation of the cornea that is caused by herpes simplex virus is:
   a. keratitis
   b. hordeolum
   c. hyperopia
   d. strabismus

7. In this condition there is destruction of the fovea centralis:
   a. macular degeneration
   b. detached retina
   c. glaucoma
   d. cataract

8. This is an infection that occurs in the middle ear cavity:
   a. otitis media
   b. otitis externa
   c. ototoxic hearing loss
   d. retrocochlear hearing loss

9. The hearing loss that can be due to a lesion on the cochlea is:
   a. conductive
   b. sensorineural
   c. ototoxic
   d. transmission

10. This condition is also known as perceptive deafness:
    a. conductive
    b. sensorineural
    c. otitis media
    d. transmission

Reimbursement Issues and Data Quality

Some of the CPT code descriptions for physician services include physician extender services. Physician extenders, such as nurse practitioners, physician assistants, and nurse anesthetists, etc., provide medical services typically performed by a physician. Within this educational material the term "physician" may include "and other qualified health care professionals" depending on the code. Refer to the official CPT® code descriptions and guidelines to determine codes that are appropriate to report services provided by non-physician practitioners.

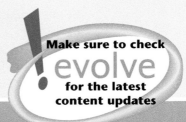
Make sure to check
evolve
for the latest
content updates

CHAPTER 14: REIMBURSEMENT ISSUES

Your Responsibility

Accurately code services that are provided and supported by documentation

Submit complete, accurate, and compliantly coded claims to obtain correct reimbursement for services rendered

Recognize upcoding (maximizing) or downcoding is never appropriate

Stay abreast of continuing changes

- Reimbursement and coverage policies, i.e., Local Coverage Determinations (LCD), or National Coverage Determinations (NCD)

- Coding guidelines from authoritative sources, i.e., AHA's *Coding Clinic for ICD-10-CM;* AHA's *Coding Clinic for HCPCS; UHDDS (Uniform Hospital Discharge Data) Guidelines;* and AMA's *CPT Assistant*

- Stay current with regulatory and Medicare Requirements. The CMS website (www.cms.gov/) offers links to many regulations for specific settings, including hospitals and physician practices. Some examples are:

Regulations such as the Health Insurance Portability and Accountability Act (HIPAA)

  - Centers for Medicare and Medicaid Policy Manuals

  - National Correct Coding Guidelines

  - MedLearn Matters Alerts and Educational Material
    www.cms.gov/Outreach-and-Education/Medicare-Learning-Network-MLN/
    MLNMattersArticles/2015-MLN-Matters-Articles.html

- Health Information Management Professionals are bound by the AHIMA Code of Ethics and the Standards of Ethical Coding (www.ahima.org/about/aboutahima?tabid=ethics)

> For the certification examination:
>   You need a working knowledge of national reimbursement and regulatory guidelines.

Population Change = Reimbursement Change

In 2012, the Administration on Aging (AOA) of the Department of Health and Human Services published a population survey (www.aoa.acl.gov/Aging_Statistics/Profile/2013/4.aspx)

- In 1900, persons 65 and older were only 4.1% of the population of the United States.

- In 2012, that same group had grown to 13%.

- By 2040, the elderly will be over 20% of the population.

Elderly compose the fastest growing segment of our population and this growth will place additional demands on health care providers and facilities.

Medicare is the primary insurance for the elderly.

■ Medicare

Getting Bigger All the Time!

According to the CMS NHE Fact Sheet (www.cms.gov/Research-Statistics-Data-and-Systems/
Statistics-Trends-and-Reports/NationalHealthExpendData/NHE-Fact-Sheet.html)

- In 2013, Medicare spending grew 3.4% to $585.7 billion, Medicare spending grew 6.1% to $449.4 billion

- By 2023 national health spending expected to reach $5.2 trillion, compared to $2.9 trillion in 2013

- Federal, state, and local governments are projected to account for 48% of national health spending by 2023

- Job security for coders!

Those Covered—Beneficiaries

Originally established in 1965 for those 65 and older, and implemented in 1966

Added coverage for disabled and permanent renal disease (end-stage renal disease or transplant) in 1972

Persons covered are called "beneficiaries"

Basic Structure

◈ Part A: Hospital and Institutional Care Coverage

Determine Service Provided

Institutional (facility) services, professional (physician or other individual) services, or supplies

- Professionals must report where services are performed with place of service code (www.cms.gov/Medicare/Coding/place-of-service-codes/Place_of_Service_Code_Set.html)

Institutional service may be inpatient (hospital bed for >24 hours) or outpatient (ambulatory surgical center, emergency room, etc.)

> For the certification examination:
> You need to know what is covered and not covered under Part A and what can be reported outside the MS-DRG payment.

Covered Inpatient Expenses Include

Room

Semiprivate room rate

- Pays the same amount whether the patient has a private room that is or is not medically necessary
- Semiprivate room
- Ward accommodations
- Accommodations must meet program standards

Patient Pays the Difference between Private and Semiprivate Room When

- Private room is not medically necessary
- Patient has requested the private room
  - Provider must inform patient of the additional charge for private room

Patient Does Not Pay the Difference between Private and Semiprivate Room When Isolation is Required to Avoid Jeopardizing the Health or Recovery of the Patient or Others

Example:

- Communicable diseases
- Heart attacks
- Cerebrovascular accidents
- Psychotic episodes
- Hospital has no semiprivate or ward accommodations available at the time of admission

Patients May be Assigned to Ward Accommodations if

- All semiprivate accommodations are occupied
- Facility has no semiprivate accommodations
- Patient requires immediate hospitalization
- Patient must be moved to semiprivate room when one is available
  - Accommodations must meet program standards

Nursing Services and Other Related Services

Defined as use of hospital facilities and medical social services ordinarily furnished by the hospital for the care/treatment of inpatients

- Meals and special diets during hospitalization

Blood transfusion

- Patient pays all costs for the first three pints of blood or equivalent units of packed red cells
  - Patient pays 20% for each additional pint
- Coverage starts with 4th pint of blood in hospital or skilled nursing facility

Drugs, Biologicals, Supplies, Appliances, and Equipment

FDA-approved drugs and biologicals for use in the hospital

- Must usually be furnished by the hospital for the care/treatment of inpatients

Supplies, appliances, and equipment

- Must be used for care/treatment solely during the inpatient hospital stay

OR

When unreasonable or impossible to limit the use to the inpatient period

> *Example:*
> - Items permanently installed in/attached to the patient's body while an inpatient, such as cardiac valves, cardiac pacemakers, and artificial limbs
> - Items that are temporarily installed in/attached to the patient's body while an inpatient and are necessary to permit the patient's release from the hospital, such as tracheotomy or drainage tubes

Hospital must have purchased the item

- A cost was incurred by the hospital for the item
  - Excluded are items given to the hospital

> *Example:*
> - Free pharmaceutical samples

Certain Other Covered Diagnostic or Therapeutic Services

Diagnostic or therapeutic items/services ordinarily furnished to inpatients by hospital

- This includes the supply by others under arrangements made by the hospital

> *Example:*
> - Diagnostic or therapeutic services of an audiologist provided off the hospital premises but billed for by the hospital
> - Surgical dressings and splints, casts, and other devices used for the reduction of fractures and dislocations

Prosthetic devices are covered that replace all/part of an organ

- The function of a permanently inoperative or malfunctioning internal body organ

> *Example:*
> - Braces, trusses, artificial replacements (legs, arms, and eyes)

Diagnostic/therapeutic inpatient services of a psychologist/physical therapist

- Must be a salaried member of the staff of a hospital

Inpatient diagnostic services furnished by an independent, certified clinical lab under arrangements with the hospital

- Lab certified under CLIA
  - CLIA = Clinical Laboratories Improvement Act

Reasonable cost of medical/surgical services of medical/osteopathic interns or residents under an approved teaching program

- Transportation services

Includes transport by ambulance to another facility for testing and/or treatment

Additionally Covered Expenses When They Meet Certain Criteria

Inpatient rehabilitation

Skilled nursing

Some personal convenience items for long-term illness/disability

Home health visit

Hospice care

Noncovered Inpatient-Hospital Expenses

Non–medically necessary services or supplies

Private-duty nurse or other private-duty attendant

Deluxe or non-medically necessary private room

Personal convenience items

- Those not routinely furnished to patients

Non-physician inpatient services that have not been provided directly or arranged for by hospital staff

Coverage Under Part A is Compulsory

Paid for by Social Security tax

Eligibility is determined by the Social Security Administration (SSA)

Reimbursement is for all covered and medically necessary services

- After annual deductible is met

ICD-10-CM diagnosis and procedure codes are basis for Part A payment

Charges are submitted electronically

Administrative Simplification Compliance Act (ASCA) prohibits payment of initial health care claims not sent electronically, except in limited situations

- Such as providers who have 25 or fewer full-time employees, or
- Claims from providers that submit fewer than 10 claims per month on average during a calendar year

Claim electronically transmitted in data "packets" over telephone line

- Medicare contractors perform series of edits
- Initial edits determine if batch of claims meets HIPAA standards
- Errors detected, entire batch of claims rejected and returned to provider to correct and resubmit
- Claims that pass initial edits are then edited against implementation guide requirements in HIPAA standards
- Errors detected, individual claims with errors rejected and returned to provider to correct and resubmit
- If first two levels of edits are passed, each claim is edited for compliance with Medicare coverage and payment policy requirements
- After successful transmission, an acknowledgment report is generated back to provider

Exempt providers may submit paper billing

◆ Part B: Supplemental

Provides Coverage for Non-Hospital Charges

Physician services

Outpatient hospital services

Home health care

Medically necessary supplies and equipment

Those services and supplies not covered under Part A that are medically necessary

Payment for the hospital stay if the patient has exhausted all Part A benefits prior to admission

Beneficiaries Purchase Coverage with Monthly Premiums
Three Coding Systems Used to Report Part B Services and Supplies
That are Medical Necessity for Services

HCPCS Level I = CPT—services

HCPCS Level II (also known as National Codes)—supplies, services, and drugs not included or covered by CPT coding system

> On the certification examination, HCPCS Level II are only on the theory portion of the examination, not on the practical portion of the examination.

ICD-10-CM—diagnoses

◆ Part C: Medicare Advantage Plans

Variety of health care options are available

- Health Maintenance Organization (HMO)
- Preferred Provider Organization (PPO)
- Private Fee-for-Service (PFFS)
- Special Needs Plans (SNPs)
- HMO Point of Service (HMOPOS)

Added after Part A and B

◆ Part D: Prescription Drug, Improvement, and Modernization Act of 2003

Prescription drug plan

Open enrollment began January 1, 2006

Premium paid by beneficiary

—Reimbursements based on the diagnoses of patients within the plan

Officiating Office

Department of Health and Human Services (DHHS)

Delegated to Centers for Medicare and Medicaid Services (CMS)

CMS runs Medicare and Medicaid

CMS delegates daily operation for Part A and Part B to Medicare Administrative Contractors (MACs)

- The Medicare Prescription Drug Improvement and Modernization Act of 2003 allowed CMS to reduce 48 fiscal intermediaries (FIs) to 15 Medicare Administrative Contractors (MACs). CMS is currently engaged in a MAC consolidation strategy, moving from 15 A/B MAC jurisdictions to 10 A/B MAC jurisdictions.

Funding for Medicare

Social security taxes

Equal match from government

CMS sends money to MACs

MACs handle paperwork and pay claims

Federal Register

Government publishes updates, revisions, deletions (changes) in *Federal Register* (Figure 14-1)

- CMS website (www.cms.gov) also contains published changes

Updates to payment systems occur throughout the year

Part A hospital inpatient payment changes are effective October 1

Hospital outpatient facility payment changes and physician payment system changes are effective January 1, published November/December

Quarterly revisions to HCPCS are published by CMS

- AMA publishes changes to CPT Category III codes effective January 1 and July 1

Electronic Transactions

HIPAA

- Created to govern health care portability

  -electronic data interchange (EDI)

  -requiring security of information and privacy of patient information

  -establishing code sets appropriate for electronic reporting

Transactions

- Activities involving transfer of health care information

Transmission

- Movement of electronic data between two entities

Today 99% of Part A and 95% Part B claims filed electronically

- Data entered electronically or onto paper CMS-1500 form
- Response is Electronic Remittance Advice (ERA) with the electronic fund transfer (EFT)

The format that supports electronic transmissions

- 5010 version

■ National Correct Coding Initiative (NCCI)

Developed by the Centers for Medicare and Medicaid Services to

- Promote national correct coding methods, to reduce/alleviate separate reporting of bundled services
- Control improper multiple procedure coding that leads to inappropriate payment of Part B physician claims and hospital outpatient claims
- Complete list may be found at www.cms.gov/NationalCorrectCodInitEd/

Unbundling

CMS defines unbundling as

- Billing separately each component of an all-inclusive procedure

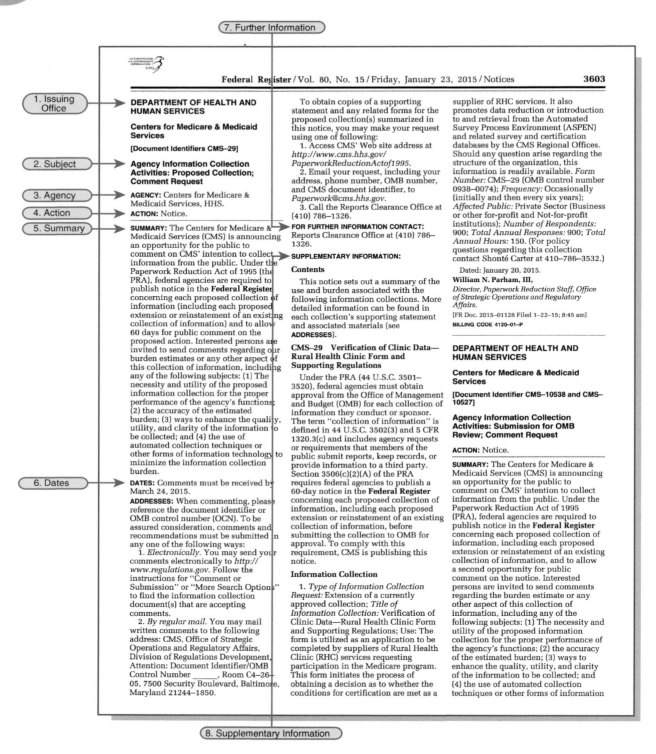

Figure **14-1** Example of page from the *Federal Register*.

Example:

Billing 15260, Full thickness graft, free, including direct closure of donor site; nose, ears, eyelids and/or lips PLUS 12016, Simple repair of superficial wounds of face, ears, eyelids, nose lips ... when code 15260 states "including direct closure of donor site"

Prospective Payment Systems (PPS)

For services provided to Medicare patients in inpatient or ambulatory surgical centers

Established by Tax Equity and Fiscal Responsibility Act (TEFRA) of 1982

Social Security amendments passed use of inpatient PPS in 1983

For services provided in

- Acute care hospitals
- Skilled nursing facilities
- Inpatient rehabilitation facilities
- Long-term care hospital settings
  - Psychiatric hospitals or exempt psychiatric units

Hospital/facility paid fixed amount for patient discharged in a treatment category

Excludes these hospitals:

- Children's
- Rehabilitation
- Cancer

Ambulatory Payment Classifications (APCs)

Omnibus Budget Reconciliation Act of 1986 (OBRA)

Prior to OBRA, Medicare hospital outpatient services paid on a cost-based system

- Also known as a retrospective system

Act Mandated

Replacement of cost-based system with a PPS (Prospective Payment System)

Medicare hospital-based outpatient facilities report services and some supplies/drugs on claims using CMS Healthcare Common Procedure Coding System (HCPCS), which includes CPT codes

- CMS uses claims data to determine future payment rates/coverage policies
- Data sources were used to develop Outpatient Prospective Payment System (OPPS)

Developed Ambulatory Patient Groups (APGs)

Grouped outpatient services

Differs from MS-DRGs because an outpatient can be assigned multiple APGs

Outpatient claims may have multiple APGs on any given day, but only one MS-DRG is paid for the entire inpatient encounter

Final Version of the Classification System Was Ambulatory Payment Classifications (APCs)

Implementation on August 1, 2000

APCs Mandatory for

- Most Medicare hospital outpatient services
  Some exceptions are lab and therapy services that are paid by a separate fee schedule
- Inpatient services covered under Part B
  - If beneficiary has exhausted Part A benefits

- Inpatient services not covered by Part A
- Partial hospitalization services
  Furnished by community mental health centers and some hospitals

APCs are Used for Reimbursement for Hospital-Based Outpatient Services
Such as:
- Outpatient surgery
- Hospital-based outpatient clinics
- Emergency departments
- Outpatient ancillary services
  Example: Radiology (Laboratory is paid on a separate fee schedule)

APC Structure

Consists of over 760 groups of services
- Each HCPCS code is assigned to an APC and has a status indicator defining how and whether separate payment is made (Figure 14-2)

Services in each APC are alike:
- Clinically
- In resources required to provide the services

APC	HCPCS	APC Description	HCPCS Description	SI	Rel. Wt.	Pay Rate	Natl. Coin.	Min. Coin.
0006		**Level I Incision & Drainage**		T	2.1836	$161.96		$32.40
0006	10060		Drainage of skin abscess					
0006	10061		Drainage of skin abscess					
0006	10080		Drainage of pilonidal cyst					
0006	10160		Puncture drainage of lesion					
0006	20950		Fluid pressure, muscle					
0006	21725		Revision of neck muscle					
0006	26010		Drainage of finger abscess					
0006	40800		Drainage of month lesion					
0006	69000		Drain external ear lesion					
0006	69020		Drain outer ear canal lesion					
0007		**Level II Incision & Drainage**		T	11.6749	$865.96		$173.20
0007	10081		Drainage of pilonidal cyst					
0007	10140		Drainage of hematoma/fluid					
0007	20103		Explore wound extremity					
0007	23931		Drainage of arm bursa					
0007	26011		Drainage of finger abscess					
0007	28001		Drainage of bursa of foot					
0007	38300		Drainage lymph node lesion					
0007	55100		Drainage of scrotum abscess					
0007	57022		I & D vaginal hematoma					

Figure **14-2** Final 2015 APC grouping of HCPCS codes (January, 2015).

APC Includes Some Items/Services That Contribute to Cost of the Service but Medicare Does Not Usually Reimburse Separately

- These incidentals are packaged into the APC payment

  Example:

  - Supplies
  - Observation services (limited exceptions)
  - Specific drugs
  - Blood
  - Medical visits on the same day of service or procedure unless separately identifiable and modified
  - Guidance services (e.g., stereoscopic x-rays)

Medicare does reimburse separately for some items and services that are not packaged, such as casting, splinting, and strapping services

Further APC information is available at www.cms.gov/HospitalOutpatientPPS/

Pass-Through Codes

Services, procedures, and/or supplies not included in APC package

Paid an additional pass-through APC payment

Payment Rate and Co-Insurance

Co-insurance amount is 20% of the median charge for all services in the APC

- This means the payment rate and co-insurance will not change until the co-insurance amount becomes 20% of the total APC payment

APC Payment Status Indicators (SI) (Fig. 14-3)

One letter or one letter followed by a number (i.e., Q1) designating a status indicator is assigned to each HCPCS/CPT code

Indicates if service, procedure, or supply is reimbursable under the Outpatient Prospective Payment System (OPPS) or other fee schedule

Also identifies if reimbursement is bundled or separately payable and/or discounted

  Example:

  - HCPCS/CPT codes under SI "A" are not paid under OPPS but are paid under a fee schedule or another payment method
  - Such as: 77057, mammogram screening (SI "A")
  - Routine Dialysis Services
  - Ambulance Services

Each APC is assigned a co-insurance amount and payment rate

- Adjusted by hospital's wage index (labor costs)

Figure 14-4 illustrates the payment rate and co-insurance amounts

  Example:

  - Drainage of skin abscess (10060) is paid at $161.96, co-insurance amount of 20% ($32.40)
  - Red blood cell deglycerolization (P9039) is paid at $463.97, co-insurance amount of 20% ($92.80)

Can receive payment for multiple services provided on the same day

Multiple procedures that have status indicator "S" are reimbursed at 100%

Indicator	Item/Code/Service	OPPS Payment Status
	ADDENDUM D1. – OPPS PAYMENT STATUS INDICATORS FOR CY 2015	
A	Service furnished to a hospital outpatient that are paid under a fee schedule or payment system other than OPPS, for example:	Not paid under OPPS. Paid by fiscal intermediaries/MACS under a fee schedule or payment system other than OPPS.
	• Ambulance Services	
	• Clinical Diagnostic Laboratory Services	Not subject to deductible or coinsurance.
	• Non-Implantable Prosthetic and Orthotic Devices	
	• EPO for ESRD Patients	
	• Physical, Occupational, and Speech Therapy	
	• Routine Dialysis Services for ESRD Patients Provided in a Certified Dialysis Unit of a Hospital	
	• Diagnostic Mammography	Not subject to deductible or coinsurance.
	• Screening Mammography	
B	Codes that are not recognized by OPPS when submitted on an outpatient hospital Part B bill type (12x and 13x).	Not paid under OPPS. • May be paid by fiscal intermediaries/MACs when submitted on a different bill type, for example, 75x (CORF), but not paid under OPPS. • An alternate code that is recognized by OPPS when submitted on an outpatient hospital Part B bill type (12x and 13x) may be available.
C	Inpatient Procedures	Not paid under OPPS Admit patient. Bill as inpatient
D	Discontinued Codes	Not paid under OPPS or any other Medicare payment system.
E	Items, Codes, and Services:	Not paid by Medicare when submitted on outpatient claims (any outpatient bill type).
	• That are not covered by any Medicare outpatient benefit based on statutory exclusion.	
	• That are not covered by any Medicare outpatient benefit for reasons other than statutory exclusion.	
	• That are not recognized by Medicare for outpatient claims but for which an alternate code for the same item or service may be available.	
	For which separate payment is not provided on outpatient claims.	
F	Corneal Tissue Acquisition; Certain CRNA Services and Hepatitis B Vaccines	Not paid under OPPS. Paid at reasonable cost.
G	Pass-Through Drugs and Biologicals	Paid under OPPS; separate APC payment.
H	Pass-Through Device Categories	Separate cost-based pass-through payment; not subject to copayment.
K	Nonpass-Through Drugs and Nonimplantable Biologicals, Including Therapeutic Radiopharmaceuticals	Paid under OPPS; separate APC payment.
L	Influenza Vaccine; Pneumococcal Pneumonia Vaccine	Not paid under OPPS. Paid at reasonable cost; not subject to deductible or coinsurance.
M	Items and Services Not Billable to the Fiscal Intermediary/MAC	Not paid under OPPS.
N	Items and Services Packaged into APC Rates	Paid under OPPS; payment is packaged into payment for other services. Therefore, there is no separate APC payment.
P	Partial Hospitalization	Paid under OPPS; per diem APC payment.
Q1	STVX-Packaged Codes	Paid under OPPS; Addendum B displays APC assignments when services are separately payable.
		(1) Packaged APC payment if billed on the same date of service as a HCPCS code assigned status indicator "S," "T," "V," or "X."
		(2) In all other circumstances, payment is made through a separate APC payment.
Q2	T-Packaged Codes	Paid under OPPS; Addendum B displays APC assignments when services are separately payable.
		(1) Packaged APC payment if billed on the same date of service as a HCPCS code assigned status indicator "T."
		(2) In all other circumstances, payment is made through a separate APC payment.
Q3	Codes That May Be Paid Through a Composite APC	Paid under OPPS; Addendum B displays APC assignments when services are separately payable.
		Addendum M displays composite APC assignments when codes are paid through a composite APC.
		(1) Composite APC payment based on OPPS composite-specific payment criteria. Payment is packaged into a single payment for specific combinations of service.
		(2) In all other circumstances, payment is made through a separate APC payment or packaged into payment for other services.
R	Blood and Blood Products	Paid under OPPS; separate APC payment.
S	Significant Procedure, Not Discounted when Multiple	Paid under OPPS; separate APC payment.
T	Significant Procedure, Multiple Reduction Applies	Paid under OPPS; separate APC payment.
U	Brachytherapy Sources	Paid under OPPS; separate APC payment.
V	Clinic or Emergency Department Visit	Paid under OPPS; separate APC payment.
X	Ancillary Services	Paid under OPPS; separate APC payment.
Y	Non-Implantable Durable Medical Equipment	Not paid under OPPS. All institutional providers other than home health agencies bill to DMERC.

Figure **14-3** Payment Status Indicators for the Hospital Outpatient Prospective Payment System Addendum.

HCPCS Code	Short Description	SI	APC	Relative Weight	Payment Rate	Minimum Unadjusted Copayment
10060	Drainage of skin abscess	T	0006	2.1836	$161.96	$32.40
10061	Drainage of skin abscess	T	0006	2.1836	$161.96	$32.40
10080	Rbc leukoreduced irradiated	R	0006	2.1836	$161.96	$32.40
10081	Drainage of pilonidal cyst	T	0007	11.6749	$865.96	$173.20
P9038	Rbc irradiated	R	9505	2.8023	$207.85	$41.57
P9039	Rbc deglycerolized	R	9504	6.2553	$463.97	$92.80
P9040	Rbc leukoreduced irradiated	R	0969	3.7139	$275.47	$55.10

Figure **14-4** Final APC payment rate and co-insurance amount (January, 2015).

Multiple significant surgical procedures performed on the same day that have a status indicator of "T" are discounted

- Full payment made for the highest reimbursed procedure APC
- Multiple procedure payment reduction applies when two or more services with status indicator "T" are billed on the same date of service

-CA Modifier

Used with status indicator "C" services, these are inpatient procedures provided on an emergency basis in the outpatient setting

- Patient expires before admission to the hospital

-CA is assigned to inpatient-only procedure

Payment is allowed for only one procedure

Transitional Pass-Through Payments for Certain Devices and Items

Payments made for certain innovative devices, drugs, and biologicals

Paid as an additional APC payment

> *Example:*

- Chemotherapeutic agents
  - Including supportive and adjunctive drugs
- Implantable devices
- Immunosuppressive drugs
- Orphan drugs
- Some new drugs
- Certain drugs given in the emergency room for heart attacks

Have co-insurance amounts that can be less than 20% of the Average Wholesale Price (AWP)

Payments for pass-throughs made for at least 2 years but not more than 3 years

Report devices and drugs with HCPCS C or J codes and SI "G," "H," or "K"

When a pass-through transitional payment has expired:

- C code removed from HCPCS and is usually given an applicable "J" code
- Separate payment is no longer made for item

Current HCPCS codes, including C codes, can be viewed and/or downloaded from the CMS website at www.cms.gov/Medicare/Coding/HCPCSReleaseCodeSets/Alpha-Numeric-HCPCS.html

Pass-through items for which separate payment expires should be reported on claim to identify cost to CMS

HCPCS codes for drugs, biologicals, devices, and radiopharmaceuticals that have a separate APC payment are listed in Final Annual Rule

Currently, very few devices are paid separately

Drugs and biologicals with final pass-through status for 2015 are displayed in Figure 14-5

Most devices have no separate APC payment because the item is packaged into APC payment for procedure. Although hospitals do not receive additional payment for these devices, they are encouraged to report HCPCS codes on claim

In some cases, hospitals are required to report device HCPCS code. (See the following section "Device-Dependent Procedures")

Most recent information concerning applications and requirements for APC payments for new technologies, additional device categories, and pass-through payments for drugs and biologicals is located on the CMS website at www.cms.gov/HospitalOutpatientPPS

Device-Dependent Procedures

When hospitals report certain procedure codes that require the use of devices

- Must also report the applicable HCPCS codes and charges for all devices used to perform the procedures
- This information is used in calculating future OPPS payment amounts

CY 2014 HCPCS Code	CY 2015 HCPCS Code	CY 2015 Long Descriptor	Final CY 2015 SI	Final CY 2015 APC
A9584	A9584	Iodine I-123 ioflupane, diagnostic, per study dose, up to 5 millicuries	N	N/A
C9285	C9285	Lidocaine 70 mg/tetracaine 70 mg, per patch	N	N/A
J0485	J0485	Injection, belatacept, 1 mg	K	9286
J9042	J9042	Injection, brentuximab vedotin, 1 mg	K	9287
J0716	J0716	Injection, centruroides immune f(ab)2, up to 120 milligrams	G	1431
J9019	J9019	Injection, asparaginase (erwinaze), 1,000 iu	K	9289
C9290	C9290	Injection, bupivicaine liposome, 1 mg	K	N/A
C9292	C9292	Injection, pertuzumab, 10 mg	N	N/A
C9293	C9293	Injection, glucarpidase, 10 units	K	9293
C9294	C9294	Injection, taliglucerase alfa, 100 units	K	9294
C9295	C9295	Injection, carfilzomib, 1 mg	G	9295
C9296	C9296	Injection, ziv-aflibercept, 1 mg	G	9296
Q4131	Q4131	EpiFix, per square centimeter	N	N/A
Q4132	Q4132	Grafix core, per square centimeter	N	N/A
Q4133	Q4133	Grafix prime, per square centimeter	N	N/A
J0131	J0131	Injection, acetaminophen, 10 mg	N	N/A
J0490	J0490	Injection, belimumab, 10 mg	K	1353
J0638	J0638	Injection, canakinumab, 1 mg	K	1311
J0712	J0712	Injection, ceftaroline fosamil, 10 mg	N	N/A

Figure **14-5** Final 2015 Drugs and Biologicals with Pass-Through Status.

If such a procedure is reported without at least one device HCPCS code, claim will be returned to provider

Procedures that require device HCPCS codes are listed in Device to Procedure Edits document

Download from CMS the device edits:

www.cms.gov/HospitalOutpatientPPS/01_overview.asp

(On left side of screen click link: "Device, Radiolabeled Product, and Procedure Edits" and on Downloads page click "Device to Procedure Edits")

Discounting

Multiple surgical procedures during the same operative procedure

- Status indicator "T" indicates multiple procedure payment reduction applied

Highest weighted procedure APC paid at 100% (after applicable co-pay and deductible)

- Multiple procedure payment reduction applies when two or more services with status indicator "T" are billed on the same date of service

Terminated surgical procedures before the induction of anesthesia paid at 50%

- Indicated by use of modifier -73 added to surgical procedure code

Outlier Adjustments

Some costs that exceed 1.75 times the payment rate and exceed the APC payment rate plus a $2,025 fixed threshold receives an adjusted higher reimbursement

Inpatient-Only Procedures with Status Indicator "C"

CMS publishes a list of procedures that are click link "inpatient-only" procedures

- Procedures that are life-threatening and require substantial mortality risks as an outpatient

www.cms.gov/HospitalOutpatientPPS and click link "Hospital Outpatient Regulations and Notices" for most current notices (Click link "Hospital Outpatient Prospective Payment- Final Rule with Comment" and next, Click link "CY2015 OPPS Addenda", when file opens, locate Addendum E)

> *Example:*
>
> Status Indicator "C" procedures are those that are not paid under OPPS

- 27258 Open treatment of spontaneous hip dislocation (developmental, including congenital or pathological), replacement of femoral head in acetabulum (including tenotomy, etc);
- 32900 Resection of ribs, extrapleural, all stages
- 33535 Coronary artery bypass, using arterial graft(s); 3 coronary arterial grafts

Ambulatory Surgical Procedures

CMS publishes a list of procedures approved for ambulatory surgery center (ASC) procedures

www.cms.gov/ASCPayment/

> *Example:*
>
> Approved ASC procedures are those that are paid under OPPS

- 10121 Incision and removal of foreign body, subcutaneous tissues; complicated
- 19340 Immediate insertion of breast prosthesis following mastopexy, mastectomy or in reconstruction
- 23155 Excision or curettage of bone cyst or benign tumor of proximal humerus; with autograft (includes obtaining graft)

Observation Status

Complete OPPS program information for 2015 was in the *Federal Register*, December 22, 2014, Volume 79, Number 245

Historically, observation services were paid only for chest pain, congestive heart failure, and asthma

Beginning in 2008, observation services were paid for any diagnosis when other observation criteria were met

Time begins when the patient is admitted to the observation unit and ends when the patient is discharged or admitted as an inpatient

Outpatient Code Editor (OCE)

General functions of the OCE system

- Reviews claim data to identify errors and returns an edit flag(s)
- Edits are based upon HCPCS and ICD-10-CM codes

Assigns an APC number to each service covered under OPPS

Medicare Severity Diagnosis-Related Groups (MS-DRGs)

System of Classifying Patients into Groups by Related Diagnoses

For payment of operating costs based on prospectively set rates

For acute care hospital inpatient stays under Medicare Part A

Each diagnosis and procedure codes are categorized into an MS-DRG

MS-DRGs have relative weights assigned based on the average resources used to treat patients in that MS-DRG

- Similar types of patients
- Similar types of illnesses or injuries
- Severity of illness
- Treatments provided
  - Similar use of resources

Each facility has its own payment rate assigned by Centers for Medicare and Medicaid Services (CMS)

Although hospitals assign MS-DRGs for internal resource and financial management, the official MS-DRG for payment is calculated by Medicare from ICD-10-CM/CD-10-PCS codes that are assigned at the hospital.

System Based on

Principal diagnosis

Principal procedure

Any qualifying complication(s) or comorbidity(ies)

Structure of MS-DRGs

Divides All Principal Diagnoses into 25 Major Diagnostic Categories (MDCs) (Figure 14-6)

Most MDCs correspond to major organ systems

Example:

- Respiratory System
- Digestive System
- Nervous System

Major Diagnostic Categories

MDC 01 Diseases & Disorders of the Nervous System
MDC 02 Diseases & Disorders of the Eye
MDC 03 Diseases & Disorders of the Ear, Nose, Mouth & Throat
MDC 04 Diseases & Disorders of the Respiratory System
MDC 05 Diseases & Disorders of the Circulatory System
MDC 06 Diseases & Disorders of the Digestive System
MDC 07 Diseases & Disorders of the Hepatobiliary System & Pancreas
MDC 08 Diseases & Disorders of the Musculoskeletal System & Connective Tissue
MDC 09 Diseases & Disorders of the Skin, Subcutaneous Tissue & Breast
MDC 10 Endocrine, Nutritional & Metabolic Diseases & Disorders
MDC 11 Diseases & Disorders of the Kidney & Urinary Tract
MDC 12 Diseases & Disorders of the Male Reproductive System
MDC 13 Diseases & Disorders of the Female Reproductive System
MDC 14 Pregnancy, Childbirth & the Puerperium
MDC 15 Newborns & Other Neonates with Conditions Originating in Perinatal Period
MDC 16 Diseases & Disorders of Blood, Blood Forming Organs, Immunologic Disorders
MDC 17 Myeloproliferative Diseases & Disorders, Poorly Differentiated Neoplasms
MDC 18 Infectious & Parasitic Diseases, Systemic or Unspecified Sites
MDC 19 Mental Diseases & Disorders
MDC 20 Alcohol/Drug Use & Alcohol/Drug Induced Organic Mental Disorders
MDC 21 Injuries, Poisonings & Toxic Effects of Drugs
MDC 22 Burns
MDC 23 Factors Influencing Health Status & Other Contacts with Health Services
MDC 24 Multiple Significant Trauma
MDC 25 Human Immunodeficiency Virus Infections

Figure **14-6** MDCs of the ICD-10-CM/PCS MS-DRGs.

Some MDCs correspond to an etiology (cause)

Example:

- Neoplasms
- Human Immunodeficiency Virus Infections

MS-DRGs are Then Further Defined by a Particular Set of Patient Attributes Defined in the Uniform Hospital Discharge Data Set (UHDDS)

By Diagnosis

Principal diagnosis Defined as "that condition established after study to be chiefly responsible for occasioning the admission of the patient to the hospital for care"

Secondary diagnosis Conditions that co-exist at the time of admission, that develop subsequently to the admission, or that affect the treatment received and/or length of stay

By Procedure

Principal procedure A procedure that is performed for definitive treatment rather than for diagnostic or exploratory purposes or that is necessary in order to take care of a complication

Significant procedure Medicare defines a significant procedure as one that is
  - Surgical in nature
  - Carries an anesthetic/procedural risk, and
  - Requires specialized training

Discharge status Condition and/or place to which the patient is being discharged, such as to home, skilled nursing facility, rehabilitation, home health care, long-term care

Birth weight: MS-DRGs for newborns may be affected by infant's birth weight

Example: MDC 15, Newborns & Other Neonates with Conditions Originating in the Perinatal Period Prematurity, Figure 14-7, illustrates DRGs 791 and 792 are affected by low birth weight and/or preterm

MS-DRGs are not affected by age

Exception: MS-DRGs for newborns

Surgical Classes in Each MDC Are Defined in a Hierarchical (Least-to-Most Resource Intense) Order

Multiple procedures related to principal diagnosis during hospital stay are assigned to only the highest surgical class in the hierarchy

- MS-DRG Grouper performs assignment
  - Grouper = Computer software

Case Study

The principal diagnosis is congestive heart failure (I50.9). Additional diagnoses are morbid obesity due to excess calories (E66.01), Type 2 diabetes without complications (E11.9), atherosclerotic heart disease (I25.10), psoriasis (L40.9), depressive disorder (F32.9), unspecified personality disorder (F60.9), pure hypercholesterolemia (E78.0), cardiomegaly (I51.7), and initial episode of acute subendocardial myocardial infarction (I21.4). If I21.4 had been listed within the top nine diagnoses, the reimbursement would have been based on MS-DRG 293 compared to 282 (for which the reimbursement is significantly greater) if the complication of subendocardial infarction had been correctly listed. Review the principal reason for admission and the principal diagnosis assignment after study for correct MS-DRG assignment.

MDC 15 Newborns & Other Neonates with Conditions Originating in Perinatal Period
Prematurity

Major Problems	DRG
Yes	791
No	792

DRG 791 PREMATURITY W MAJOR PROBLEMS
DRG 792 PREMATURITY W/O MAJOR PROBLEMS

PREMATURITY
PRINCIPAL OR SECONDARY DIAGNOSIS

P0700	Extremely low birth weight newborn, unspecified weight
P0710	Other low birth weight newborn, unspecified weight
P0714	Other low birth weight newborn, 1000-1249 grams
P0715	Other low birth weight newborn, 1250-1499 grams
P0716	Other low birth weight newborn, 1500-1749 grams
P0717	Other low birth weight newborn, 1750-1999 grams
P0718	Other low birth weight newborn, 2000-2499 grams
P0726	Extreme immaturity of newborn, gestational age 27 completed weeks
P0730	Preterm newborn, unspecified weeks of gestation
P0731	Preterm newborn, gestational age 28 completed weeks
P0732	Preterm newborn, gestational age 29 completed weeks
P0733	Preterm newborn, gestational age 30 completed weeks
P0734	Preterm newborn, gestational age 31 completed weeks

MAJOR PROBLEMS
See Major Problem Diagnoses Listed under DRG 793

Figure **14-7** MDC 15, Newborns & Other Neonates with Conditions Originating in the Perinatal Period, Prematurity.

MS-DRGs MCC and CC

- All diagnoses were reviewed to determine if they qualify as a CC or non-CC
- Key criterion being the increase in hospital resources
- All diagnoses were divided into three severity levels:
  - Major complications or comorbidities (MCC)
  - Complications or comorbidities (CC)
  - Non-CCs—do not affect MS-DRG assignment

The MS-DRG system is 001-998 with allowances for future changes

Chronic conditions may have to be decompensated or in exacerbation to qualify as a CC for MS-DRGs

The following codes are MCCs only if patient is discharged alive:

I46.2	Cardiac arrest due to underlying cardiac condition
I46.8	Cardiac arrest due to other underlying condition
I46.9	Cardiac arrest, cause unspecified
I49.01	Ventricular fibrillation
R09.2	Respiratory arrest
R57.0	Cardiogenic shock
R57.1	Hypovolemic shock
R57.8	Other shock

A hospital's reimbursement depends even more on complete documentation and accurate coding with MS-DRGs

MS-DRGs are affected by the CC exclusions list

- Lists certain diagnoses that would not be considered CCs when coded as a secondary diagnosis with a certain principal diagnosis
- Example: J82 (Eosinophilic pneumonia) is excluded as a CC when most of the pneumonia codes are assigned as principal diagnosis
- Good documentation and accurate coding will be even more important to obtain the optimum reimbursement for the hospital

Challenges for coding staff include:

- It may take more time to review and code a record resulting in decreased productivity
- Greater specificity in code assignment is necessary with ICD-10-CM/PCS and MS-DRGs
- There will be an increase in physician queries and communications
- Assigning POA (present on admission) indicators requires extra attention and may decrease productivity
- The coder must have a strong knowledge base about clinical conditions and disease to effectively use the MS-DRG system

MS-DRG Classification

Begins with diagnosis and pre-MDC (Figure 14-8)

Pre-Major Diagnostic Categories (Pre-MDCs)
Pre-MDC MS-DRGs are very resource intensive

Services for these MS-DRGs may be performed for diagnoses in many different MDCs

Assigned independently of the MDC to indicate the procedure performed

Cases are assigned to these MS-DRGs before they are assigned a MDC

DRG	DRG Description
001	Heart transplant or implant of heart assist system w MCC
002	Heart transplant or implant of heart assist system w/o MCC

See Figure 14-9 for the Pre-MDC table for DRG 001 and DRG 002.

There are 2 MDCs based on **both** principal diagnosis and secondary diagnosis

- MDC 24   Multiple Significant Trauma
- MDC 25   Human Immunodeficiency Virus Infections

Pre-MDC

ALL PATIENTS

Heart Transplant or Implant of Heart Assist System

MCC	DRG
Yes	001
No	002

ECMO or Tracheostomy with MV 96+ Hours or PDX Except Face, Mouth and Neck

ECMO	Tracheostomy	Major O.R. Procedure	DRG
Yes	n/a	n/a	003
No	Yes	Yes	003
No	Yes	No	004

Liver or Intestinal Transplant

Intestinal Transplant	MCC	DRG
Yes	n/a	005
No	Yes	005
No	No	006

Allogeneic Bone Marrow Transplant

Lung Transplant

Simultaneous Pancreas/Kidney Transplant

Autologous Bone Marrow Transplant

MCC	DRG
Yes	016
No	017

Pancreas Transplant

	DRG
	010

Tracheostomy for Face, Mouth and Neck Diagnoses

MCC	CC	DRG
Yes		011
No	Yes	012
No	No	013

Figure **14-8** Pre-MDC in ICD-10-CM/PCS MS-DRG.

Pre-MDC
Heart Transplant or Implant of Heart Assist System

MCC	DRG
Yes	001
No	002

DRG 001 HEART TRANSPLANT OR IMPLANT OF HEART ASSIST SYSTEM W MCC
DRG 002 HEART TRANSPLANT OR IMPLANT OF HEART ASSIST SYSTEM W/O MCC

HEART TRANSPLANT
OPERATING ROOM PROCEDURES

02HA0QZ	Insertion of Implantable Heart Assist System into Heart, Open Approach
02HA3QZ	Insertion of Implantable Heart Assist System into Heart, Percutaneous Approach
02HA4QZ	Insertion of Implantable Heart Assist System into Heart, Percutaneous Endoscopic Approach
02YA0Z0	Transplantation of Heart, Allogeneic, Open Approach
02YA0Z1	Transplantation of Heart, Syngeneic, Open Approach
02YA0Z2	Transplantation of Heart, Zooplastic, Open Approach

02RK0JZ	Replacement of Right Ventricle with Synthetic Substitute, Open Approach
with	
02RL0JZ	Replacement of Left Ventricle with Synthetic Substitute, Open Approach

IMPLANT OF HEART ASSIST SYSTEM

One of

02HA0RS	Insertion of Biventricular External Heart Assist System into Heart, Open Approach
02HA0RZ	Insertion of External Heart Assist System into Heart, Open Approach
02HA3RS	Insertion of Biventricular External Heart Assist System into Heart, Percutaneous Approach
02HA3RZ	Insertion of External Heart Assist System into Heart, Percutaneous Approach
02HA4RS	Insertion of Biventricular External Heart Assist System into Heart, Percutaneous Endoscopic Approach
02HA4RZ	Insertion of External Heart Assist System into Heart, Percutaneous Endoscopic Approach
02WA0QZ	Revision of Implantable Heart Assist System in Heart, Open Approach
02WA0RZ	Revision of External Heart Assist System in Heart, Open Approach
02WA3QZ	Revision of Implantable Heart Assist System in Heart, Percutaneous Approach
02WA3RZ	Revision of External Heart Assist System in Heart, Percutaneous Approach
02WA4QZ	Revision of Implantable Heart Assist System in Heart, Percutaneous Endoscopic Approach
02WA4RZ	Revision of External Heart Assist System in Heart, Percutaneous Endoscopic Approach
with one of	
02PA0RZ	Removal of External Heart Assist System from Heart, Open Approach
02PA3RZ	Removal of External Heart Assist System from Heart, Percutaneous Approach
02PA4RZ	Removal of External Heart Assist System from Heart, Percutaneous Endoscopic Approach

Figure **14-9** Pre-MDCs in ICD-10-CM/PCS MS-DRG, DRG 001 and 002.

Example: Patient with HIV (B20), admitted for treatment of pneumonia due to pseudomonas (J15.1). The principal diagnosis is HIV with secondary diagnosis of pneumonia. The assignment of MS-DRG 976 HIV with Major Related Condition without CC/MCC is affected by the secondary diagnosis of J15.1.

Use surgical procedure MS-DRG if surgery was performed

- Surgical procedures pay more than nonsurgical MDCs

Figure 14-10 illustrates MDC 1, Diseases and Disorders of the Nervous System

MDC 1 Diseases & Disorders of the Nervous System
Intracranial Vascular Procedures with PDX Hemorrhage

MCC	CC	DRG
Yes		020
No	Yes	021
No	No	022

DRG 020 INTRACRANIAL VASCULAR PROCEDURES W PDX HEMORRHAGE W MCC
DRG 021 INTRACRANIAL VASCULAR PROCEDURES W PDX HEMORRHAGE W CC
DRG 022 INTRACRANIAL VASCULAR PROCEDURES W PDX HEMORRHAGE W/O CC/MCC

INTRACRANIAL VASCULAR PROCEDURES
OPERATING ROOM PROCEDURES

031H09J   Bypass Right Common Carotid Artery to Right Extracranial Artery with Autologous Venous Tissue, Open Approach
031H0AJ   Bypass Right Common Carotid Artery to Right Extracranial Artery with Autologous Arterial Tissue, Open Approach
031H0JJ   Bypass Right Common Carotid Artery to Right Extracranial Artery with Synthetic Substitute, Open Approach
031H0KJ   Bypass Right Common Carotid Artery to Right Extracranial Artery with Nonautologous Tissue Substitute, Open Approach
031H0ZJ   Bypass Right Common Carotid Artery to Right Extracranial Artery, Open Approach
031J09K   Bypass Left Common Carotid Artery to Left Extracranial Artery with Autologous Venous Tissue, Open Approach
031J0AK   Bypass Left Common Carotid Artery to Left Extracranial Artery with Autologous Arterial Tissue, Open Approach
031J0JK   Bypass Left Common Carotid Artery to Left Extracranial Artery with Synthetic Substitute, Open Approach
031J0KK   Bypass Left Common Carotid Artery to Left Extracranial Artery with Nonautologous Tissue Substitute, Open Approach

Figure 14-10 MDC 1 Diseases & Disorders of the Nervous System. Surgical DRGs.

- Contains DRGs 020-036 with selection based on
  with or without a major complication or comorbidity (MCC)
  with or without complication or comorbidity (CC)

Figure 14-11 illustrates MDC 1, DRGs 020-022.

- Surgical procedures with or without MCC or CC

Use principal diagnosis to select MS-DRG if no surgery was performed

MS-DRG Selection if No Surgical Procedure is Performed is Based on:

- Qualifying MCC/CC
  - An MCC/CC is likely to result in increased use of hospital resources
  - Pneumonia is an MCC; benign hypertension is not an MCC or a CC
  - Discharge disposition may make a difference in the MS-DRG assigned
- **May be excluded as MCC/CC**
  - Chronic and acute manifestations of the same disease (not CCs for one another)
  - Is closely related to the principal diagnosis
  - *Example:*
  - Cardiomyopathy is not considered a CC with congestive heart failure
  - Urinary tract infection is considered a CC with congestive heart failure

MDC 1 Diseases & Disorders of the Nervous System

MDC 1 Assignment of Diagnosis Codes

Surgical DRGs. O.R. Procedure of ...

Intracranial Vascular Procedures with PDX Hemorrhage

MCC	CC	DRG
Yes		020
No	Yes	021
No	No	022

Craniotomy

Major Device Implant or Acute Complex CNS PDX	Chemotherapy Implant	MCC	CC	DRG
	Yes			023
Yes	No	Yes		023
Yes	No	No		024
No	No	Yes		025
No	No	No	Yes	026
No	No	No	No	027

Spinal Procedures

MCC	CC	Spinal Neurostimulator Combinations	DRG
Yes			028
No	Yes		029
No	No	Yes	029
No	No	No	030

Ventricular Shunt Procedures

MCC	CC	DRG
Yes		031
No	Yes	032
No	No	033

Carotid Artery Stent Procedures

MCC	CC	DRG
Yes		034
No	Yes	035
No	No	036

Figure **14-11** MDC 1 Diseases & Disorders of the Nervous System. DRG 020, 021, and 022.

Certain ICD-10-CM diagnosis codes include both an acute manifestation or complication with the underlying condition in one code.

Example:

- Exacerbation of Crohn's disease of small intestine with abscess: K50.014 (MS-DRG 386 Inflammatory Bowel Disease w CC)

MCC/CCs for MS-DRGs

CMS publishes a list of ICD-10-CM codes that are MCCs and CCs

Post Acute Transfer

CMS thought it was overpaying the acute care hospital for these patients at the full MS-DRG rates, so a reduction in payment formula was implemented

- Medicare developed special rules that apply to particular MS-DRGs in which patients are frequently discharged immediately to a rehab hospital, skilled nursing facility, a long-term care hospitals or home health care
- Termed transfer MS-DRGs
- Part of the Balanced Budget Act of 1997

Payment is adjusted when the covered days preceding the "transfer" are less than the Geometric Mean Length of Stay (GMLOS) of the assigned MS-DRG

- The facility is reimbursed on a per diem rate that is calculated by taking the Hospital's normal reimbursement for the MS-DRG divided by the GMLOS

There are three types of transfers that are affected:

- Transfers to another acute care hospital
  - The transferring hospital receives double the per diem rate for the first day plus the per diem rate for each subsequent day prior to the transfer
  - Not to exceed the total MS-DRG payment
- Designated MS-DRGs transferred to a post acute care setting
  - The same formula as a transfer to another acute care hospital
- Designated special pay MS-DRGs transferred to a post acute care setting
  - The transferring hospital receives the per diem rate for the first day plus one-half the per diem rate for each subsequent day prior to the transfer

Present on Admission Indicator (POA)

Hospitals submit Medicare inpatient claims with a Present On Admission (POA) indicator for nearly every diagnosis

Exempt are:

- Critical access hospitals
- Maryland waiver hospitals*
- Long-term care hospitals
- Cancer and inpatient psychiatric hospitals
- Inpatient rehabilitation facilities
- Children's inpatient facilities
- Rural health clinics
- Federally qualified health centers
- Religious non-medical health care institutions
- Veterans Administration/Department of Defense hospitals

Medicare returns claims without POA codes

- Hospitals must correct and resubmit a claim

POA guidelines are provided in Appendix I of the *ICD-10-CM Official Guidelines for Coding and Reporting*

POA defined as present at the time the order for inpatient admission occurs

---

*No longer exempt from reporting requirements, but report does not calculate into payment.

- Conditions that develop during an outpatient encounter are considered as Present On Admission
  - Example: Emergency room, observation, outpatient surgery

The reporting options are:

Y Yes (this diagnosis was present at the time of admission)

N No (this diagnosis was not present at the time of admission)

U Unknown (documentation is insufficient to determine if condition was present at time of inpatient admission)

- N and U indicators report as Not Present on Admission (NPOA) and do not cause an increased payment at the CC/MCC level

W Clinically undetermined (provider is unable to clinically determine whether the condition was present at the time of admission or not)

Unreported/Not used – (Exempt from POA reporting)

Hospitals report ICD-10-CM/CD-10-PCS codes for procedures and diagnoses, and CMS determines the MS-DRG and payment

Hospitals also calculate MS-DRGs to estimate accounts receivable, occupancy rates, and case mix

Hospital-Acquired Conditions (HAC)

Medicare will not reimburse a higher-payment MS-DRG if one of the following hospital-acquired or preventable conditions occurs after the patient's admission to the hospital:

*No longer exempt from reporting requirements, but report does not calculate into payment

- Foreign object retained after surgery
- Air embolism
- Blood incompatibility
- Pressure ulcer stages 3 and 4
- Falls and trauma
- Catheter-associated urinary tract infection
- Vascular catheter-associated infection
- Manifestations of poor glycemic control
- Surgical site infection following surgery
  - Coronary artery bypass graft (CABG)
  - Orthopedic procedures
  - Bariatric surgery
  - Cardiac electronic device implant
- Deep vein thrombosis and pulmonary embolism following certain orthopedic procedures
- Iatrogenic pneumothorax with venous catheterization

These diagnoses will not qualify as MCC/CC if not present at the time of admission, thus reducing facility reimbursement

- Proposal for HAC Reduction Program for 2016 that will adjust payment when HAC occurs

72-Hour Rule

Also known as the "3-day window"

Part of Medicare's Prospective Payment System (PPS)

- IRF (Inpatient Rehabilitation Facilities) and PPS providers not subject to 72-hour rule

States that reimbursement for any hospital outpatient diagnostic or other services provided for the same diagnosis occasioning the admission 3 days prior to admission is included in the MS-DRG payment for that hospital stay.

- Hospitals must demonstrate with supporting documentation that the services (outpatient) were unrelated to the diagnoses/reason for admission to report these services as an outpatient account.

Monitoring MS-DRG Reimbursement

Accounts Receivable (AR)

List of high-dollar cases

List of unbilled accounts/claims

Remittance Advice

Sent by MACs listing amounts paid to hospital

Always verify correct MS-DRG was paid based on MS-DRG initially submitted

Audit for underpayments of transfer MS-DRGs

Resource Utilization Groups (RUGs)

Reimbursement system used in long-term skilled health care settings

- Long-term care hospitals (LTCH) are defined as those with average stays greater than 25 days

Based on resources

Utilizes information from the minimum data set (MDS)

- Rehabilitation services
- Special care needs
- Clinical requirements
- Activity of daily living
- Cognitive function
- Behavioral symptoms and resident's distressed mood

Assessment of patient must be on days 5, 14, 30, 60, and 90

- Defined by federal law

Home Health Prospective Payment System (HHPPS)

Reimbursement system used in home care agencies

Based on information in Outcome and Assessment Information Set (OASIS)

Payment based on visit

Home Assessment Validation and Entry (HAVEN) is the CMS free-data entry software utilized by most Home Health Agencies (HHA)

Inpatient Rehabilitation Facility (IRF) Prospective Payment System

Paid on a per-discharge basis

Utilizes information from an Inpatient Rehabilitation Facility Patient Assessment Instrument (IRF PAI)

- Classifies patients into distinct groups based on clinical characteristics and expected resource needs

Inpatient Psychiatric Facility (IPF) Prospective Payment System

- Originally excluded from PPS
- Also excluded were rehabilitation, children's, cancer, and long-term care hospitals, rehabilitation and hospitals located outside the 50 states and Puerto Rico
- Referred to as TEFRA (Tax Equity and Fiscal Responsibility Act) facilities. Paid on a per diem amount
- Adjusted based on:
  1. Diagnosis-Related Group classification
  2. Patient age
  3. Length of stay
  4. Any comorbidities

Revenue Codes

Four digit classification system that
- Identifies services/procedures
- Identifies location where services were rendered
- Begins with 0 (zero)

Three Main Categories

1. Billing revenue codes

   Example:
   - 0137, replacement of a prior claim for a hospital outpatient charge
2. Accommodation revenue codes

   Example:
   - 0120, semiprivate room and board for obstetrical patient
3. Ancillary revenue codes

   Example:
   - 0314, laboratory pathological services for a biopsy

The Digits and Their Placement Further Define Elements of the Revenue Code

Example:

Revenue code for laboratory pathological service is 031X

The fourth digit (X) is assigned from one of five subcategory digits
- Subcategory identifies type of service/procedure within category

Example:
- Fourth digit (4) identifies biopsy services (0314)

Medicare Determines Included and Excluded Services Based on Revenue Codes

Under the OPPS, Medicare requires use of HCPCS codes by hospital outpatient departments when a code for that service is available

Example:

- *Services that require HCPCS codes:*

Revenue Code	Description	HCPCS Codes
0274	Prosthetic and orthotic devices	L9900, Orthotic
0331	Injected chemotherapy	96401, Chemotherapy administration
0481	Cardiac catheterization laboratory	93460, Combined heart cath
0623	Surgical dressing	G0168, Wound closure
0636	Pharmacy	J1645, Dalteparin sodium
0901	Electroshock treatment	90870, Electroconvulsive therapy

■ Data Quality

Charge Description Master

Database used by hospitals

Includes all services, procedures, supplies, and drugs with a

- Corresponding internal numbered description of everything utilized by the patient
- Revenue code
- CPT/HCPCS codes
- Charge (Figure 14-12)

Elements of a Charge Description Master

- Unique department code number
- Description number (charge code) that is internally assigned to identify each procedure, supply, drug, and service
- The charge code is a unique alpha or alphanumeric code that remains constant year after year
- Procedure/service description
- CPT/HCPCS codes—HCPCS code may change based on code changes and changes in payer requirements
- Revenue code—may change based on payer requirements
- Cost/Charge—generally evaluated and changed annually
- Hard-coded modifiers when applicable
- Charge master automatically enters appropriate modifier

Should be Reviewed Regularly and Updated as Needed to Assist in

- Reduction of claim denials
- Accurate reimbursement
- Compliance

HCPCS	Description	Active Date	Revenue Code	Charge
Q2017	Teniposide, 50mg	01/01/2014	0636	$825.50
96413	Chemotherapy admin Infusion, up to one hour	01/01/2007	0261	$285.11
P9016	Red blood cells, leukocytes reduced, each unit	01/01/1994	0380	$189.45
96360	Infusion therapy, not chemotherapy drugs, 1 hr	01/01/2009	0450	$108.24
J0207	Amifostine, 500mg	01/01/1994	7000	$475.05

Figure **14-12** Example of basic charge description master.

- Better data management and quality
- Tracking of services and supplies

Review for

Invalid/inaccurate codes

- Unclear/incorrect descriptions
- Omitted procedures or supplies
- Correct service/supply and revenue code linkage
- Appropriate fees

Beneficiary signatures on file

- Service, charges submitted without need for patient signature

Things that may be perceived as fraudulent

Fraud

Intentional deception to benefit

> *Example:* Submitting for services not provided

Anyone who submits for Medicare services can be violator, such as

- Physicians
- Hospitals
- Laboratories
- Billing services
- YOU

Fraud Can be

Billing for services not provided

Misrepresenting diagnosis, CPT, or HCPCS code(s)

Kickbacks

Unbundling services

Falsifying medical necessity

Systematic waiver of co-payment

Fraud Examples

Patient presents with chest pain and is treated.
   Progress note indicates myocardial infarction (MI) is to be ruled out.
   Laboratory tests do not suggest or indicate MI.
   Coder assigns MI as PDx as the reason for encounter/admission.
Chest pain pays less than MI.
This is fraud!

Other Examples of Fraud

Upcoding is using a higher-level code for a lower-level service

Misrepresenting the diagnosis for a patient to justify the service or equipment furnished

Unbundling or exploding charge

> *Example:* Reporting multichannel lab tests (many tests in one process) to appear as if the individual tests were performed

Billing noncovered services

Example: Routine foot care reported as more involved form of foot care that is paid under the Medicare program

Applying for duplicate payment

Example: Patient has Medicare and another insurance and both are billed without indicating that there is another third-party payer

Office of the Inspector General (OIG)

Develops and publishes Work Plan annually

Outlines Medicare monitoring program

MACs monitor those areas identified in plan

Complaints of Fraud or Abuse

Submitted orally or in writing to MACs or OIG

Allegations made by anyone against anyone

Allegations followed up by MACs and/or OIG

www.oig.hhs.gov/reports-and-publications/workplan/index.asp

Abuse

Generally involves

- Impropriety
- Lack of medical necessity for services reported

Review takes place after claim is submitted

- MACs go back and do historical review of claims

Kickbacks

Bribe or rebate for referring patient for any service covered by Medicare

Any personal gain kickback

A felony

- $25,000 fine or
- 5 years in jail or
- Both

Protect Yourself

Use your common sense

Submit only truthful and accurate claims

If you are unsure about charges, services, or procedures check with physician or supervisor

Managed Health Care

Network health care providers and facilities that offer health care services under one organization

Group hospitals, physicians, or other providers

Majority of people with health care coverage are covered by a managed care organization (e.g., HMO, PPO, POS)

Managed Care Organizations

Responsible for health care services to an enrolled group or person

Coordinate various health care services

Negotiate with facilities and providers

Capitation method common in managed care

- Prepaid, fixed amount for each person in the plan
  - Regardless of resource use

Preferred Provider Organization (PPO)

Providers and facilities form network to offer health care services as group

Enrollees who seek health care outside PPO pay more

Point of Service (POS)

In-network or out-of-network providers may be used

Benefits are paid at a higher rate to in-network providers

Subscribers are not limited to providers, but to amount covered by plan

Health Maintenance Organization (HMO)

Total package health care

Out-of-pocket expenses minimal

Assigned physician acts as gatekeeper to refer patient outside organization

ABBREVIATIONS

AMLOS	Arithmetic Mean Length of Stay
APCs	Ambulatory Patient Classifications
APGs	Ambulatory Patient Groups
AWP	Average Wholesale Price
CC	Complications and Co-morbidities
CCI	Correct Coding Initiative (AKA, NCCI)
CLIA	Clinical Laboratories Improvement Act
DCN	Document Control Number
DME	Durable Medical Equipment
DRG	Diagnosis-Related Groups
EDI	Electronic Data Interchange
EIN	Employer Identification Number
EOB	Explanation of Benefits
ESRD	End Stage Renal Disease
FL	Field Locators
FUD	Follow-up Days

GMLOS	Geometric Mean Length of Stay
GPN	Group Provider Number
HAC	Hospital-Acquired Condition
HAVEN	Home Assessment Validation and Entry
HCPCS	Healthcare Common Procedural Coding System
HHA	Home Health Agencies
HHPPS	Home Health Prospective Payment System
HICN	Health Insurance Claim/Identification Number
HIPAA	Health Insurance Portability and Accountability Act
HMO	Health Maintenance Organization
HOPPS	Hospital Outpatient Prospective Payment System
HPMP	Hospital Payment Monitoring Program
ICN	Internal Control Number
IPF	Inpatient Psychiatric Facility
IRF	Inpatient Rehabilitation Facility
IRF PAI	Inpatient Rehabilitation Facility Patient Assessment Instrument
LCD	Local Coverage Determination
LMRP	Local Medical Review Policies, replaced by LCD, Local Coverage Determination
MCC	Major Complication/Comorbidity
MDCs	Major Diagnostic Categories
NCCI	National Correct Coding Initiative
NCD	National Coverage Decisions
NCHS	National Centers for Health Statistics
NPI	National Provider Identifier
OASIS	Outcome and Assessment Information Set
OBRA	Omnibus Budget Reconciliation Act of 1986
OCE	Outpatient Code Editor
OIG	Office of the Inspector General
OR	Operating Room
PDx	Principal Diagnosis

PIN	Provider Identification Number
POA	Present on Admission
PPO	Preferred Provider Organization
PPS	Prospective Payment System
PRO	Peer Review Organization, now QIO
QIO	Quality Improvement Organization
RBRVS	Resource-Based Relative Value Scale
RUGs	Resource Utilization Groups
SI	Status Indicators
UCR	Usual, Customary, and Reasonable
UHDDS	Uniform Hospital Discharge Data Set
WHO	World Health Organization

REIMBURSEMENT TERMINOLOGY

Advance Beneficiary Notice	ABN, notification in advance of services that Medicare may not pay for them, including the estimated cost to the patient
Ancillary Service	A service that is supportive of care of a patient, such as laboratory services
APC	A classification system used to group like services based upon clinical similarities and resources utilized
Assignment	A legal agreement that allows the provider to receive direct payment from a payer and the provider to accept payment as payment in full for covered services
Attending Physician	The physician legally responsible for oversight of an inpatient's care
Beneficiary	The person who benefits from insurance coverage; also known as subscriber, dependent, enrollee, member, or participant
Birthday Rule	When both parents have insurance coverage, the parent with the birthday earliest in the year is the primary coverage for a dependent
Certified Registered Nurse Anesthetist	CRNA, an individual with specialized training and certification in nursing and anesthesia
Charge Description Master	Record of services, procedures, supplies, and drugs with corresponding codes, descriptions, and charges billed
Co-insurance	Cost-sharing of covered services
Compliance Plan	Written strategy developed by medical facilities to ensure appropriate, consistent documentation within the medical record and ensure compliance with third-party payer guidelines
Concurrent Care	More than one physician providing care to a patient at the same time

Coordination of Benefits	COB, management of multiple third-party payments to ensure overpayment does not occur
Co-payment	Cost-sharing between beneficiary and payer
Correct Coding Initiative	CCI, developed by CMS to control improper unbundling of CPT codes leading to inappropriate payment; also known as NCCI (National Correct Coding Initiative)
Deductible	That portion of covered services paid by the beneficiary before third-party payment begins
Denial	Statement from the payer that reimbursement is denied
Documentation	Detailed chronology of facts and observations regarding a patient's health
Diagnosis-Related Groups	DRGs, a case mix classification system established by CMS consisting of classes of patients who are similar clinically and in consumption of hospital resources; replaced with MS-DRGs
Durable Medical Equipment	DME, medically related equipment that is not disposable, such as wheelchairs, crutches, and vaporizers
Electronic Data Interchange	EDI, computerized submission of health care insurance information exchange
Employer Identification Number	EIN, an Internal Revenue Service (IRS)–issued identification number used on tax documents
Encounter Form	Medical document that contains information regarding a patient visit for health care services
Explanation of Benefits	EOB, written, detailed listing of medical service payments by third-party payer to inform beneficiary and provider of payment
Fee Schedule	Established list of payments for medical services, i.e., lab, physician services
Follow-up Days	FUD, established by third-party payers and listing the number of days after a procedure for which a provider must provide normal uncomplicated related services to a patient for no fee (also known as global days, global package, or global period)
Group Provider Number	GPN, numeric designation for a group of providers that is used instead of the individual provider number
Hospital Payment Monitoring System	HPMS, an inpatient PPS audit system used by CMS to reduce improper payments
Invalid Claim	Claim that is missing necessary information and cannot be processed or paid
Inpatient	CMS defines an inpatient as a person who has been formally admitted to a hospital with the expectation that he or she will remain at least overnight and occupy a bed even if it later develops that the patient can be discharged or transferred to another hospital and not actually use a hospital bed overnight
Medical Record	Documentation about the health care of a patient
Medicare Administrative Contractors	MACs replaced Fiscal Intermediaries (FIs)

Medicare Severity Diagnosis-Related Groups	MS-DRG, classification system implemented October 2007 that is based on the principal diagnosis and the medical or surgical service provided to the Medicare inpatient in which the hospital/facility is paid a fixed amount for each patient discharged in a treatment category
National Correct Coding Initiative	Developed by CMS to control improper unbundling of CPT codes leading to inappropriate payment; also known as CCI (Correct Coding Initiative)
Noncovered Services	Any service not included by a third-party payer in the list of services for which payment is made
National Provider Identifier	NPI, 10-digit number assigned to provider and used for identification purposes when submitting services to third-party payers
Hospital Outpatient	An individual who is not an inpatient of a hospital but who is registered as an outpatient at the hospital
Prior Authorization	Also known as preauthorization, which is a requirement by the payer to receive written permission prior to patient services if the service is to be considered for payment by the payer
Provider Identification Number	PIN, or UPIN, assigned by the third-party payer to providers to be used for identification purposes when submitting services to third-party payers
Rejection	A claim that does not pass edits and is returned to the provider as rejected
Reimbursement	Payment from a third-party payer for services rendered to a patient covered by the payer's health care plan
State License Number	Identification number issued by a state to a physician who has been granted the right to practice in that state
Usual, Customary, and Reasonable	UCR, used by third-party payers to establish a payment rate for a service in an area with the usual (standard fee in area), customary (standard fee by the physician), and reasonable (as determined by payer) rate

CHAPTER 14: REIMBURSEMENT QUIZ

(Quiz Answers are located in Appendix B)

1. Any person who is identified as receiving life insurance or medical benefits:
   a. primary
   b. beneficiary
   c. participant
   d. recipient

2. TEFRA of 1982 established the _____, which pays a fixed amount intended to cover the cost of treating a typical patient for a particular DRG.
   a. OPPS
   b. NPI
   c. DRG
   d. PPS

3. The set of patient attributes that is used to define each MS-DRG consists of:
   a. principal diagnosis, secondary diagnosis, insurance policy rules, principal procedure, and patient age
   b. principal procedure, discharge status, patient age and sex, and principal diagnosis
   c. principal and secondary diagnosis, principal procedure, patient age and sex, and discharge status
   d. principal diagnosis, secondary diagnosis, medical or surgical service (principal or significant), and any qualifying complication(s)/comorbidity(ies), discharge status

4. A four-digit classification system that identifies and explains services or procedures and the location in which they were rendered is called a(n):
   a. ancillary code
   b. revenue code
   c. billing code
   d. accommodation code

5. CMS delegates the daily operation of the Medicare program to:
   a. DHHS
   b. QIO
   c. RVU
   d. MACs

6. The Omnibus Budget Reconciliation Act of 1986 required a PPS-based payment system to replace the one based on existing outpatient hospital cost. This system is what classification system?
   a. MS-DRGs
   b. APCs
   c. CPT
   d. ICD-10-CM

7. This part of Medicare covers the inpatient hospital portion:
   a. Part A
   b. Part B
   c. Part C
   d. Part D

8. This issue of the *Federal Register* contains major outpatient facility changes for CMS programs for the coming year:
   a. October/November
   b. November/December
   c. December/October
   d. November/August

9. This is the number of MS-DRGs:
   a. 001-502
   b. 001-999
   c. 001-998
   d. 001-604

10. Entity responsible for development of the plan that outlines monitoring of the Medicare program:
    a. MACs
    b. OIG
    c. DHSS
    d. HEW

CPT and HCPCS Coding

Some of the CPT code descriptions for physician services include physician extender services. Physician extenders, such as nurse practitioners, physician assistants, and nurse anesthetists, etc., provide medical services typically performed by a physician. Within this educational material the term "physician" may include "and other qualified health care professionals" depending on the code. Refer to the official CPT® code descriptions and guidelines to determine codes that are appropriate to report services provided by non-physician practitioners.

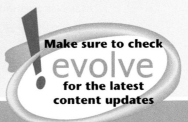

Make sure to check
evolve
for the latest
content updates

■ Introduction to Medical Coding

Translates services/procedures/supplies/drugs into CPT/HCPCS/ICD-10-PCS procedural codes

Translates diagnosis(es) into ICD-10-CM codes

Two Levels of Service Codes

1. Level I CPT
2. Level II HCPCS, National Codes

Diagnosis Codes, ICD-10-CM

ICD-10-CM, *International Classification of Diseases,* 10th Edition, Clinical Modification

- Classification system
- The diagnosis explains why service was provided
- Specific in nature and may be up to seven characters
- Example: Diabetes becomes E11.9

CHAPTER 15: INTRODUCTION TO CPT

Developed by the AMA in 1966

Five-digit codes to report services provided to patients

Updated each November for use January 1

Resequencing was a 2010 new initiative for CPT

- Historically in numerical order
- Not the case for more than 100 codes
- Pound symbol (#) appears before the resequenced codes

    Example: In the 51725-51798 range, code 51797 follows 51729 (in numeric order). Code 51797 also appears in correct numeric order in the CPT, but next to the code a note states, "Code is out of numerical sequence. See 51725-51798."

See Appendix N of the CPT for a complete list of the resequenced codes.

Incorrect Coding

Results in providers being paid inappropriately (either overpayment or underpayment)

Inpatient Services

Reported on standardized insurance form

- CMS-1450/Universal Billing Form 04 (UB-04) (see Figure 19-1 on page 386 of this text), or electronically with 837I

Outpatient Services

Reported on CMS-1500 paper form or electronically via 837P

- Payer determines claim form

■ CPT/HCPCS Level I Modifiers

Indicates anatomical site of procedure or service

Alters CPT or HCPCS code

- Does not alter original intent of CPT code

Full list, CPT, Appendix A

- Two separate lists
   1. One for physicians to use
   2. One for hospital outpatient facilities to use

Modifier Functions

Altered services (i.e., more or less)

Altered circumstances (return/discontinued)

Bilateral

Multiple

Only portions of service (i.e., professional service only)

More than one surgeon

ASC Modifiers

-25 Significant, Separately Identifiable E/M Service, by Same Physician or Other Qualified Health Care Professional on the Same Day of the Procedure or Other Service

Documentation must support service

> *Example:* Patient seen for sinus congestion; hospital-based physician performs H&P, prescribes decongestant, notes lesion on back, and removes it

Code: E/M-25 + Procedure

-27 Multiple Outpatient Hospital E/M Encounters on the Same Date

Separate and distinct E/M encounters

Performed in multiple outpatient hospital settings

Used only with E/M services

-50 Bilateral Procedure

Organs that are bilateral

> *Example:* Procedure on hands

Caution: Some codes describe bilateral procedures

Typically not used on integumentary codes when reporting services

NOTE: Modifier -51 is not used when reporting facility services

-52 Reduced Services

Services reduced from those in code description

There is no other code that accurately reflects the service actually provided

Physician directed reduction

Documentation substantiates reduction

Procedure discontinued after IV sedation administered

Not for patient unable to pay

-58 Staged or Related Procedure or Service by the Same Physician or Other Qualified Health Care Professional During the Postoperative Period

Subsequent procedure planned at time of initial surgery

- During postoperative period of previous surgery in series

  Example: Multiple skin grafts completed in several sessions

- Do not use when code describes a session

  Example: 67208 lesion destruction of retina, one or more sessions

- Therapeutic procedure performed during the global period of a diagnostic procedure

  Example: Surgical biopsy of breast followed by subsequent mastectomy

-59 Distinct Procedural Service

Used to report non-E/M services not normally reported together

- Different session or encounter
- Different procedure
- Different site

Separate incision, excision, lesion, injury

  Example: Physician removes several lesions from patient's leg, also notes a suspicious lesion on torso and biopsies the torso lesion

- Excision code for lesion removal + biopsy code for torso lesion with -59
- Indicates biopsy as distinct procedure, not part of lesion removal

In January of 2015 CMS introduced four HCPCS subset modifiers:

- referred to as –X {EPSU} modifiers
- more descriptively define modifier -59
- payer specific

For more details see page 266.

-73 Discontinued Outpatient Hospital/Ambulatory Surgery Center (ASC) Procedure Prior to the Administration of Anesthesia

Procedure stopped due to patient's condition

After surgical preparation and sedation

Prior to administration of anesthesia

-74 Discontinued Outpatient Hospital/Ambulatory Surgery Center (ASC) Procedure after Administration of Anesthesia

Procedure stopped due to patient's condition

After administration of anesthesia

May be after procedure begins

  Example: Intubation started or incision was made

-76 Repeat Procedure or Service by Same Physician or Other Qualified Health Care Professional

Assigned to indicate medically necessary service

  Example: X-rays before and after fracture repair

-77 Repeat Procedure by Another Physician or Other Qualified Health Care Professional

Performed by one individual, repeated by another individual

Submitted with written report to establish medical necessity

- Do not append to E/M codes

-78 Unplanned Return to the Operating/Procedure Room by the Same Physician or Other Qualified Health Care Professional Following Initial Procedure for a Related Procedure During the Postoperative Period

For complication of first procedure

> *Example:* Patient has outpatient procedure in morning, returned to operating room in afternoon with severe hemorrhage

Indicates charge is not typographical, technical, or medical error

- Medical record must specifically document need for service provided

-79 Unrelated Procedure or Service by the Same Physician or Other Qualified Health Care Professional During the Postoperative Period

Example: Several days after discharge for procedure, patient returns for unrelated problem

- Diagnosis code would also be different

-91 Repeat Clinical Diagnostic Laboratory Test

Repeat same laboratory tests on same day for multiple test results

- e.g., serial troponin levels for acute MI confirmation

No tests rerun to confirm original test results

No malfunction of equipment or technician error

■ HCPCS Level II Modifiers

Examples of Anatomical Modifiers

-LT	Left side
-RT	Right side
-E1	Upper left, eyelid
-E2	Lower left, eyelid
-E3	Upper right, eyelid
-E4	Lower right, eyelid
-FA	Left hand, thumb
-F1	Left hand, second digit
-F2	Left hand, third digit
-F3	Left hand, fourth digit
-F4	Left hand, fifth digit
-F5	Right hand, thumb
-F6	Right hand, second digit
-F7	Right hand, third digit
-F8	Right hand, fourth digit
-F9	Right hand, fifth digit

-TA   Left foot, great toe

-T1   Left foot, second digit

-T2   Left foot, third digit

-T3   Left foot, fourth digit

-T4   Left foot, fifth digit

-T5   Right foot, great toe

-T6   Right foot, second digit

-T7   Right foot, third digit

-T8   Right foot, fourth digit

-T9   Right foot, fifth digit

-LC   Left circumflex coronary artery

-LD   Left anterior descending coronary artery

-RC   Right coronary artery

Anatomical modifiers are not used with skin procedures

> **Example:** Removal of skin tags, any area

Exception is with codes for procedures on sites including sweat glands, eyelids, and breasts

HCPCS Modifiers for Selective Identification of Subsets of Distinct Procedural Services (-59 modifier)

-XE Separate Encounter

A service that is distinct because it occurred during a separate encounter

-XS Separate Structure

A service that is distinct because it was performed on a separate organ/structure

-XP Separate Practitioner:

A service that is distinct because it was performed by a different practitioner

-XU Unusual Non-Overlapping Service

The use of a service that is distinct because it does not overlap usual components of the main service

Example: -XE

- Patient seen in the morning for a cardiovascular stress test and then later in the day patient returns for a rhythm ECG

- Patient is seen in the outpatient infusion center at 8:00 a.m. and seen again in the outpatient infusion center for another treatment at 6:00 p.m.

Example: -XS

- Patient seen for destruction and during procedure unrelated to the destruction the physician obtains tissue for pathologic examination

- Patient undergoes a laparoscopy, surgical, ablation of one or more liver tumor(s) and during the surgery, patient has ultrasonic guidance for needle placement

Example: -XP

- Patient undergoes a hernia repair at 7:00 a.m. Later in the day the patient develops acute abdominal pain and returns for another physician to perform a surgical laparoscopic appendectomy

Example: -XU

- Patient seen for two separate lesions; a lipoma is excised on upper thigh region (3 cm), and a separate lipoma excised lipoma excised on the lower leg region (less than 3 cm)

The Index

Used to locate service/procedure terms and codes

Speeds up code location

Serves as a dictionary

- First entries and last entries on top of page
- Code display in index
  - Single code: 38115
  - Multiple codes: 26645, 26650
  - Range of codes: 22305-22325

Location Methods

Service/procedure: Repair, excision

Anatomical site: Meniscus, knee

Condition or disease: Cleft lip, clot

Synonym: Toe and interphalangeal joint

Eponym: Jones Procedure, Heller Operation

Abbreviation: ECG, PEEP (positive end-expiratory pressure)

"See" in index

Cross-reference terms: "Look here for code"

Index: Stem, Brain: *See* Brainstem

Appendices of CPT

Appendix A: Modifiers

Appendix B: Summary of Additions, Deletions, Revisions

Appendix C: Clinical Examples (E/M Codes)

Appendix D: Summary of CPT Add-on Codes

Appendix E: Summary of CPT Codes Exempt from Modifier -51

Appendix F: Summary of CPT Codes Exempt from Modifier -63

Appendix G: Summary of CPT Codes That Include Moderate (Conscious) Sedation

Appendix H: Alphabetical Clinical Topics Listing (moved to AMA website)

Appendix I: Genetic Testing Code Modifiers (Deleted)

Appendix J: Electrodiagnostic Medicine Listing of Sensory, Motor, and Mixed Nerves

Appendix K: Products Pending FDA Approval

Appendix L: Vascular Families

Appendix M: Deleted CPT Codes

Appendix N: Summary of Resequenced CPT codes

Appendix O: Multianalyte Assays with Algorithmic Analyses

Be certain to review information in CPT appendices before the examination

CHAPTER 16: EVALUATION AND MANAGEMENT (E/M) SECTION (99201-99499)

■ Outpatient

One who has not been admitted to a health care facility

Example: Patient receives services at clinic, ED, or same-day surgery center

■ Inpatient

One who has been formally admitted to a health care facility

Example: Patient admitted to hospital or nursing home

Physician dictates

- Admission orders
- H&P (history and physical)
- Requests for consultations

Type A Emergency Department (ED) Services (99281-99285)

No distinction between new and established patients

To qualify as a Type A ED (ER), facility must be open 24 hours a day, 7 days a week

Five ED codes do not report all ED services

- The codes report only physician evaluation and management services during an encounter, not all interventions may be provided during encounter (Figure 16-1)
- Services provided in addition to the interventions are reported separately

Professional and ancillary services that impact facility resources

All documentation utilized to determine service

- Physician documentation
- Nursing notes
- Ancillary notes

No standard guideline for reporting facility services

Per OPPS final rule each facility sets own guidelines

Guidelines must meet certain criteria

- Services are medically necessary
- Methodology is accurate
- Coding is reproducible
- Coding correlates with intensity of services provided

Example:

1. One ED may develop method in which two elements in Level 3 are provided and one element in Level 4 is provided, Level 4 (99284) is reported
2. Second ED may develop method in which two elements in Level 3 are provided and one element in Level 4 is provided, Level 3 (99283) is reported

For the purposes of the worktext, the level is assigned based on the highest level of service provided, as in Example 1

Critical Care (99291, 99292, 99466-99476, 99485, 99486) and ED Codes

ED services often require additional codes from Critical Care Services

Example: Multiple organ failure

Level 1—99281	Level 2—99282	Level 3—99283
1. Initial (triage) assessment 2. Suture removal 3. Wound recheck 4. Note for work or school 5. Simple discharge information	Interventions from previous level plus any of the following: 1. OTC med administration 2. Tetanus booster 3. Bedside diagnostic tests (stool hemoccult, glucometer) 4. Visual acuity 5. Orthostatic vital signs 6. Simple trauma not requiring x-ray 7. Simple discharge information	Interventions from previous level plus any of the following: 1. Heparin/saline lock 2. Crystalloid IV therapy 3. X-ray, one area 4. RX med administration 5. Fluorescein stain 6. Quick cath 7. Foley cath 8. Receipt of ambulance patient 9. Mental health emergencies (mild) not requiring parenteral medications or admission 10. Moderate complexity discharge instructions 11. Intermediate layered and complex laceration repair

Level 4—99284	Level 5—99285	Critical Care 99291, 99292
Interventions from previous level plus any of the following: 1. X-ray, multiple areas 2. Special imaging studies (CT, MRI, ultrasound) 3. Cardiac monitoring 4. Multiple reassessments of patient 5. Parenteral[1] medications (including insulin) 6. Nebulizer treatment (1 or 2) 7. NG placement 8. Pelvic exam 9. Mental health emergencies (moderate). May require parenteral medications but not admission 10. Administration of IV medications [1]*not through the alimentary canal but rather by injection through some other route, such as subcutaneous, intramuscular, intraorbital, intracapsular, intraspinal, intrasternal, or intravenous*	Interventions from previous level plus any of the following: 1. Monitor/stabilize patient during in hospital transport and/or testing (CT, MRI, ultrasound) 2. Vasoactive medication 3. Administration (dopamine, dobutamine, multiple) nebulizer treatments (3 or more) 4. Conscious sedation 5. Lumbar puncture 6. Thoracentesis 7. Sexual assault exam 8. Admission to hospital 9. Mental health emergency (severe) psychotic and/or agitated/combative 10. Requires admission 11. Fracture/dislocation reduction 12. Suicide precautions 13. Gastric lavage 14. Complex discharge instructions	Interventions from any previous level plus any of the following: 1. Multiple parenteral medications 2. Continuous monitoring 3. Major trauma care 4. Chest tube insertion 5. CPR 6. Defibrillation/cardioversion 7. Delivery of baby 8. Control of major hemorrhage 9. Administration of blood or blood products

Figure **16-1** Example of ED acuity sheet.

Critical Care Services are provided to patients in life-threatening (critically ill or injured) situations

- Both Critical Care codes (99291 & 99292) are included in Critical Care and reimbursed at $656.94 (not a time-based payment)

Trauma Team Activation (G0390) and ED Critical Care Codes

Certified trauma centers

Must provide ED and CC services

APC = 0618 (Trauma Response with Critical Care)

■ APC (Ambulatory Patient Classification) Levels of Service

Facilities report ED services for non-OPPS patients using CPT codes

- There are 10 ED codes only under OPPS; these codes are represented by 11 APCs
- 99281-99285 are each represented by a corresponding APC
- Facility determines what services are provided under each APC

Type A, Emergency Department Visits

99281 = APC 0609

99282 = APC 0613

99283 = APC 0614

99284 = APC 0615 or APC 8003 (when certain SI "Q3" criteria apply)

99285 = APC 0616 or APC 8003 (when certain SI "Q3" criteria apply)

Type B Emergency Room Visits

24-hour rule doesn't apply

Facility is licensed by the state as an Emergency Department

One third of all outpatient visits for treatment of emergent medical conditions on an urgent basis

G0380 = APC 0626 (SI "V")

G0381 = APC 0627 (SI "V")

G0382 = APC 0628 (SI "V")

G0383 = APC 0629 (SI "V")

G0384 = APC 0630 (SI "Q3")

Each APC is reimbursed at different rates by CMS

- For example

APC 0609 = $60.49	APC 0626 = $62.72
APC 0613 = $112.79	APC 0627 = $69.51
APC 0614 = $198.39	APC 0628 = $112.97
APC 0615 = $333.80	APC 0629 = $198.98
APC 0616 = $492.69	APC 0630 = $304.38

Each APC includes a baseline level of service

- Baseline services are
  - Registration
  - Initial Nursing Assessment
  - Periodic Vital Signs
  - Discharge Instructions
  - Exam Room setup/cleanup
  - Limited intervention using minimal resources (10 minutes or less staff contact)

  Examples:
  - Administration of oral medications
  - Initiation of oxygen therapy
  - Obtaining lab specimens

Levels of service ascend based upon

- Increase in staff time
- Additional interventions

  Examples:
  - Extended initial nursing assessment or discharge
  - Starting an IV
  - Insertions of tubes (catheters, Foley, or nasogastric)

Each hospital creates its own set of internal guidelines to determine what services are included in each Critical Care and ED CPT code

- CMS directs only that the system is reasonable and relates to resource intensity

Critical care codes collapse into 2 APCs

- APC 0617 Critical Care or APC 0168 (when certain SI "S" criteria apply)

Uses of Anesthesia

Relieve pain

Manage unconscious patients, life functions, and resuscitation

Analgesia

Relief of pain

Some Methods of Anesthesia

Endotracheal: Through mouth

Local: Application to area (injection or topical)

Epidural: Between vertebral spaces—injection into epidural space

Regional: Field or nerve

MAC: Monitored anesthesia care (service provided by an anesthesiologist or CRNA)

Patient is monitored, and if necessary, sedation (including general anesthesia) may be provided

Patient-Controlled Analgesia (PCA)

Patient administers drug

Used to relieve chronic pain or temporarily for severe pain following surgery

Moderate (Conscious) Sedation

Codes in Medicine Section of CPT

To be used when the surgeon or another physician administers the sedation

- No anesthesia personnel are present

Decreased level of consciousness

Report with 99143-99145 (Medicine)

Presence of trained observer, such as a nurse, is required

Second physician administered sedation, report 99148-99150

PRACTICE EXERCISES

Using Figure 16-1, ED acuity sheet, complete the following Practice Exercises.

Practice Exercise 16-1: Neck Pain

Assign an external cause code to indicate how the accident occurred.

LOCATION: Emergency Department

PATIENT: Betsey Anderson

PATIENT COMPLAINT: Neck pain.

PHYSICIAN: Paul Sutton, MD

HISTORY OF PRESENT ILLNESS: This is a 23-year-old woman who was involved in a motor vehicle accident today. She was a restrained front seat passenger in a car that had air bags that did deploy. She had a little bit of sharp neck pain after this accident. It has progressed a little bit more. It is actually in her upper shoulders. There is no numbness or tingling. She did not strike her head against anything and she has been doing well, but here at the emergency department she is placed in a C-collar and she is being evaluated in the presence of her mother.

PAST MEDICAL HISTORY: Her past medical history is negative.

PAST SURGICAL HISTORY: Her past surgical history is negative.

CURRENT MEDICATIONS: She is on no medications.

SOCIAL HISTORY: She does not smoke.

REVIEW OF SYSTEMS: Review of systems is as stated.

PHYSICAL EXAM: Temperature is 37.0, pulse rate is 109, respirations 61, blood pressure is 149/92. O_2 saturations are 99%. General appearance: Awake, alert, 23-year-old. HEENT: Head is normocephalic. C-collar is removed. I examined her posterior C-spine. There is no midline C-spine step-offs or crepitus or bony deformity. She is able to move her head through pain-free range of motion. She has some tightness in her upper shoulders. Only paraspinal tenderness is present. Neural exam: She is awake and alert. No dullness or tingling. She has excellent grip strength in her upper extremities.

EMERGENCY DEPARTMENT COURSE: The patient certainly will not need to have x-rays performed. She simply has a neck strain. I feel we can manage her as an outpatient with pain medications. She is provided Lorcet, Motrin, and also Norflex for pain control. She is agreeable with this plan.

ASSESSMENT: Acute neck strain, secondary to motor vehicle accident.

PLAN: The patient will be discharged. She is agreeable with the plan for follow-up. She understands my treatment regimen and again she understands that I do not believe she is a good candidate for an x-ray. I do not feel this will help her symptoms. She is aware that she may worsen tomorrow and she has appropriate instructions on how to deal with this.

CPT Code(s): _____

ICD-10-CM Code(s): _____

Abstracting Questions

1. Since this trauma case did not require x-rays, what level of service would it be according to the chart of levels at the front of this chapter? _____

2. What was the final diagnosis for the patient? _____

3. Does the patient's location in the vehicle affect diagnosis code assignment when reporting the accident? _____

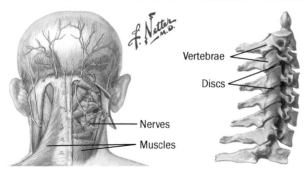

Vertebrae

Discs

Nerves

Muscles

Spinal cord

The neck is made up of vertebrae, spinal cord with nerves, discs between vertebrae, and tissues such as muscles and tendons. Neck strains are injuries in which muscles and tendons tear. Anyone can have one.

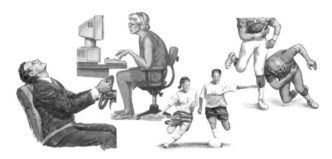

Contact in sports (such as in football and heading in soccer) can lead to neck strains. Other causes include falls, auto accidents (whiplash), poor posture, trauma, and overuse of neck muscles.

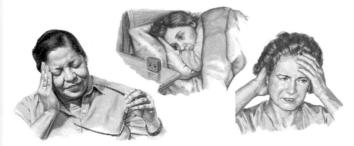

Cramping, dull, aching pain can occur in the back or sides of the neck. Neck strain can cause headaches, stiffness, spasms, and problems looking from side to side, driving, reading, and sleeping.

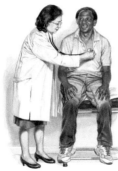

Your doctor makes a diagnosis from your medical history, physical examination, and other tests (x-rays, MRI, myelography, radionuclide scanning, and maybe EMG).

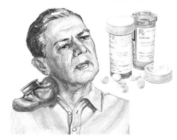

Treatment depends on the cause. For an injury, the doctor may suggest using ice on the area for 2 to 3 days and then heat. NSAIDs and maybe stronger medicines may help the pain. A muscle relaxant may help muscle spasms.

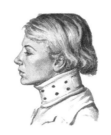
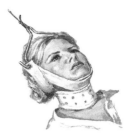

Short-term rest, gentle stretching, and short-term immobilization (with a soft collar) are also used. Physical therapy may reduce pain with deep heat treatments, traction, and exercise.

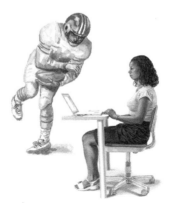

Wear the right sports equipment, such as a good, protective helmet. Practice the right techniques (such as in tackling and blocking). Use good sitting and standing postures. Do your neck exercises every day.

Call your doctor if you continue to have neck pain or headaches, you have numbness or tingling in your arms, or you need a referral to a physical therapist.

Practice Exercise 16-2: Back and Abdominal Pain

LOCATION: Emergency Department

PATIENT: Jodie Dvorak

PHYSICIAN: Paul Sutton, MD

SUBJECTIVE: This is a 32-year-old female in today for assessment of right low back pain and right-sided abdominal pain. The right flank pain started last night. It is hard to get comfortable. No prior similar symptoms. Standing up is actually a little better. No slips or falls. No trauma. No numbness or tingling. No nausea, vomiting, or diarrhea. Last normal menstrual period was several months ago. No abdominal pain was noted until my examination. No other significant symptomatology. She has no dysuria, hematuria, urgency, or frequency. No diarrhea, constipation, hematochezia. No upper GI symptoms. No respiratory tract symptoms.

PAST MEDICAL HISTORY: Reveals hyperprolactinemia. No other medical or surgical problems. No medications. No known drug allergies.

SOCIAL HISTORY: No tobacco utilization.

REVIEW OF SYSTEMS: Complete review of systems was undertaken and was negative.

OBJECTIVE: On examination today, temperature is 36, pulse 57, respirations 14; blood pressure 110/65, O_2 saturations 99% on room air. She is in no acute distress. Head and neck exam reveals normal TMs, canals, and ears. Nasal mucous membranes are slightly boggy. Oropharynx is unremarkable. Neck is supple. No cervical adenopathy. Chest is clear to auscultation and percussion with good air entry throughout. No rubs. No crackles. No wheezes. Heart sounds are normal. Rate and rhythm are normal. No rubs, clicks, or murmurs. No CVA tenderness. She is tender over the thoracolumbar junction on the right on palpation externally. It is reproducible, same place each time, about 1 inch to $1\frac{1}{2}$ inches lateral to the midline, just above the level of the thoracolumbar junction. Abdomen is tender throughout the right side. No guarding. No rebound. Good bowel sounds. No obvious organomegaly. Pelvic and rectal exam were deferred at this time. Skin is normal with no rash and no lesions. Hydration status is normal. KUB does not reveal any stones or lesions. It does reveal a lot of stool on the right-hand side. Urinalysis was completely negative. CBC reveals a white count of 8.5, normal differential cell count, and hemoglobin of 14. Normal indices. Platelet count of 350. HCG beta subunit was negative. Comprehensive metabolic panel to look at liver and gallbladder and electrolytes was all within normal limits, except for total protein being a little bit elevated.

IMPRESSION

1. Mechanical back pain. Treatment is steroid anti-inflammatories.

2. Abdominal pain secondary to constipation.

PLAN: Push fluids. Stool softeners. Follow up if signs or symptoms worsen or if any new problems are encountered or if symptom resolution is not forthcoming in a timely fashion.

CPT Code(s): _____

ICD-10-CM Code(s): _____

Abstracting Questions

1. What was the highest level of service provided for this patient? _____

2. Were more definitive diagnoses established from the presenting problems? _____
   _____

Practice Exercise 16-3: Chest Pain

LOCATION: Emergency Department

PATIENT: Frances Miley

PHYSICIAN: Paul Sutton, MD

CHIEF COMPLAINT: Chest pain.

SUBJECTIVE: This is a 74-year-old female who presents to the emergency department complaining of chest pain. Apparently, this evening, she was talking to her son about his divorce. She then developed pain up her back, into her left arm and chest. She describes it as sharp and severe. Her Nitro did not help. One Nitro from our medics took the pain from a 10 to almost a 0. She has a history of chest pain and was placed on some p.r.n. Nitro. She was scheduled for a stress test, but she canceled it. She describes the pain as moderately severe, sharp in nature. It lasted approximately 1 hour.

PAST HISTORY: Significant for:

1. Degenerative joint disease.

2. Hypertension.

PAST SURGICAL HISTORY: Hip repair.

ALLERGIES: Sulfa.

FAMILY HISTORY: Negative for premature coronary artery disease.

SOCIAL HISTORY: She is a rare tobacco user and is not an alcohol user.

REVIEW OF SYSTEMS: Remarkable for the chest pain, as noted above, into the back and the arm, associated with diaphoresis and nausea. No vomiting. No fever, chills, or sweats.

CARDIOVASCULAR: As noted above.

RESPIRATORY, GI and GU: Negative.

OBJECTIVE: VITAL SIGNS: Stable. She generally appears well. She is nondiaphoretic. HEENT: Grossly benign and deferred. LUNGS: Mostly clear without rales, rhonchi, or wheezing. CARDIOVASCULAR EXAM: S1, S2 without obvious S3, murmur, or rub. CHEST WALL: Nontender. ABDOMEN: Soft. Bowel sounds are active. No masses, rebound, or rigidity.

LABORATORY: We did obtain an electrocardiogram, which is without hyperacute ST-T wave change. Blood work is remarkable for hemoglobin of 11.6. Basic metabolic panel is normal. CK and troponin are negative.

ASSESSMENT:

1. Chest pain.

2. Anemia.

PLAN: I have notified the patient's primary physician and he has graciously agreed to assume care and will be admitting the patient presently.

CPT Code(s): _____

ICD-10-CM Code(s): _____

Abstracting Questions

1. What was the level and point of this service? _____

2. How does the admission to the hospital affect Facility Services? _____

3. Was there a definitive diagnosis for the presenting problem of chest pain? _____
_____

4. Would any other diagnoses be reported? _____

Practice Exercise 16-4: Foot Injury

Assign an external cause code to indicate how the accident occurred.

LOCATION: Emergency Department

PATIENT: Tanner Gray

PHYSICIAN: Paul Sutton, MD

SUBJECTIVE: This is a 4-year-old male who has history of reactive airway disease; he is on Singulair. He has no known allergies. He is up to date for immunizations. He presents to the emergency department with a history of injury to his left third and fourth toes when a bedroom TV dropped on his foot accidentally.

NEUROMUSCULOSKELETAL REVIEW OF SYSTEMS: He is not describing any paresthesias. Range of motion has been uncomfortable due to pain and the injury.

OBJECTIVE: He is afebrile, pulse 108, respiratory rate 30. Examination reveals a slight injury to the distal third toe with a possible slight fracture of the nail. This is minimal, however. The fourth toe has a partial nail avulsion. There is full range of motion, and the toes are neurovascularly intact.

X-ray of the left foot with emphasis on the distal third and fourth toe injuries is negative for gross bony abnormality.

ASSESSMENT: Left fourth and third toe injuries as described above with partial nail avulsion of the left fourth toe.

PLAN: These injuries were dressed with Bacitracin nonadherent dressing, 4 × 4s, and Kling wrap. We recommend ice, elevation, ibuprofen or Tylenol, and a follow-up for dressing change and wound check on Thursday or Friday with Dr. Lewis. His condition was stable at the time of discharge.

CPT Code(s): _____

ICD-10-CM Code(s): _____

Abstracting Questions

1. What was the highest level of intervention provided for this patient? _____

2. Would the different types of injuries be reported for each toe? _____

3. Was more than one external cause code required? _____

Practice Exercise 16-5: Left Lower Quadrant Pain

LOCATION: Emergency Department

PATIENT: Loretta Striker

PHYSICIAN: Paul Sutton, MD

SUBJECTIVE: The patient is a 65-year-old woman who presents to the emergency department. She initially saw my partner, and then care was turned over to me. We are just waiting for urinalysis results. Working diagnosis at this point was possible renal colic. The patient has stated the pain started this afternoon and worsened. She describes it mainly in the left lower quadrant. It radiates a little bit toward the left flank, sort of on the top of her left hip area on her side. She had two episodes of diarrhea today. She also carries a history of spastic colon for numerous years. She states that when that flares she usually has a little bit of low mid-back pain before she has a bowel movement. A lot of times it is mostly water, and then the pain goes away with that. This therefore does not feel like that. Her spastic colon has been flaring the last three weeks she tells me. She has had one ovary removed and she does not know which one. She has also had an appendectomy in the past. She has not noticed any discoloration to her urine. No dysuria, hematuria, or frequency.

EXAMINATION: Examination reveals pain to palpation in the left lower quadrant. No focal mass. No guarding. No CVA tenderness; we did review the KUB and it showed no obvious stones. However, there is a small radial opaque density across from L5, maybe 10 cm laterally. I think that is too far out to be the ureter. Some scattered stool and gas. Urinalysis showed 4 to 5 white cells, no red cells, and 2+ bacteria; this was on a sample with 1 to 2 epithelial cells. She had been given Tordal 60 mg IM. I checked on her and she states she still has pain, although it was better. I talked to her at length about possible diagnoses, including renal colic. I also talked about diverticulitis, which is difficult to say if she has that at this point. Also, possibly ovarian related such as a cyst, but I think that is not as likely either.

I talked to the patient about giving her some more pain medicine here and monitoring this, but she wanted to leave. I did request that she drink plenty of fluids, strain her urine, and follow up with her doctor this week. She said she was going to call him tomorrow. I told her that if her pain in any way changes or worsens tonight she should return. I sent her home with some Lorcet.

CPT Code(s): _____

ICD-10-CM Code(s): _____

Abstracting Questions

1. What was the highest level of intervention provided for this patient? _____

2. Were more definitive diagnoses confirmed after evaluation of the presenting problems? _____

_____

CHAPTER 17: SURGERY SECTION (10021-69990)

Largest CPT section

Each year CMS publishes a list of CPT surgery codes that are paid only as an inpatient procedure

- For example, 33300-33335, repair of wounds of the heart and great vessels, are inpatient procedures
  - Whereas 33282-33284, implantation or removal of cardiac event recorders, are paid as outpatient procedures
- Inpatient procedures reported with Volume 3 procedure codes
- Outpatient procedures reported with CPT surgery codes

Section Format
Divided by subspecialty (e.g., integumentary, cardiovascular)

Notes and Guidelines
Throughout section

Information varied and extensive

"Must" reading

Subsection notes apply to entire subsection

Subheading notes apply to entire subheading

Category notes apply to entire category

Parenthetical information (Figure 17-1)

Unlisted Procedure Codes
Used only when more specific code not found in Category I or Category III

Written report accompanies submission

Each unlisted code service paid on case-by-case basis

Separate Procedures
"(Separate procedure)" follows code description

Usually minor surgical procedure

Incidental to more major procedure

- Breast biopsy
- Biopsy before radical mastectomy would not be coded unless results of biopsy resulted in mastectomy
- Modifier -59 appended to biopsy code
- Appendectomy performed incidentally when other abdominal surgery is performed

Separate procedures reported when

- Only procedure performed

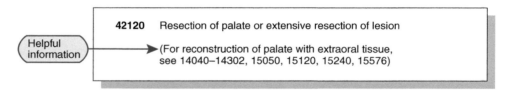

Helpful information

42120   Resection of palate or extensive resection of lesion

(For reconstruction of palate with extraoral tissue, see 14040–14302, 15050, 15120, 15240, 15576)

Figure **17-1** Parenthetical information in the CPT manual.

- With another procedure
  - On different site
  - Unrelated to major procedure

General Subsection (10021, 10022)

Fine needle aspirations with or without (w/wo) imaging guidance

Pathology 88172, 88173, and 88177 are for evaluation of fine needle aspirate

Integumentary System Subsection (10030-19499)

Often used in all specialties of medicine

Used not just by surgeons or dermatologists but by a wide range of physicians

Subheadings of Integumentary Subsection

- Skin, Subcutaneous and Accessory Structures
- Nails
- Pilonidal Cyst
- Introduction
- Repair (Closure)
- Destruction
- Breast

Skin, Subcutaneous and Accessory Structures (10030-11646)

Introduction and Removal (10030-10036)
Report percutaneous image-guided fluid drainage of a catheter collection from soft tissue

- Example: Abscess, seroma, cyst, hematoma, or lymphocele

Reported once for each individual collection drained

Report codes 10035, 10036 for placement of soft tissue markers

Incision and Drainage (10040-10180)
I&D of abscess, carbuncle, boil, cyst, infection, hematoma, pilonidal cyst

- Lancing (cutting of skin)
- Aspiration (removal by puncturing lesion with a needle and withdrawing fluid)

Gauze or tube may be inserted for continued drainage

Excision—Debridement (11000-11047)
Dead tissue cut away

11000, 11001 Eczematous or infected skin

11004-11006 Debridement of infected area based on location and **depth** of necrotizing tissue (subcutaneous, muscle, fascia)

+11008 Removal of prosthetic material or mesh from abdominal wall

11010-11012 Foreign material with open fracture or dislocation

- Skin, subcutaneous tissue, muscle fascia, muscle, and bone

11042-11044 Subcutaneous tissue, muscle, bone

- Debridement partial thickness based on 20 square centimeters or less

11045-11047 Based on each additional 20 square centimeters

Paring or Cutting (11055-11057)
Removal by scraping or peeling (e.g., removal of corn or callus)

Codes indicate number: 1, 2-4, 4+

Biopsy (11100, 11101)

Skin, subcutaneous tissue, or mucous membrane biopsy

Not all of lesion removed

- All of lesion removed = excision

Codes indicate number: 1 or each additional

Tissue that is removed during excision, shave, etc., and submitted to pathology is NOT reported separately as a biopsy

- Rather, it is included in the code for the excision

Skin Tag Removal (11200, 11201)

Benign lesions

Removed with scissors, blade, chemicals, cryosurgery, electrosurgery, etc.

Codes indicate number: Up to and including 15 lesions and each additional 10 lesions

Shaving of Lesions (11300-11313)

Removed by transverse incision or sliced horizontally

Based on

- Size (e.g., 1.1-2 cm)
- Location (e.g., arm, hand, nose)

Does not require suture closure

Benign/Malignant Lesions (11400-11646)

Codes divided: Benign or malignant

Physician assesses or pathologist confirms lesion as benign or malignant

Codes include local anesthesia and simple closure

Report each excised lesion separately

Lesion size

- Taken from physician's notes
- Includes greatest diameter plus narrowest margins of 2 sides (Figure 17-2)

    Example: A benign lesion measuring 0.5 cm at widest point is removed with 0.5-cm margin at narrowest point (each side, 0.5 + 0.5 = 1.0 cm). Reported as 1.5-cm lesion excision (11402)

    - Do not take size from pathology report—storage solution shrinks tissue
    - Margins (healthy tissue) are also taken for comparison with unhealthy tissue

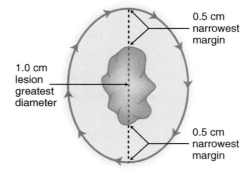

Figure **17-2** Calculating the size of a lesion.

Example: 1-cm lesion with 2-cm margin left and right of lesion

1 + 2 + 2 = 5 cm

- Re-excisions following initial excision of malignant lesion coded as excision of malignant lesion

All excised tissue pathologically examined

Codes 11400-11646 report excision of lesion

Destroyed lesions have no pathology samples

Example: Laser, cryosurgery, or chemical destruction (lysis)

Lesion closure

- Simple or subcutaneous closure included in removal
- Reported separately
  - Layered or intermediate, 12031-12057 (Repair—Intermediate)
  - Complex, 13100-13153 (Repair—Complex)

Nails (11719-11765)

Includes toes and fingers

Types of services

- Trimming, debridement, removal, biopsy, repair

Introduction (11900-11983)

Types of Services

- Lesion injections (therapeutic or diagnostic), tattooing, tissue expansion, contraceptive insertion/removal, hormone implantation services, and insertion/removal of nonbiodegradable drug-delivery implant

Repair (Closure) (12001-13160)

Repair Factors in Wound Repair

As types of wounds vary, types of wound repair also vary

Length, complexity (simple, intermediate, complex), and site must be documented

- Length measured in centimeters
- Measured prior to closure

Types of Wound Repair

Simple: Superficial, epidermis, dermis, or subcutaneous tissue

- One-layer closure
- Dermabond closure
- Medicare patients report Dermabond closure with CPT repair codes or G0168

Intermediate: Layered closure of deeper layers of subcutaneous tissue and superficial fascia with skin closure

- Single-layer closure can be coded as intermediate if extensive debridement is required

Complex: Greater than layered; may include multiple layers of tissue and fascia or extensive debridement

Example: Scar revision, complicated debridement, extensive undermining, stents, extensive retention sutures

Included in Wound Repair Codes

Simple ligation of vessels in an open wound

Simple exploration of nerves, blood vessels, and exposed tendons

Normal debridement

- Additional codes for debridement can be used when
  - Gross contamination requires prolonged cleaning
  - Appreciable amounts of devitalized/contaminated tissue are removed to expose healthy tissue
  - Debridement is provided without immediate primary closure

Grouping of Wound Repair

Add together lengths by

- Complexity of wound
  - Simple, intermediate, complex
- Location of wound
  - e.g., face, ears, eyelids, nose, lips

1 inch = 2.54 cm

> *Example:* **Same complexity, same codes description location:** Intermediate repairs of 2.9-cm laceration of leg and 1.1-cm laceration of buttocks. 2.9 + 1.1 = 4.0 cm (12032)

> *Example:* **Different complexity:** Intermediate repair of 2.9-cm laceration of leg and simple repair of 1.1-cm laceration of buttocks. 2.9-cm intermediate repair (12032) and 1.1-cm simple repair (12001)

> *Example:* **Same complexity, different code description locations:** Intermediate repair of 2.9-cm laceration of leg and intermediate repair of 1.1-cm laceration of nose. 2.9-cm intermediate repair of leg (12032) and 1.1-cm intermediate repair of nose (12051)

Do Not Group Wound Repairs That Are

Different complexities

> *Example:* Simple repair and complex repair

Different locations as stated in the code description

> *Example:* Simple repairs of scalp (12001) and nose (12011)

Adjacent Tissue Transfer, Flaps, and Grafts (14000-15778)

Information Needed to Code Graft

Type of graft—adjacent, free, flap, etc.

Donor site (from)

Recipient site (to)

Any repair to donor site

Size of graft

Adjacent Tissue Transfer/Rearrangement (14000-14350)

Includes excision and/or repair (e.g., Z-plasty, W-plasty, V-plasty, Y-plasty, rotation flap, advancement flap)

Codes based on size and location of graft

Measure site of defect from excision plus size of defect from flap design for total size

Skin Replacement Surgery (15002-15431)

15002-15005 Site preparation based on size and site

15040-15261 Autografts/Tissue Cultured Autografts

- 15050-15431 Autograft codes by type and size
- 15271-15278 Skin substitute grafts

Split-thickness: Epidermis and some dermis (Figure 17-3)

Full-thickness: Epidermis and all dermis

Allograft: Donor graft

Xenograft: Nonhuman donor

Code is based on recipient site, not donor site

Flaps (15570-15777)

Some skin left attached to blood supply

- Keeps flap viable

Donor site may be far from recipient site

Flaps may be in stages

Codes divided by location and size

Formation of flap (15570-15576)

- Based on recipient location: Trunk, scalp, nose, etc.

Transfer of flap (15650): Previously placed flap released from donor site

- Also known as walking or walk up of flap
- 15777 is an add-on code to report soft tissue reinforcement with biological implants

Muscle, Myocutaneous, or Fasciocutaneous Flaps (15732-15738)

- Based on recipient location: head and neck, trunk, upper or lower extremity
- Repairs made with
  - Muscle
  - Muscle and skin
  - Fascia and skin
- Flaps rotated from donor to recipient site
- Includes closure donor site unless skin graft or local flaps are necessary

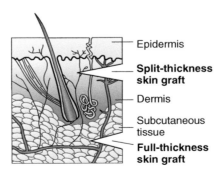

Figure **17-3** Split-thickness and full-thickness skin grafts.

Other Procedures (15780-15879)

Many cosmetic procedures including:

- Dermabrasion
- Chemical peel
- Blepharoplasty
- Rhytidectomy
- Excessive skin excision

Pressure (Decubitus) Ulcers (15920-15999)

Excision and various closures

- Primary, skin flap, muscle, etc.

Many codes "with ostectomy"

- Bone removal

Locations

- Coccygeal (end of spine)
- Sacral (between hips)
- Ischial (lower hip)
- Trochanteric (outer hip)

Site preparation only: 15936, 15937, 15946, 15956, or 15958

- Defect repair of donor site reported separately

Burns Treatment (16000-16036)

Codes for small, medium, and large

Must calculate percentage of body burned using the Rule of Nines for adults (Figure 17-4)

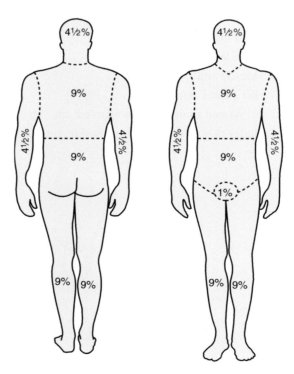

Figure **17-4** The Rule of Nines is used to calculate burn area on an adult.

- <5% = small
- 5% to 10% = medium
- >10% = large

Lund-Browder for children (Figure 17-5)

- Proportions of children differ from those of adults
- Heads are larger

Often require multiple debridements and redressing

Based on

- Initial treatment of 1st-degree burn (16000)
- Size

Report percent of burn and depth (Refer to Figure 17-3)

Destruction (17000-17286)

Ablation (destruction) of tissue

- Laser, electrosurgery, cryosurgery, chemosurgery, etc.
- Benign/premalignant or malignant tissue
- Malignant tissue is based on location and size
- Benign/premalignant is based on the number of lesions removed or size (sq cm)

Mohs Micrographic Surgery (17311-17315)

Surgeon acts as pathologist and surgeon

Removes one layer of lesion at a time, examines under microscope

Continues until no malignant cells can be detected by microscopy

Based on stages and number of specimens per stage indicated in medical record

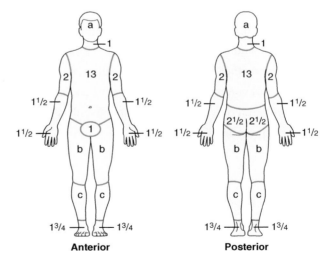

Relative percentage of body surface areas (% BSA) affected by growth

	0 yr	1 yr	5 yr	10 yr	15 yr
a – 1/2 of head	9^1/2	8^1/2	6^1/2	5^1/2	4^1/2
b – 1/2 of 1 thigh	2^3/4	3^1/4	4	4^1/4	4^1/2
c – 1/2 of lower leg	2^1/2	2^1/2	2^3/4	3	3^1/4

Figure **17-5** Lund-Browder chart for estimating the extent of burns on children.

Other Procedures (17340-17999)

Treatment of acne

- Cryotherapy
- Chemical exfoliation
- Electrolysis
- Unlisted procedures

Breast Procedures (19000-19499)

Divided based on procedure

- Incision
- Excision
- Introduction
- Mastectomy Procedures
- Repair and/or Reconstruction

Use excision of lesion codes if entire lesion is removed during incisional biopsy

Use additional codes for placement of radiological markers

- Code each marker placement separately

Mastectomies based on extent of procedure

- Wide excision
  - Removal of neoplasm, capsule, and surrounding margins
- Radical
  - Wide excision and anatomical structure surrounding neoplasm
  - *Example:* Muscle or fascia
  - Performed on an inpatient basis
- Conservative partial mastectomy in which lesion is removed with adequate margins, 19301
- Axillary dissection and partial mastectomy, 19302
- Radical and modified radical, 19305, 19306, and 19307, based on extent

Confirm whether pectoral muscles, axillary, or internal lymph nodes were removed

19307 most common and includes breast and axillary lymph node removal

Code removal of lymph nodes separately unless included in code description

Bilateral procedures, use -50

Biopsy/Removal of Lesion

Incisional biopsy: Incision made into lesion and small portion of lesion removed

Excisional biopsy: Entire lesion removed

Open incisional biopsy most complex (19101)

Percutaneous needle core biopsy without imaging guidance (19100)

- Same procedure with imaging guidance based on guidance method:
  - 19081, 19082 stereotactic
  - 19083, 19084 ultrasound
  - 19085, 19086 magnetic resonance

Complete, simple removal of a mass is reported with 19120

Lesion may be preoperatively marked with localization devices (clip, metallic pellet, wire, needle, radioactive seed) based on guidance method:

- 19281, 19282, mammographic
- 19283, 19284, stereotactic
- 19285, 19286, ultrasound
- 19287, 19288, magnetic resonance

PRACTICE EXERCISES

Practice Exercise 17-1: Excision, Basal Cell Carcinoma

LOCATION: Outpatient, Hospital

PATIENT: Dana Kelley

PREOPERATIVE DIAGNOSIS: Basal cell carcinoma, right side of nose.

POSTOPERATIVE DIAGNOSIS: Same.

SURGICAL FINDINGS: Healing 5-mm ulcer, right side of nose, with surrounding inflammatory response.

SURGICAL PROCEDURE: Excision of basal cell carcinoma, right side of nose, with reconstruction by 3 × 2.5 cm bilobed flap.

SURGEON: Gary Sanchez, MD

ANESTHESIA: Standby sedation with 5 cc of 1% Xylocaine with 1 : 100,000 epinephrine.

DESCRIPTION OF PROCEDURE: The patient's face was prepped with Betadine scrub and solution, and draped in a routine sterile fashion. The lesion and the surrounding tissue for the flap were both anesthetized with a total of 5 cc of 1% Xylocaine with 1 : 100,000 epinephrine. The lesion was excised circumferentially with a 5-mm margin. It was submitted for frozen section with a tag on the inferior aspect. The lesion was clear on all margins. Bleeding was electrocoagulated. We developed a 3 × 2.5 cm bilobed flap based on the left side, rotating it in place and insetting it with 5–0 Prolene. Antibiotic ointment and Surgicel were applied followed by a 4 × 4. The patient tolerated the procedure well and left the area in good condition.

Pathology Report Later Indicated: Basal cell carcinoma.

CPT Code(s): _____

ICD-10-CM Code(s): _____

Abstracting Questions

1. Was the nasal lesion intranasal (within the nose) or extranasal (on the nose)? _____
   _____

2. Was the repair performed with an adjacent tissue transfer or a free graft? _____

3. Are both the excision and the repair reported? _____

CLINICAL AND HISTOLOGICAL EVALUATION OF BASAL CELL CARCINOMA

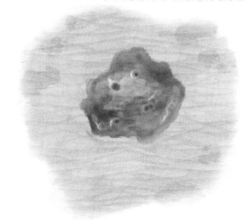

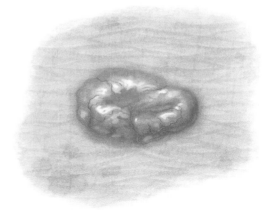

Superficial basal cell carcinoma. Slightly scaly pink to red patch. These tumors are slow growing and occur on chronically sun-exposed skin.

Nodular basal cell carcinoma. Pearly plaque with telangiectatic central ulceration, and rolled border

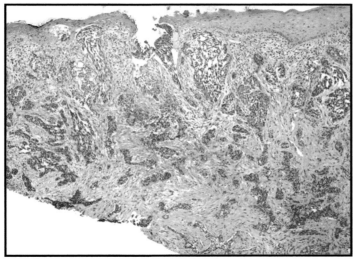

Basophilic tumor lobules and strands extending from the epidermis into the dermis

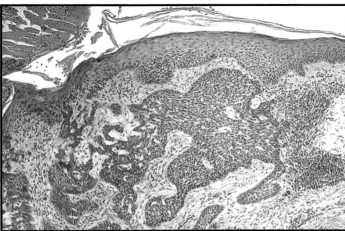

Basophilic tumor lobules within the dermis showing slight retraction artifact and peripheral palisading

Practice Exercise 17-2: Ulcer Repair

OPERATIVE REPORT

LOCATION: Outpatient, Hospital

PATIENT: Andy Green

PREOPERATIVE DIAGNOSES

1. Chronic ulcer of the left ischium.

2. Status post debridement of left ischial ulcer.

POSTOPERATIVE DIAGNOSES: Same.

SURGICAL FINDINGS: Approximately 8-cm diameter open wound, left ischium with large clot.

SURGICAL PROCEDURE: Minimal debridement, left ischial ulcer with complex closure.

SURGEON: Gary Sanchez, MD

ANESTHESIA: General endotracheal.

DESCRIPTION OF PROCEDURE: The patient was intubated and turned in the prone position, the ischial area was prepped with Betadine scrub and solution, and draped in routine sterile fashion. Following preparation of Betadine scrub and solution, the old clot was removed from the wound and more necrotic tissue was removed. The wound was closed in layers with interrupted 2–0 Monocryl and interrupted 0 Prolene for the skin using vertical mattress sutures. A #10 Jackson-Pratt drain was placed at the wound and brought out through a separate stab wound incision. It was sutured to the wound with 0 Prolene. Tegaderm was applied to the actual wound itself to prevent fecal contamination; Kerlix fluffs were placed on top of this with an Elastoplast dressing. Estimated blood loss was negligible. The patient tolerated the procedure well and left the area in good condition.

Pathology Report Later Indicated: Benign tissue.

CPT Code(s): _____

ICD-10-CM Code(s): _____

Abstracting Questions

1. Are both excision of the lesion and the repair reported separately? _____

2. Was the repair simple, intermediate, or complex? _____

3. Does the size of the open wound affect the coding? _____

4. How many codes are required to report the closure of the open wound? _____

5. Does the location of the wound repair affect coding? _____

Practice Exercise 17-3: Ulcer Debridement

OPERATIVE REPORT

LOCATION: Outpatient, Hospital

PATIENT: Eric Crest

PREOPERATIVE DIAGNOSIS: Large necrotic pressure ulcer of the right lateral leg.

POSTOPERATIVE DIAGNOSIS: Large necrotic pressure ulcer of the right lateral leg.

SURGEON: Gary Sanchez, MD

PROCEDURE: Sharp debridement of soft tissues, tendon, and fascia down to muscle of the right lateral leg. Measures approximately 4–5 cm in length × 3 cm in width × 1 cm in depth.

DESCRIPTION OF PROCEDURE: He basically has no sensation in his lower extremities. Then using sharp dissection, we sharply debrided all the necrotic tissue. This included some tendinous tissues. This was down into some muscle in a couple of spots. This was getting down to fairly close to the fibular head. There was not a lot of tissue between here and the fibular head. We debrided all the necrotic tissue. There were a few areas along the periphery that actually had hypergranulation tissue. These were treated with silver nitrate. Hemostasis was achieved. We ended up with a fair amount of necrotic debris and things cleaned up pretty well here. Could be looking at placing a TransiGel dressing at this time. The patient tolerated the procedure well.

Pathology Report Later Indicated: Benign ulcerative tissue.

CPT Code(s): _____

ICD-10-CM Code(s): _____

Abstracting Questions

1. Was a repair of the ulcer documented for this procedure? _____

2. What was the deepest level of debridement of the ulcer: skin, subcutaneous tissue, muscle fascia, muscle, or bone? _____

3. When referencing the Index of the ICD-10-CM at the main term "Pressure ulcer," the coder is directed to: _____

Practice Exercise 17-4: Split-Thickness Skin Graft

OPERATIVE REPORT

LOCATION: Outpatient, Hospital

PATIENT: Manny Hartwell

PREOPERATIVE DIAGNOSES

1. Ulcer of the right lateral foot.

2. Superficial ulcer of the right anterior ankle.

POSTOPERATIVE DIAGNOSES: Same.

SURGEON: Gary Sanchez, MD

PROCEDURES PERFORMED

1. Split-thickness skin graft to right lateral foot, 7 cm × 5 cm.

2. Split-thickness skin graft to right anterior ankle ulcer, 2 cm × 3 cm.

INDICATIONS: The patient is a 75-year-old male who has developed wounds to his feet. He has been revascularized. These wounds have started to show signs of healing. The main concern was on the right lateral foot. He also developed an ulcer to the anterior ankle. We examined this today in the holding room before surgery and this wound was also clean, but it sloughed off the epithelialization of the skin/blister over this. I recommended to him that we also skin graft this at the same time. We discussed the procedure again. We reviewed the risks again. He understands and wishes to proceed with this.

ANESTHESIA: General.

PROCEDURE: This was done under a general anesthetic. The right lateral foot and right anterior ankle wound sites were prepped and debrided of the granulation. There was fair bleeding but neurovascularization of bleeding underneath this. The beds were cleaned. The skin graft was then taken from his right anterior thigh using a dermatome set at 0.012 inch. This was meshed at a ratio of 1:1.5. The one segment that was raised was used to cover both of the wound sites. These were stapled in place and Adaptic, gauze, mineral oil, wet cotton batting, and Fluffs were applied over this and secured in place with an Ace wrap in a snug but not tight manner. He has a small superficial heel ulcer, which was covered with a wet-to-dry dressing, and this was also covered with the above dressing. The patient tolerated the procedure well and went to the recovery room in stable condition.

CPT Code(s): _____

ICD-10-CM Code(s): _____

Abstracting Questions

1. Were the right foot and the ankle reported with separate codes or reported collectively? ____
   _____

2. Are the wounds reported separately or would they be added together and reported with one CPT code? _____

3. Was the wet-to-dry dressing applied to the small, superficial heel ulcer reported separately?
   _____

4. Are diagnosis codes required for both ulcer areas? _____

Practice Exercise 17-5: Lesion Excision

OPERATIVE REPORT

LOCATION: Outpatient, Hospital

PATIENT: Dave Schroeder

INDICATIONS: This patient has a mole of the left chest wall that has been changing in character for the past two months. When we saw this in the office, it was originally dark with surrounding erythema, but now it has lost some of its pigmentation. Nevertheless, there is still a definite lesion present.

PREOPERATIVE DIAGNOSIS: Changing compound nevus of the left chest wall.

POSTOPERATIVE DIAGNOSIS: Pending.

SURGEON: Gary Sanchez, MD

SURGICAL FINDINGS: A 5-mm diameter, lightly pigmented lesion on the left lateral chest wall, benign.

SURGICAL PROCEDURE: Excision of lesion of left chest wall with 5-mm proximal and distal margins and 2-mm lateral margins.

ANESTHESIA: 1% Xylocaine and 1:100,000 Epinephrine, 3 cc.

DESCRIPTION OF PROCEDURE: Chest wall was prepped in Betadine solution and draped in sterile fashion. The lesion was anesthetized with a total of 3 cc of 1% Xylocaine and 1:100,000 epinephrine. The lesion was excised elliptically with 5-mm proximal and distal margins and 2-mm lateral margins. Bleeding was electrocoagulated. The wound was closed with subcuticular 4–0 Monocryl in interrupted twists of 4–0 Monocryl. Steri-Strips were applied. The patient tolerated the procedure well and left the area in good condition.

Pathology Report Later Indicated: Benign neoplastic nevus.

CPT Code(s): _____

ICD-10-CM Code(s): _____

Abstracting Questions

1. Does the benign/malignant status of the excised lesion affect code selection? _____
   _____

2. Does the size of the lesion affect CPT code selection? _____

3. Does the location of the lesion on the body affect CPT code selection? _____

4. Does the number of excised lesions affect CPT code selection? _____

■ Musculoskeletal System Subsection (20005-29999)

Subsection divided: Anatomical site, then service (e.g., excision)

Used extensively by orthopedic surgeons

- Many codes commonly used by variety of physicians

Extensive notes

Most common

- Fracture and dislocation treatments
- "General" subheading
- Arthroscopic procedures
- Casting and strapping

Eponyms are "things" named after "people"

> *Example:* Barr procedure is a tendon transfer of the lower leg (27690-27692), and Mitchell Chevron procedure is a complex metatarsal osteotomy (bunion correction) (28296)

- Procedures are often referred to with eponyms
- Check the index of the CPT manual for directions to eponym codes

Fracture Treatment

Type of treatment depends on type and severity of fracture

Diagnosis codes must support the procedure codes and document the medical necessity

Open: Surgically opened to view or remotely opened to place nail across fracture site

- Open reduction with internal fixation is ORIF

Closed: Not surgically opened

Percutaneous: Insertion of devices through skin. Percutaneous fracture treatment neither open nor closed

Treatment terms should not be confused with **types** of fractures:

- Open fracture: Fractured bone penetrates skin
- Closed fracture: Fractured bone does not penetrate skin

Traction

- Application of force to align bone
- Force applied by internal device (e.g., wire, pin) inserted into bone (skeletal fixation)
- Application of force by means of adhesion to skin (skin traction)

Manipulation

Use of force to return bone back to normal alignment by manual manipulation (reduction) or temporary traction

Codes often divided based on whether manipulation was or was not used

Dislocation

Bone displaced from normal joint position

Treatment: Return bone to normal joint location

Subheading "General"

Incision" (20005)

Depth determines between Integumentary or Musculoskeletal incision codes

Musculoskeletal code used when underlying bone or muscle is involved or procedure is deep subcutaneous

Wound Exploration (20100-20103)

Traumatic penetrating wounds

Divided on wound location

Includes

- Surgical exploration
- Enlargement
- Debridement
- Removal of foreign body (bodies)
- Ligation
- Repair of tissue and muscle

Use additional code for repair of major structures or blood vessels

Not used for integumentary repairs

- Unless the repair requires extension, enlargement, or exploration

Repair of major structure is reported instead when exploration leads to repair

Excision (20150-20251)

Biopsies for bone and muscle

Divided by

- Type of biopsy (bone/muscle)
- Depth
- Some by method

Can be percutaneous needle or excisional

Does not include tumor excision, which is coded separately

Biopsy with excision: Code only excision

Introduction or Removal (20500-20697)

Codes for

- Injections
- Aspirations
- Insertions
- Applications
- Removals
- Adjustments

Therapeutic sinus tract injection procedures

- Not nasal sinus
- Abscess or cyst with passage (sinus tract) to skin
- Antibiotic injected with use of radiographic guidance

Removal of foreign bodies lodged in muscle or tendon sheath

Integumentary removal codes for removal from skin

Injection into

- Tendon sheath
- Tendon origin
- Ligament
- Ganglion cyst
- Trigger points

Placement of needles or catheters into muscle and/or soft tissue

- For interstitial radioelement application

Arthrocentesis injection "and/or" aspiration of a joint

- Both aspiration and injection reported with one code (20600-20611)
- Codes based on joint size: Small, intermediate, major and with or without guidance
- Do not unbundle and report aspiration/injection with two codes

External Fixation (20690-20697)

Device that holds bone in place

- Application, adjustment, removal under anesthesia

Code fracture treatment and external fixation

- Unless treatment and fixation both included in fracture care code description
- Adjustment to (20693) and removal of (20694 [under anesthesia]) EFD are coded separately

Replantation (20802-20838)

Used to report reattachment of amputated limb

Code by body area

Performed only on an inpatient basis

Grafts (or Implants) (20900-20938)

Autogenous Grafts

Used to report harvesting through separate incision of

- Bone
- Cartilage
- Tendon
- Fascia lata
- Tissue

Fascia lata grafts: From upper lateral thigh where fascia is thickest

Some codes include obtaining grafting material (then, not coded separately)

Some grafts are add-on codes for spine surgery only (20930-20938)

Other Procedures (20950-20999)

Monitoring interstitial fluid pressure (interstitial for compartment syndrome, etc.)

- Pressure increases due to increased accumulation of fluids, causing blood supply to be compromised

Bone grafts identified by donor site

Free osseocutaneous flaps: Bone grafts

- Taken along with skin and tissue overlying bone

Electrical stimulation
- Used to speed bone healing
- Placement of stimulators externally or internally
- Ultrasound also used externally

Soft Tissue Tumors

Codes identify excision of soft tissue and subfascial (intramuscular) tumors
- Subcutaneous soft tissue tumors: Below skin but above deep fascia
- Fascial or subfascial soft tissue tumors: Within or below deep fascia (not bone)
- Soft tissue tumors: May involve resection from one or more layer (i.e., subcutaneous, subfascial)

    Example: 21011-21016 to report subcutaneous, subfascial, and soft tissue tumors

Arthrodesis

Fixation of joint (arthro = joint, desis = fusion)
- Boney structures of joint fused together to form one solid bone
- Fixation with pins, wires, rods, etc. to hold the joint immobile

Often performed with other procedure such as fracture repair
- Arthrodesis of the spine is also called spinal fusion

Subsequent Subheadings

After General subheading, divided by anatomical location
- Anatomical subheadings divided by type of procedure

    Example: Subheading "Head" divided by procedure
- Incision
- Excision
- Manipulation
- Head Prosthesis
- Introduction or Removal
- Repair, Revision, and/or Reconstruction
- Fracture and/or Dislocation
- Other Procedures

Spine and Spinal Instrumentation

Insertion of spinal instrumentation reported in addition to arthrodesis (fusion)

Many codes are add-on and are reported in addition to definitive procedure

Spine (Vertebral Column), 22010-22899, divided by repair location
- Cervical (C1-C7)
  - C1 = Atlas
  - C2 = Axis
- Thoracic (T1-T12)
- Lumbar (L1-L5)
- Sacral (S1-S5)
- Coccyx (tailbone)

Vertebral segment: Single complete vertebral bone with articular processes and laminae

Vertebral interspace: Non-bony compartment between two vertebral bodies which contains the disc

Single level = two vertebrae and the disc that separates them

Percutaneous vertebroplasty

- Use of polymethylmethacrylate injected into the vertebral space
- Polymethylmethacrylate is a type of bone glue applied when doughlike and then hardening into a clear cement
- Adheres bone fragments together
- Fills vertebral body defects

Types of Spinal Instrumentation

Segmental: Devices at each end of repair area plus at least one other attachment

Nonsegmental: Devices at each end of defect only

Approach: Pay special attention to the approach used to perform the surgery

- Several different approaches to spine: Most common anterior (front) and posterior (back)
- Most spinal instrumentation codes divided based on approach

Spinal instrumentation procedures are performed only on an inpatient basis

Casts and Strapping (29000-29799)

Replacement procedure or initial placement to stabilize when provided without additional restorative treatment

> *Example:* Application of wrist splint or cast for wrist sprain

Initial fracture treatment includes placement and removal of first cast

- Subsequent cast applications coded separately
- Payers have strict individual reimbursement policies for subsequent casting

Application not coded when part of surgical procedure

> *Example:* Repair of radial fracture includes application of cast or splint

Ace bandage applications not billed separately

Removal bundled into surgical procedure

Supplies reported separately

Endoscopy/Arthroscopy (29800-29999)

Surgical arthroscopy always includes diagnostic arthroscopy

Codes divided by joint

- Subdivided by procedure
- Be aware of subterms and bundled procedures within code descriptions

NOTE: Parenthetical information following codes indicates codes to use if procedure was an open procedure

PRACTICE EXERCISES

Practice Exercise 17-6: Closed Reduction

OPERATIVE REPORT

LOCATION: Outpatient, Hospital

PATIENT: Patrick Jutes

PREOPERATIVE DIAGNOSIS: Displaced intra-articular distal left radius fracture.

POSTOPERATIVE DIAGNOSIS: Same.

SURGEON: Mohomad Almaz, MD

PROCEDURE PERFORMED: Closed reduction and external fixator application, distal left radius fracture.

ANESTHESIA: General anesthesia.

PROCEDURE: The patient was brought to the operating room, and general anesthetic was induced. The left upper extremity was hung in finger-trap traction with 5 pounds of counterweight. We then exsanguinated the limb, and tourniquet was inflated to 250 mm Hg for 35 minutes. We manipulated the distal radius fracture and used the C-arm in AP (anterior/posterior views) and lateral planes to confirm excellent reduction of the articular surface and restitution of length of the distal radius. We therefore prepped the arm with Betadine and draped it in a sterile fashion. We proceeded with application of an external fixator, applying two pins into the base of the index metacarpal and two pins in the radial shaft more proximally and connected these with stacked external carbon fiber bars. The appearance of the pins and reduction of the fracture was excellent on the C-arm views. We cut off excess pin length. We then applied Xeroform about the pins and applied a compression long-arm Robert–Jones dressing with plantar splints immobilizing the arm at 90-degree flexion. The patient tolerated the procedure well. The tourniquet was released prior to this, and good circulation returned to the arm. He went to the recovery room in excellent condition. He will be dismissed as an outpatient today with plans for follow-up back in the office in 2 weeks. Discharge medication included Lorcet, 30 tablets.

CPT Code(s): _____

ICD-10-CM Code(s): _____

Abstracting Questions

1. Was the fracture of the radius open or closed? _____

2. Does the specific bone involved affect the diagnosis code assignment? _____

3. What other terms indicated that there were other factors that affected the diagnosis code? ___
   _____

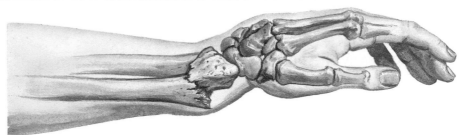

Colles fracture

Lateral view of Colles fracture demonstrates characteristic silver fork deformity with dorsal and proximal displacement of distal fragment. Note dorsal instead of normal volar slope of articular surface of distal radius.

Barton fracture

Dorsal Barton more common. Note dorsal intra-articular lip fracture of distal radius and associated subluxation of the carpus.

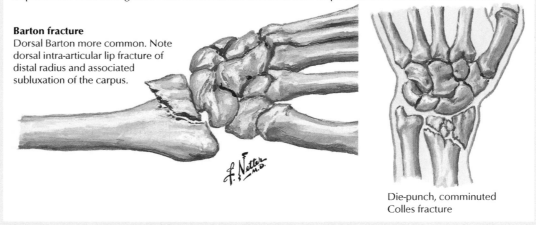

Die-punch, comminuted Colles fracture

Practice Exercise 17-7: Synovectomy

OPERATIVE REPORT

LOCATION: Outpatient, Hospital

PATIENT: Theodore Schumer

PREOPERATIVE DIAGNOSES

1. Left knee medial femoral condyle fracture.

2. Retained metal, left knee.

POSTOPERATIVE DIAGNOSES: Same.

SURGEON: Mohomad Almaz, MD

PROCEDURE PERFORMED: Left knee arthroscopy with synovectomy and metal removal and manipulation under general anesthesia.

ANESTHESIA: General.

ESTIMATED BLOOD LOSS: Minimal.

DRAINS: None.

PROCEDURE: A 28-year-old male 6 weeks status post medial femoral condyle fracture on the left. He underwent open reduction internal fixation. He was taken back to surgery. After appropriate level of anesthesia was achieved, the left knee was appropriately prepped and draped in orthopedic manner. We made two portals in the knee, one medial and the other lateral to the patellar tendon. Sharp dissection was carried through the skin and blunt dissection was carried into the joint space. On examination of the knee we appreciated that the patient had extensive scarring in the suprapatellar area and the medial gutter. This was debrided with a shaver. We appreciated some scarring in the femoral notch area but this was debrided. The patient had a nonfunctioning anterior cruciate ligament tear. The medial and lateral meniscus were probed and felt to be intact. The fracture site was identified. We could appreciate no gross motion with palpation or range of motion across the fracture site.

We manipulated the knee but we could not get more than 45 degrees of flexion. For fear of suffering a fracture or rupture, we did not do any further aggressive manipulation. There was appreciated a metal staple in the femoral notch area. This appeared to be loose. We went ahead and pulled it out through the scope. We repaired the portal sites with interrupted nylon sutures and dressed the wound sterilely. The patient was placed in an Ace wrap. The patient appeared to tolerate the procedure well and left the operating room in good condition.

CPT Code(s): _____

ICD-10-CM Code(s): _____

Abstracting Questions

1. Was the synovium actually excised? _____

2. Would the removal of the retained loose staple be reported separately? _____

3. Removal of the staple is classified as a _____.

Practice Exercise 17-8: Anterior Cruciate Ligament Reconstruction

OPERATIVE REPORT

LOCATION: Outpatient, Hospital

PATIENT: Morris Valley

PREOPERATIVE DIAGNOSIS: Status post right knee meniscal repair now secondary staged anterior cruciate ligament reconstruction.

POSTOPERATIVE DIAGNOSIS: Anterior cruciate ligament deficit, right knee.

SURGEON: Mohomad Almaz, MD

PROCEDURE PERFORMED: Anterior cruciate ligament reconstruction.

ANESTHESIA: General.

PROCEDURE: After satisfactory level of general anesthesia, the patient was placed in a supine position and the extremity was prepped and draped in routine sterile manner. Exam at this time under anesthesia showed that he has continuation of a grade 2+ ACL deficiency positive pivot shift.

Upon entering the joint through routine established arthroscopic portals, it was significant to note the suprapatellar pouch was unremarkable. Patella had areas of grade 1 osteoarthritic change similar to the type of changes of grade 1 to 2 varieties about the intercondylar notch.

Medial gutter was unremarkable. Medial compartment was significant for documented and demonstrated excellent repair and healing of the medial meniscus. The articular surface had scant areas of diffuse grade 1 osteoarthritic change. The notch proper at this time was addressed, completing a more formal definitive notch plasty, and with completion of this the lateral compartment was well visualized and unremarkable in its appearance. The articular surfaces and the meniscus were pristine in their character.

Through the arthroscopic portals, I simply proceeded at this time with the advancement of a guide pin and simultaneous to this we also created an anterior-based incision sharply dissecting down to the prepatellar fascia. The fascia was then further incised. Also, at this interval in time, we proceeded with harvesting of the central of ⅓ the patellar tendon with use of bone-tendon-bone construct of 10 mm in width, 25 mm in length from both the tibia and the tibial tubercle. This was then further prepared on the back table. The prior placed tibial guide pin was in excellent position in the remnant stump of the ACL. I then simply proceeded to over-ream about the guide pin, creating a 10-mm channel. This was then further followed by advancement of a Beeth needle in the 11-o'clock position. The needle was advanced, and over advanced needle use of acorn reamer created a 40-mm × 10-mm channel within the femoral advanced.

The Beeth needle was then used to advance the prior prepared reconstruction ACL graft. The advancement of this within the femoral tunnel and with use of counter distraction, a guide pin, was placed through guide pin. A bioabsorbable screw was used to fixate the femoral elements of the graft. This was then further followed by advancement of a bioabsorbable interference screw about the tibial tunnel in the graft. At this setting, the knee was without encumbrance to movement other than that limited by the table at approximately 115 degrees of flexion. At this time there was no demonstration as to positive Lachman's test findings and/or pivot shift through limited arcs of movement as above. There was no abutment, as noted arthroscopically.

After completion of this element of the procedure, the knee was evacuated of irrigating material, donor site closed in an interrupted manner, followed by whipstitch closure of the fascia. Portal sites were also closed. Indwelling Stryker pain pump was placed.

Estimated blood loss was minimal. Tourniquet time for the procedure was 62 minutes. Sponge and needle counts were correct. There were no noted complicating events. The patient tolerated the procedure well. Intraoperative photos were obtained as well for documentation.

CPT Code(s): _____

ICD-10-CM Code(s): _____

Abstracting Questions

1. Was the procedure an open or arthroscopic procedure? _____

2. Does the specific ligament repaired affect CPT code selection? _____

3. Was the harvest of the tendon graft reported separately? _____

Practice Exercise 17-9: Mosaicplasty

OPERATIVE REPORT

LOCATION: Outpatient, Hospital

PATIENT: Jason Black

PREOPERATIVE DIAGNOSES

1. Internal derangement of right knee.

2. Known area of grade 4 arthritic change of the medial femoral condyle.

POSTOPERATIVE DIAGNOSES: Same.

SURGEON: Mohomad Almaz, MD

PROCEDURE PERFORMED: Mosaicplasty.

PROCEDURE: At this time in this regard under sterile technique, the patient underwent establishment of routine arthroscopic portals about the knee. Upon entering the knee proper, the patella and its tracking were only significant in that there were some scanty areas of grade 2 arthritic change with subtle fissuring of the mid cistern of the patella. The articular notch was otherwise unremarkable. There was some remnant of a plical type entity, which was trimmed back at this time for the sake of visualization. At this setting there was a focal area of approximately 1 cm^2 about the medial femoral condyle, which had a loose redundant flap-type tear and some overlaying very frail fibrous-type tissue. At this time in this regard the meniscus was propalpated and otherwise unremarkable. There was no reciprocating wear about the medial tibial plateau other than some scant areas of grade 1 arthritic change. The intra-articular notch had an A-frame–type notch. Cruciate structures were otherwise unremarkable. In the lateral compartment, the meniscus was propalpated and unremarkable other than some scant fraying about the circumferential inner one-third, but this is nonpathologic. He also had frank fissuring of grade 2/3 qualities about the medial tibial plateau, but this was without abnormal excursion or redundancy and required no definitive other management. At this time in this regard, I had some difficulties in trying to inflate the patella through a very limited mini-arthrotomy procedure. We simply proceeded with the harvesting of one 6.5-mm graft. The graft was then further prepared on the back table, and at this time we debrided the margins of the defect, medial and femoral condyle followed by drilling, dilating, and implanting arthroscopically the graft. This restored the contour and profile of the articular surfaces. It was confirmed arthroscopically. There was some light debris from the shavings, which was also removed at this time, and with propalpation demonstrated that the defect of the condyle was restored to approximately 90% of its full weight-bearing surface being covered with articular cartilage. The minimal areas of exposed bleeding bone were basically a non–weight-bearing entity. I filled the defects in an excellent manner and created no eburnate type of abutment throughout its course of range of movement. On completion of this, portal sites were simply closed. Limited mini-arthrotomy portal site was closed. The patient was transported to the recovery room in a stable manner.

CPT Code(s): _____

ICD-10-CM Code(s): _____

Abstracting Questions

1. Was the procedure performed open or closed? _____

2. Was the harvesting of the autograft included in the procedure code? _____

Practice Exercise 17-10: Arthroscopy

Assign an external cause code to indicate how the injury occurred.

OPERATIVE REPORT

LOCATION: Outpatient, Hospital

PATIENT: Kristine Millermann

PREOPERATIVE DIAGNOSIS: Right shoulder possible biceps tendon injury, possible labral injury, possible rotator cuff tear.

POSTOPERATIVE DIAGNOSIS: Right shoulder biceps tendon tear.

SURGEON: Mohomad Almaz, MD

PROCEDURES PERFORMED

1. Right shoulder arthroscopy.

2. Open right biceps tenodesis.

CLINICAL HISTORY: This 26-year-old lady presents with a history of a right shoulder impingement type syndrome from several years ago. This had been operated on with an arthroscopy and had done well. About 2 months ago she began having increasing pain after sustaining a popping sensation within the shoulder. She had pain with continued supination. Biceps tests preoperatively were positive. An arthrogram was negative. After the risks and benefits of anesthesia and surgery were explained to the patient, a decision was made to undertake this procedure.

ANESTHESIA: Regional.

PROCEDURE: Under regional anesthetic, the patient was laid in the beach chair position on the operating table. The right shoulder was prepped and draped in usual fashion. The patient was given 1 gram of Cefazolin intravenously prior to surgery. A standard posterior arthroscopic portal was created and the camera introduced to the back of the joint. We had excellent visualization. An anterior portal was created using a switching stick technique, and the 7-mm cannula was then brought in from the front along with a blunt probe. Inspection of the articular surfaces showed no damage on the humerus or glenoid surfaces. There was some minor fraying of the anterior glenoid labrum. The biceps tendon was inspected and was found to have tearing through approximately 50% of the fiber structure. The biceps was then brought into the joint with the use of the probe and we could see that this extended through an area of approximately 2 cm. It was believed that this was the fundamental pathology. The rotator cuff was inspected. No further abnormalities could be identified on the humeral surface. The subacromial space was then entered through the posterior portal, and we could not see any damage to the rotator cuff on this surface.

Instruments were then removed from the joint. A lateral incision approximately 4 cm in length was made centered over the anterior aspect of the greater tuberosity. It was deepened through subcutaneous tissue to expose the deltoid fascia, which was then incised longitudinally and the deltoid bluntly split to expose the area of the bicipital groove. The biceps tendon was easily identified. The biceps tendon was then isolated and a suture was passed through it to hold its position. An arthroscopy camera was then placed into the posterior portal. The anterior portal was once again opened and the biceps was then transected using a scissors just near its attachment on the superior glenoid. The biceps was then brought in to the open wound laterally.

A drill hole was then made in the groove and two smaller drill holes proximally. A series of #5 Ethibond sutures were then woven through the biceps tendon. The four strands of suture were then brought in to the larger central hole and then two out on each side. The sutures were then tied onto themselves, pulling the biceps tendon into the large central hole to hold its position.

Once this was completed, the wound was irrigated with normal saline. The deltoid fascia was then repaired with 3–0 Vicryl suture. The skin was closed with Monocryl suture, and then the wound was dressed with Steri-Strips.

The wounds were then dressed with Mepore dressing and the arm placed in a Cryocuff sling. The patient was then awakened and placed on her hospital bed and taken to the recovery room in good condition. Estimated blood loss for the procedure was negligible. Sponge and needle counts were correct.

CPT Code(s): _____

ICD-10-CM Code(s): _____

Abstracting Questions

1. Would the diagnostic arthroscopy be reported in this case? _____

2. Was the tendon repair performed with an endoscope, or was it an open procedure? _____
   _____

3. According to the ICD-10-CM Index "Tear, tendon," you are to *see* this main term. _____
   _____

■ Respiratory System Subsection (30000-32999)

Anatomical site arrangement; such as:

- Nose
- Accessory Sinuses
- Larynx
- Trachea and Bronchi
- Lungs and Pleura

Further subdivided by procedure; such as:

- Incision
- Excision
- Endoscopy
- Repair

Endoscopy

Endoscopy in all subheadings except Nose

Each preceded by "Notes"

Endoscopy Rule One
Code full extent

> *Example:* Procedure begins at mouth and ends at bronchial tube

Bronchial tube = full extent

Endoscopy Rule Two
Code correct approach

> *Example:* For removal:
> - Interior lung lesion via endoscope inserted through mouth
> - Exterior lung lesion via endoscope inserted through skin into chest

Incorrect approach = incorrect code = incorrect reimbursement

Endoscopy Rule Three
Diagnostic endoscopy always included in surgical endoscopy

> *Examples:*
> - Diagnostic bronchial endoscopy begins
> - Identifies foreign body
> - Removed foreign body (surgical endoscopy)
> - Only surgical endoscopy reported

Multiple Procedures

Frequent in respiratory coding

- **Watch for bundled services**

Sequence primary procedure first, no modifier

Sequence secondary procedures next

Bilateral procedures often performed, use -50

Remember: Modifier -51 is not used in facility coding

Format for reporting chosen by payer

Example: Bilateral nasal lavage

- 31000-50

Nose (30000-30999)

Used extensively by otorhinolaryngologists (ear, nose, and throat [ENT] specialists)

Also wide variety of trained physicians in other specialties

Approach to nose

- External approach, use Integumentary System
- Internal approaches, use Respiratory System

Incision (30000, 30020)

Bundled into Incision codes are drain or gauze insertion and removal

Supplies reported separately

Excision (30100-30160)

Contains intranasal biopsy codes

Polyp excision coded by complexity

- Excision includes any method of destruction, even laser
- Use -50 (bilateral) for both sides

Turbinate excision and resection

- Three turbinates: Superior, middle, inferior as illustrated in Figure 17-6
- Excision of inferior turbinate, 30130
- Excision of superior or middle turbinate, 30999
- Submucous resection of inferior turbinate, 30140
  Reduction of inferior turbinates, 30140-52
- Submucous resection of superior or middle turbinate, 30999

Introduction (30200-30220)

Common procedures

> *Example:* Injections to shrink nasal tissue or displacement therapy (saline flushes) to remove mucus

Displacement therapy performed through nose

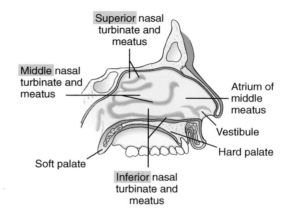

Figure **17-6** Superior, inferior, and middle nasal turbinates.

Removal of Foreign Body (30300-30320)

Distinguished by the site of removal, whether at office or in hospital (requires general anesthesia)

Repair (30400-30630)

Many plastic procedures, e.g.,

- Rhinoplasty (reshaping nose internal and/or external)
- Septoplasty (rearrangement or repair of nasal septum)

Destruction (30801-30802)

Use of ablation (removing by cutting)

Used for removal of excess nasal mucosa or to reduce inferior turbinate inflammation

Based on intramural or superficial extent of destruction

- **Intramural:** Deeper mucosa
- **Superficial:** Outer layer of mucosa

Other Procedures (30901-30999)

Control of nasal hemorrhage

- Packing
- Ligation
- Cauterization

Anterior packing for less severe bleeding

Posterior packing for more severe bleeding

Accessory Sinuses, Incision, Excision, Endoscopy (31000-31297)

Codes for lavage (washing) of sinuses

- Cannula (hollow tube) placed into sinus
- Sterile saline solution flushed through

Codes are divided by surgical approach: Incision, Excision, or Endoscopy

Procedures may involve multiple codes when multiple locations are accessed

> ***Example:*** 31020, sinusotomy, maxillary, can be coded with 31050 sinusotomy, sphenoid, and 31070 sinusotomy, frontal

Repair of fractures occurring during procedure may be coded separately if not included in code description

Use -50 (bilateral) for both sides

Maxillary sinusotomy may use an external and intranasal approach to creating passage between sinus and nose

- Used to clear blocked or infected sinus
- Intranasal sinusotomy, 31020
- External sinusotomy, radical (such as Caldwell-Luc)

  Access through mouth

  Incision above eyetooth

  Sinus is cleaned

  New opening created or existing opening enlarged

Larynx (31300-31599)

Excision (31300-31420)

Laryngotomy: Open surgical procedure to expose larynx

- For removal procedure (e.g., tumor)

May be confused with Trachea/Bronchi codes for tracheostomy used to establish air flow

Introduction (31500-31502)

Used to establish, maintain, and protect air flow

Endotracheal intubation, establishment of airway

Based on planned (ventilation support) or emergency procedure

Laryngoscopic (Endoscopy) Procedures (31505-31579)

Uses terms *indirect* and *direct*

- **Indirect:** Tongue depressor with mirror used to view larynx
- **Direct:** Endoscope passed into larynx, physician directly views vocal cords

Repair (31580-31590)

Several plastic procedures and fracture repair

Laryngoplasty procedures based on purpose

Fracture code is open reduction code

Trachea and Bronchi (31600-31899)

Incision (31600-31614)

Tracheostomy divided by

- Planned (ventilation support), based on age
- Emergency

Divided by type

- Transtracheal or cricothyroid (location of incision)

Endoscopy (31615-31661)

Bronchoscopy tube may be inserted into nose or mouth

Rigid endoscopy may be performed under general anesthesia

Flexible endoscopy usually performed under local or moderate (conscious) sedation

Bronchial Thermoplasty (31660, 31661)

- Treatment for severe asthma in which radiofrequency is utilized to produce heat in the airways that results in the reduction of the airway smooth muscles

Introduction (31717-31730)

Catheterization

Instillation

Aspiration

Tracheal tube placement

Excision/Repair (31750-31830)

Repairs of the trachea and bronchi

Lungs and Pleura (32035-32999)

Incision (32035-32225)
Thoracotomy
Surgical opening of chest to expose to view; used for

- Biopsy
- Cyst
- Foreign body removal
- Cardiac massage, etc.

Excision/Removal (32310-32540)
Biopsy codes in both Excision and Incision categories

- Excisional biopsy with percutaneous needle
- Incisional biopsy with chest open

Also services of pleurectomy, pneumocentesis, and lung removal

- **Segmentectomy:** 1 segment
- **Lobectomy:** 1 lobe
- **Bilobectomy:** 2 lobes
- **Total Pneumonectomy:** 1 lung

Introduction and Removal (32550-32557)
Thoracentesis
Needle inserted into pleural space for aspiration (withdrawal) of fluid and/or air (32554, 32557)

Pleural Drainage
Permanent catheter for drainage placed

- Insertion of indwelling tunneled pleural catheter (removal 32552)
- Tube thoracostomy
- Placement of interstitial device(s) for radiation therapy guidance
- Thoracentesis and percutaneous pleural drainage

Destruction (32560-32562)

- Chemical pleurodesis
- Fibrinolysis, initial day, subsequent day

▪ Cardiovascular System Subsection (33010-37799)

Cardiology Coding Terminology

Both Medicine and Surgery sections contain invasive procedures

Invasive: Enters body by the following methods

- Incision

  Example: Opening chest for removal (e.g., tumor on heart)
- Percutaneous
  - Wire threaded through needle placed through skin into vessel and catheter placed over wire

  Example: PTCA (percutaneous transluminal coronary angioplasty) procedure
  - Cut down—small nick made into vessel under direct vision and catheter inserted

  Example: Catheter inserted into femoral or brachial artery

Common catheters are

- Broviac
- Hickman
- HydroCath
- Arrow multi-lumen
- Groshong
- Dual-lumen
- Triple-lumen

Noninvasive: Procedures that do not break skin

Example: Electrocardiogram

Electrophysiology (EPS): Study of electrical system of heart

Example: Study of irregular heartbeat (arrhythmia)

Nuclear Cardiology: Diagnostic and treatment specialty; uses radioactive substances to diagnose cardiac conditions

Example: Myocardial perfusion and cardiac blood pooling imaging studies

Codes for Procedures

Heart/Pericardium (33010-33999)

- Pacemakers, valve disorders

Arteries/Veins (34001-37799)

◆ Heart/Pericardium (33010-33999)

Both percutaneous and open surgical

- Cardiologists often use percutaneous intervention; cardiovascular or thoracic surgeons often use open surgical procedures

Extensive notes throughout

Frequent changes with medical advances

Examples of categories of Heart/Pericardium subheading

- Pericardium
- Cardiac Tumor
- Pacemaker or Implantable Defibrillator

Examples of services

- Pericardiocentesis: Percutaneous withdrawal of fluid from pericardial space (pericarditis) (33010-33011)
- Cardiac Tumor: Open surgical procedure for removal of tumor on heart (33130)

Pacemaker and Implantable Defibrillator (33202-33273)

Devices that assist heart in electrical function

- Differentiate between temporary and permanent devices
- Differentiate between one-chamber and dual-chamber devices

Divided by where pacer placed, approach, and type of service

Patient record indicates revision or replacement

- Pacemaker pulse generator is also called a battery
- Pacemaker leads are also called electrodes
- Usual follow-up 90 days (global period)

Placed

Atrium (single chamber)

- Pulse generator and one or more electrodes in atrium (single-chamber pacemaker)

Ventricle (single chamber)

- Pulse generator and one or more electrodes in ventricle (single-chamber pacemaker)

Both (dual chamber)

- Pulse generator and one electrode in right ventricle and one electrode in right atrium

Biventricular, right ventricle and coronary sinus

- Pulse generator and one electrode(s) in right ventricle, one electrode(s) may be placed in right atrium, and one electrode in the coronary sinus over left ventricle

Approach

Epicardial: Open procedure to place electrodes on heart

Transvenous: Through vein to place in heart (endoscopic)

Type of Service

Initial placement or replacement of all or part of device

Number of leads placed is important in code selection

Electrophysiologic Operative Procedures (33250-33266)

Surgeon repairs defect causing abnormal rhythm

Chest opened to full view

- Cardiopulmonary (CP) bypass usually used

Endoscopy procedure

- Without cardiopulmonary bypass

Codes based on reason for procedure and if CP bypass used (inpatient only)

Patient-Activated Event Recorder (33282, 33284)

Also known as cardiac event recorder or loop recorder

Internal surgical implantation required

Divided based on whether device is being implanted or removed

Cardiac Valves (33361-33478)

Divided by valve

- Aortic, mitral, tricuspid, pulmonary

Subdivided by whether replacement, repair, or resection and use of bypass machine

33361-33369 report transcatheter aortic valve replacement and implant

Coronary Artery Bypass Graft (CABG)

CABG performed for bypassing severely obstructed coronary arteries (atherosclerosis or arteriosclerosis)

Performed only on an inpatient basis

Determine what was used in repair

- Vein (33510-33516)
- Artery (33533-33548)
- Both artery and vein (33517-33530)

Based on number of bypass grafts performed and if combined venous and arterial grafts are used

Venous Grafting Only for Coronary Artery Bypass (33510-33516)

Based on number of grafts being replaced

> *Example:* Three venous grafts = 33512

Combined Arterial-Venous Grafting (33517-33530)

Divided based on number of grafts and whether initial procedure or reoperation

Procuring saphenous vein included, unless performed endoscopically

These codes are never used alone

Arterial-Venous codes (33517-33523) report only **venous** graft portion of procedure

Always used with Arterial Grafting codes (33533-33536)

> *Example:* 3 vein grafts and 2 arterial grafts = 33519 and 33534

Open procurement of saphenous vein is included in procedure (not coded separately)

Code harvesting of saphenous vein graft separately when endoscopic video-assisted procurement is performed (33508)

Code harvesting separately for upper extremity or femoral vessels

Arterial Grafting for Coronary Artery Bypass (33533-33548)

Divided based on number of grafts

Obtaining artery for grafting included in codes, except

- Procuring upper-extremity artery (i.e., radial artery), coded separately (35600)

Several codes (33542-33548) for myocardial resection, repair of ventricular septal defect (VSD), and ventricular restoration

Endovascular Repair of Descending Thoracic Aorta (33880-33891)

Placement of an endovascular aortic prosthesis for repair of descending thoracic aorta

- Less invasive than traditional approach of chest or abdominal incision

Synthetic aortic prosthesis placed via catheter

- Report fluoroscopic guidance separately (75956-75959)

Fluoroscopic guidance codes include diagnostic imaging prior to placement and intraprocedurally

Stent-graft (endoprosthesis) is deployed to reinforce weakened area

Extracorporeal Membrane Oxygenation and Extracorporeal Life Support Services (33946-33989)

Cardiac and/or respiratory support to the heart and/or lungs

- Provide cardiac and respiratory support for patients whose heart and lungs are diseased or damaged beyond function

Arteries and Veins Subheading (34001-37799)

Only for noncoronary vessels

- Divided based on whether artery or vein involved

  > *Example:* Different codes for embolectomy, depending on whether artery or vein involved

Catheters placed into vessels for monitoring, removal, repair

Nonselective or selective catheter placement

- **Nonselective:** Direct placement without further manipulation
- **Selective:** Place and then manipulate into further order(s)
  - Selective placement includes nonselective placement

Catheter placement example

- **Nonselective:** 36000, Introduction of needle into vein
- **Selective:** 36012, Placement of catheter into second-order venous system

Vascular Families Are Like a Tree

First-order (main) branch (tree trunk)

Second-order branch (tree limb)

Third-order branch (tree branch)

Brachiocephalic vascular family (Figure 17-7)

- Report farthest extent of catheter placement in a vascular family; labor intensity is increased with the extent of catheter placement

Embolectomy and Thrombectomy (34001-34490)

Embolus: Dislodged thrombus

Thrombus: Mass of material in vessel located in place of formation

- May be removed by dissection or balloon

Balloon: Threaded into vessel, inflated under mass, pulled out with mass

- Codes are divided by site of incision and artery/vein

Venous Reconstruction (34501-34530)

Types of Repairs

- Valve of the femoral vein
- Vena cava
- Saphenopopliteal vein anastomosis

Aneurysm

Aneurysm: Weakened arterial wall causing a bulge or ballooning

Repair by removal, bypass, or coil placement

Endovascular repair (34800-34900) from inside vessel

Direct (35001-35152) from outside vessel

Endovascular Repair of Abdominal Aortic Aneurysm (34800-34834)

Performed only on an inpatient basis

Fenestrated Endovascular Repair of the Visceral and Intrarenal Aorta (34839-34848)

A perforated stent that improves anastomosis to other vessels

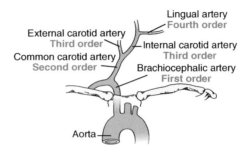

Figure **17-7** Brachiocephalic vascular family with first-, second-, third-, and fourth-order vessels.

Repair Arteriovenous Fistula (35180-35190)

Abnormal passage from artery or vein

Divided based on fistula type

- Congenital, acquired/traumatic, by site

Angioplasty (35450-35476)

Divided by whether open or percutaneous and by vessel

- **Transluminal:** By way of vessel
- **Transluminal Angioplasty:** Catheter passed into vessel and a balloon is inflated to crush/flatten fatty deposits in vessel
  - Placement of eluting or non-eluting stents coded in addition to catheter placement

Noncoronary Bypass Grafts (35500-35671)

Divided by

- Vein
- In Situ Vein (veins repaired in their original place)
- Other Than Vein

Code by type of graft and vessels being used to bypass

> *Example:* 35506, Bypass graft, with vein; carotid-subclavian

- Graft attached to carotid and to subclavian, bypassing defect of subclavian

Procurement of saphenous vein graft is included and not reported separately

Harvesting of upper-extremity vein (35500) or femoropopliteal vein (35572) is reported separately

Vascular Injection Procedures (36000-36598)

Divided into

- Intravenous
- Intra-Arterial—Intra-Aortic
- Venous
- Central Venous Access Procedures

Used for many procedures, including

- Local anesthesia
- Introduction of needle
- Injection of contrast material
- Preinjection and postinjection care related to injection procedure
  > *Example:* Injection of opaque substance for venography (radiography of vein)
- Bypass grafts are performed only on an inpatient basis
- Harvesting of veins for bypass grafts can be performed on outpatient basis

Central Venous Access (CVA) Procedures

Long-term use for medication/chemotherapy administration and short-term use for monitoring

Approach

Central: jugular, subclavian, femoral vein, or vena cava

Peripheral: basilic or cephalic vein

Categories

1. Insertion
2. Repair

3. Replacement, partial or complete

4. Removal

5. Other central venous access procedures

6. Guidance for vascular access

Insertion (36555-36571)

Insertion of newly established venous access

- Tunneled under skin (e.g., Hickman, Broviac, Groshong)
- Nontunneled (e.g., PICC)
- Central (e.g., subclavian, internal jugular, femoral, inferior vena cava)
- Peripheral (basilic or cephalic vein)

Codes divided by tunneled/non-tunneled, with port or without port, central/peripheral, and age

Repair (36575, 36576)

Repair of malfunction without replacement with or without subcutaneous port or pump

Repair of central venous access device

No differentiation between age of patient or central/peripheral insertion

Replacement (Partial or Complete) (36578-36585)

Partial (36578) is replacement of catheter only

Complete (36580-36585) is replacement through same venous access site

Differentiated by tunneled/non-tunneled, central/peripheral, and with or without subcutaneous port or pump

Removal (36589, 36590)

To be used for tunneled catheter

Removal of non-tunneled catheter is not reported separately

Other Central Venous Access Procedures (36591-36598)

Collection of blood specimen

Declotting of catheter or access device by thrombolytic agent

Mechanical removal of obstructive material from around catheter or within lumen

Guidance for Vascular Access

77001, fluoroscopic guidance for central venous access device placement, replacement, or removal

Reported in addition to primary procedure

76937, ultrasound guidance for vascular access

Reported in addition to primary procedure

Transcatheter Procedures (37184-37218)

Arterial mechanical thrombectomy (37184-37186)

- Removal of thrombus by means of mechanical device

    From artery or arterial bypass graft

Venous mechanical thrombectomy (37187-37188)

- Removal of a thrombus by means of a mechanical device

    From vein

Arterial and venous mechanical thrombectomy may be performed as primary procedure or add-on

- Includes

  Introduction of device into thrombus

  Thrombus removal

  Injection of thrombolytic drug(s), if used

  Fluoroscopic and contrast guidance, and interpretation

  Follow-up angiography

- Report separately

  Diagnostic angiography

  Catheter placement(s)

  Diagnostic studies

  Pharmacologic thrombolytic infusion before or after (37211-37214, 75898)

  Other interventions

Other Procedures (37195-37218)

- Used to report a variety of transcatheter procedures

  Example: Transcatheter biopsy therapy infusion for thrombolysis or antispasmotic treatment of a vessel, retrieval of foreign object, occlusion or embolization, and intravascular stents

  Endovascular Revascularization (Open or Percutaneous, Transcatheter) (37220-37325)

■ Hemic and Lymphatic System Subsection (38100-38999)

Divisions

- Spleen
- General
- Lymph Nodes and Lymphatic Channels

Spleen Subheading (38100-38200)

Spleen easily ruptured, causing massive and potentially lethal hemorrhage

- Excision

Splenectomy: Total or partial/open or laparoscopic

Often done as part of more major procedure and bundled into major procedure

- Repair
- Laparoscopy

General (38204-38243)

Bone Marrow

Codes divided based on

- Preservation
- Preparation
- Purification
- Aspiration
- Biopsy
- Harvesting
- Transplantation

Hematopoietic Progenitor Cell (HPC)

- Obtained from bone marrow, peripheral blood apheresis, umbilical cord blood

Types of Stem Cells

Allogenic: Same species (38240)

Autologous: Patient's own (38241)

Lymph Nodes and Lymphatic Channels Subheading (38300-38999)

Two types of lymphadenectomies

- **Limited:** For example, lymph nodes only for staging
- **Radical:** For example, lymph nodes and surrounding tissue

Often bundled into more major procedure (e.g., prostatectomy)

Do not unbundle and report lymphadenectomy separately

Mediastinum and Diaphragm Subsection (39000-39499)

Mediastinum (39000-39499)

Incision codes for foreign body removal, biopsy, or drainage

Excision codes for removal of cyst or tumor

All procedures, except for 39401, 39402 (mediastinoscopy), are performed on an inpatient basis

Diaphragm (39501-39599)

Only two categories: Repair and Other Procedures

Includes hernia and laceration repairs

PRACTICE EXERCISES

Practice Exercise 17-11: Aspiration and Biopsy

OPERATIVE REPORT

LOCATION: Outpatient, Hospital

PATIENT: Oliver Ganz

INDICATION:

1. Hypoproliferative anemia.

2. Development of lymphoma.

3. Aplastic anemia.

4. Myelodysplastic syndrome versus effective medications.

SURGEON: Edward Riddle, MD

PROCEDURE PERFORMED: Bone marrow aspiration and biopsy.

The need to perform the procedure, benefits, risks, and associated side effects were explained to the patient. Questions and concerns were answered. Informed consent has been obtained.

PROCEDURE: The patient was placed on his right lateral side. The left posterior iliac crest area was prepped by sterilizing the skin with Betadine. Local anesthesia with lidocaine was given. In addition, he received Versed 5 mg and fentanyl 50 mcg. After local anesthesia with lidocaine, a Jamshidi needle was inserted and approximately 4 mL of bone marrow aspirate and about 1.5 cm core biopsy were obtained. The patient tolerated the procedure well without any significant side effects. The specimen will be evaluated for morphology, flow cytometry, and cytogenetics.

Pathology Report Later Indicated: Nonmalignant cells found in bone marrow.

CPT Code(s): _____

ICD-10-CM Code(s): _____

Abstracting Questions

1. Were the aspiration and biopsy reported separately? _____

2. What conditions are reported to support the medical necessity for this biopsy? _____
_____

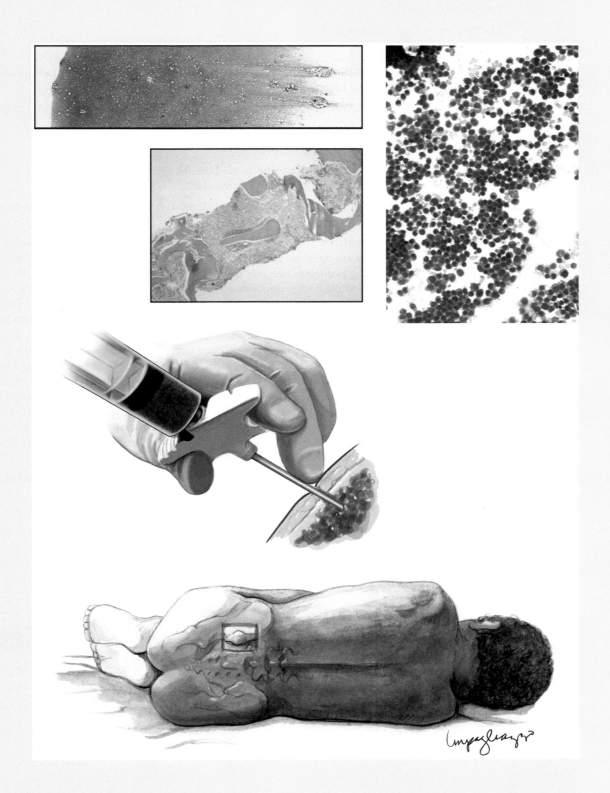

Practice Exercise 17-12: Bronchoscopy

OPERATIVE REPORT

LOCATION: Outpatient, Hospital

PATIENT: Anthony Radel

PREOPERATIVE DIAGNOSIS: Bilateral lower lobe ground-glass opacities and infiltrates consistent with possible interstitial lung disease.

POSTOPERATIVE DIAGNOSIS: Same.

SURGEON: Gregory Dawson, MD

PROCEDURE PERFORMED: Bronchoscopy.

Informed consent was obtained prior to the procedure. The patient was explained the risks, benefits, complications, and other options of the procedure.

Prior to the procedure, the patient was given codeine along with atropine to decrease the heart rate and suppress the cough reflex.

PROCEDURE: Topical anesthesia was applied with local lidocaine spray and also intranasal cocaine mix for the local vasocongestion and for local anesthesia. The procedure was performed in the fluoroscopy unit. The bronchoscope was introduced through the nostril and negotiated into the upper airway. The vocal cords were visualized. Vocal cords were moving equally with phonation and respiration. There was no abnormality found in the upper airway. Then the bronchoscope was negotiated through the vocal cords into the trachea and along the major airways. The airways all seemed to be pretty normal actually. There was no inflammation there. There were no endobronchial lesions. All the major bronchi to tertiary branches were visualized, and no endobronchial lesions were noted. Right upper, middle, and lower lobe bronchi and right main to the subsegmental branches were visualized, and no endobronchial lesions were noted. Again, the left main, left upper lingula, and lower lobe branches of the subsegmental branches were visualized, and no endobronchial lesions noted. Airway mucosa was completely normal. The bronchoscope was wedged into the right lower lobe; specimens were collected with brushings, washings, and bronchioalveolar lavage; and transbronchial biopsies were performed from the right lower lobe and the right middle lobe in one side.

The patient tolerated it pretty well; actually, it was an uneventful procedure. He will be monitored in the recovery room for a couple of hours and then will be discharged.

During the procedure, blood pressure, oxygen saturation, and EKG were continuously monitored and were uneventful. There was minor oozing in the first lobe, but was able to be controlled with local epinephrine instillation. It was an uneventful procedure.

Pathology Report Later Indicated: Benign specimens from the right lower lobe.

CPT Code(s): _____

ICD-10-CM Code(s): _____

Abstracting Questions

1. What procedures were performed during the bronchoscopy? _____

2. What was the approach for the biopsies? _____

3. Would the actual lobe biopsied affect CPT code selection? _____

Practice Exercise 17-13: Pulmonary Function Study

LOCATION: Outpatient, Hospital

PATIENT: Brad Nord

PHYSICIAN: Gregory Dawson, MD

ENTRANCE DIAGNOSIS: Hypoxia, short of breath walking more than 100 yards, wheezes, 58.5 pack-year history of smoking, gave good effort; however, because he has a hip fracture, we could not get him in the body box, so we could not get most of the test.

INTERPRETATION

1. Flow volume loop shows significant concavity toward the volume axis, well-preserved inspiratory limb, and reduced flow rates of a significant degree.

2. There is no statistical significant change after bronchodilator.

3. Plethysmographic lung volumes could not be done.

4. Single-breath lung volumes are normal.

5. There is evidence of dynamic airway collapse (air trapping), which can be seen with obstructive disease.

6. DLCO was only 24% of predicted, which is quite reduced, suggesting reduced alveolar capillary membrane surface area and/or V/Q mismatching.

7. Pre-bronchodilator flow rates show a pattern consistent with obstructive disease of a moderate degree.

8. Post-bronchodilator values show no significant change and the same conclusions can be reached.

9. The MVV is actually normal pre- and post-bronchodilator and between that and only a mildly abnormal FEV_1, I would expect only a mildly abnormal exercise tolerance.

10. Airway resistance could not be done.

The DLCO is reduced way out of proportion to reduction in flow rates, as is the patient's complaint of being short of breath walking less than 100 yards. It does not match the patient's defects seen on spirometry. Other causes should be looked for. Clinical correlation should, of course, be used.

CPT Code(s): _____

ICD-10-CM Code(s): _____

Abstracting Questions

1. Would this study be reported with only one CPT code? _____

2. Would the pre- and post-bronchodilator administration affect the spirometry code selection? _____

3. What do the following represent?

   a. DLCO _____

   b. MVV _____

   c. FEV _____

4. Would the measurement of the carbon monoxide be reported separately from the spirometry? _____

5. Was there evidence of air trapping, determined via thoracic gas volume testing? _____

6. How would the "could not be done" procedures affect coding? _____

7. Was there a definitive diagnosis established and reported? _____

Practice Exercise 17-14: Right Chest Tube Placement

LOCATION: Outpatient, Hospital

PATIENT: Peter Nelson

EXAMINATION OF: Ultrasound-guided placement of a right chest tube.

PHYSICIAN: Gregory Dawson, MD

CLINICAL SYMPTOMS: Right pleural effusion.

ULTRASOUND-GUIDED PLACEMENT OF RIGHT CHEST TUBE: Informed consent was obtained. The patient was sat upright and his right back was prepped and draped in the usual sterile fashion. Skin and subcutaneous tissues were infiltrated with 1% lidocaine. Under ultrasound guidance, a 5 French Yueh catheter was placed into the right pleural fluid. Sixty milliliters of fluid was aspirated and sent to the lab for requested analysis. Over a 0.035 Amplatz guidewire, the Yueh catheter was exchanged for an 8.5 French Dawson-Mueller pigtail catheter. The catheter was secured to the skin with 2–0 Ethilon suture. The drainage catheter was placed to Pleur-evac suction.

The patient received conscious sedation. Signs were monitored throughout the exam. He tolerated the procedure well and left in stable condition.

Pathology Report Later Indicated: Normal right pleural fluid.

CPT Code(s): _____

ICD-10-CM Code(s): _____

Abstracting Questions

1. Could the procedure performed in this case be considered a thoracostomy? _____
   _____

2. Does the utilization of a water seal affect the CPT code reported? _____

3. Was the ultrasound guidance reported separately? _____

Practice Exercise 17-15: Central Venous Placement

OPERATIVE REPORT

LOCATION: Outpatient, Hospital

PATIENT: Harriet Smith

SURGEON: George Orbitz, MD

PROCEDURE PERFORMED: Tunneled triple-lumen central venous catheter.

ANESTHESIA: 1% lidocaine was used as a local anesthetic.

INDICATION: Intravascular access for dialysis because of acute renal failure.

PROCEDURE: After the procedure and its possible complications were explained and consent was obtained from the patient (age 46), she was prepped for left internal jugular tunneled triple-lumen catheter placement.

The area was sterilized using a standard Chloraprep solution. Sterile drapes were then applied around the area in the usual fashion. Under direct ultrasonographic guidance, an introducer needle was used to cannulate the patient's left internal jugular: Once in place, the J-tipped guidewire was inserted through the needle and advanced without any difficulty. The needle was subsequently removed. A small skin incision was made at the insertion site. A peel-away sheath with an internal dilator was then inserted over the guidewire using Seldinger technique. The guidewire was subsequently removed. The tunnel was created about 3 inches away from the internal jugular insertion site, below the left clavicle using a Hawkins needle. Once the tunnel was created, then the J-tipped guidewire was placed through the Hawkins needle. The Hawkins needle was subsequently removed. The preflushed 30-cm triple lumen Arrow catheter was then inserted through the tunnel over the guidewire. Once the catheter was through the tunnel, the guidewire was removed. The tip of the catheter was then inserted into the peel-away sheath up to the 23-cm mark. The peel-away sheath was then subsequently removed. The triple-lumen catheter was then secured into place using 2–0 sutures. Steri-Strips were then applied to the internal jugular insertion site.

The patient tolerated the procedure well. A subsequent chest x-ray showed that the tip of the catheter was well into the left atrium. The catheter was then subsequently withdrawn about 2 cm so that the tip was within the area of the superior vena cava.

There was minimal bleeding. There were no acute complications.

CPT Code(s): _____

ICD-10-CM Code(s): _____

Abstracting Questions

1. Was the procedure performed in this case a tunneled catheter placement? _____
   _____

2. Does the age of the patient affect the CPT code selection? _____

3. Does the site of the catheter placement affect the CPT code selection? _____

4. What was the medical condition treated that required placement of the central line? _____
   _____

■ Digestive System Subsection (40490-49999)

Divided by anatomical site from mouth to anus + organs that aid digestive process

Example: Liver and gallbladder

Many bundled procedures

Endoscopy

Diagnostic endoscopy is always bundled into a surgical endoscopy

Code to furthest extent of procedure

Endoscopy Terminology

Notes define specific terminology

Code descriptions are specific regarding

- Technique and depth of scope

  Esophagoscopy: Esophagus only

  Esophagogastroscopy: Esophagus and past diaphragm

  Esophagogastroduodenoscopy: Esophagus and beyond pyloric channel

- Proctosigmoidoscopy: Rectum and sigmoid colon (6-25 cm)

- Sigmoidoscopy: Entire rectum, sigmoid colon, and may include part of descending colon (26-60 cm)

- Colonoscopy: Entire colon, rectum to cecum, and may include terminal ileum (greater than 60 cm)

Laparoscopy and Endoscopy

Some subheadings have both laparoscopy (outside) and endoscopy (inside) procedures

Example: Subheading Esophagus

- Endoscopy views inside

- Laparoscopy—scope inserted through umbilicus; views from outside

- Adjustment during 90-day post-op period included in surgery

Hemorrhoidectomy and Fistulectomy Codes (46200-46320)

Divided by

- Location
  - Internal
  - External
- Complexity
  - Simple: No repair procedure involved
  - Complex: Includes repair procedure and fissurectomy
- Anatomy
  - Subcutaneous: No muscle involvement
  - Submuscular: Sphincter muscle
  - Complex fistulectomy involves excision/incision of multiple fistulas

Hernia Codes (49491-49659)

Divided by

- Type of hernia

Example: Inguinal, femoral, incisional, ventral

- Initial or subsequent repair
- Age of patient
- Clinical presentation:
  - **Strangulated:** Blood supply cut off
  - **Incarcerated:** Cannot be returned to cavity (not reducible)

Additional code is used for implantation of mesh or prosthesis for incisional or ventral hernias only

- Open or laparoscopic surgical approaches

PRACTICE EXERCISES

Practice Exercise 17-16: Colonoscopy with Polypectomy

OPERATIVE REPORT

LOCATION: Outpatient, Hospital

PATIENT: Mark Hall

INDICATION: Colon polyps noted on screening flexible sigmoidoscopy.

POSTOPERATIVE DIAGNOSES

1. Colon polyps.

2. Diverticular disease.

SCOPE USED: Pentax video colonoscope.

SURGEON: Daniel Olanka, MD

PREOPERATIVE MEDICATIONS: Demerol 50 mg IV; Versed 3 mg IV.

Informed consent was obtained after the patient was explained the risks, benefits, and alternatives to the procedure.

PHYSICAL EXAMINATION: Blood pressure is 163/82. Pulse is 58. Abdomen is nondistended and nontender. Neurologic: The patient is alert and oriented. No focal signs. Lungs are clear to auscultation. Respirations are unlabored. Coronary: Regular rate and rhythm.

FINDINGS: The scope was passed under direct vision and advanced through the colon to the cecum. The ileocecal valve and appendiceal orifice were well visualized. The cecum, ascending colon, and transverse colon were all found to be normal. There was moderately severe diverticular disease in the descending and sigmoid colon. There was a very large, 3-cm pedunculated mass in the mid-descending colon. Most of this was removed by snare electrocautery. The rest of the rather broad base of the polyp was then injected with saline and again removed by snare technique. The rest of the descending colon was normal. In the sigmoid colon, there was a 5-mm sessile polyp removed by hot biopsy. Sigmoid colon is otherwise unremarkable. Rectum was normal.

IMPRESSION

1. Mid-descending colon polyp measuring approximately 3 cm in diameter. This was removed by piecemeal by snare electrocautery after the base of the polyp was injected with saline.

2. Five-millimeter sessile polyp of the sigmoid colon removed by hot biopsy.

3. Moderately severe diverticular disease.

RECOMMENDATIONS

1. Follow up the results of the biopsy to ensure that there is no invasion of the stock of the polyp. Repeat the biopsies. There was no stock invasion. Next colonoscopy in 3 years' time.

2. Metamucil or Citrucel one tablespoon daily for diverticular disease.

3. The patient education and handout on diverticular disease.

Pathology Report Later Indicated: Benign tissue.

CPT Code(s): _____

ICD-10-CM Code(s): _____

Abstracting Question

1. What techniques were used for polyp removal in this case? _____
_____

Polyps of Colon

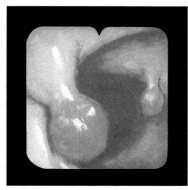

Multiple pedunculated polyps

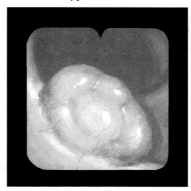

Sessile polyp
(may be multiheaded)

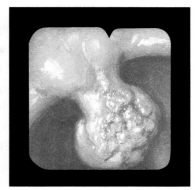

Polyp with area of
malignant transformation

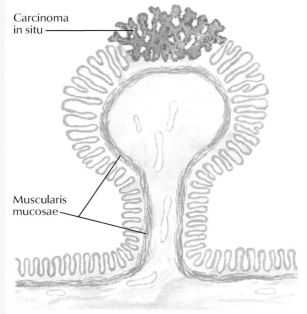

Carcinoma
in situ

Muscularis
mucosae

If carcinomatous involvement of polyp has not
penetrated muscularis mucosae, it is classified
as "carcinoma in situ," and simple endoscopic
removal by fulgurating snare is believed adequate

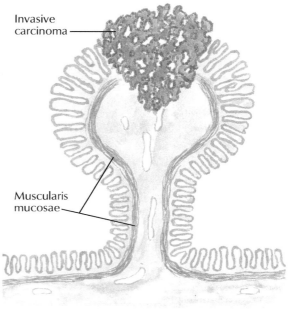

Invasive
carcinoma

Muscularis
mucosae

If pathologic examination of specimen shows
tumor to have penetrated muscularis mucosae,
it is classified as "invasive carcinoma," and more
extensive surgery is indicated

Pedunculated polyps are
removed endoscopically
by encircling pedicle
with wire snare and
applying fulgurating
current

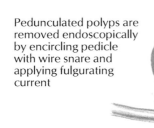

Sessile polyps may be
removed by successive
bites with snare and
fulgurating current in
one or more sessions

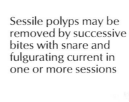

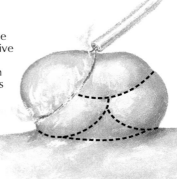

Practice Exercise 17-17: Sigmoidoscopy

OPERATIVE REPORT

LOCATION: Outpatient, Hospital

PATIENT: Lorretta Hatfield

PREOPERATIVE DIAGNOSIS: Diarrhea.

POSTOPERATIVE DIAGNOSIS: Mild resolving patchy colitis, nonspecific, probably infectious. The patient should still be worked up for fever as the colitis may not be the cause of the fever.

SURGEON: Larry Friendly, MD

PROCEDURE PERFORMED: Flexible sigmoidoscopy.

INDICATIONS: 42-year-old white female with SLE and chronic renal failure on hemodialysis who has had diarrhea since returning from her vacation where she was hospitalized. Her stools were negative. She did well, but on the day of discharge she began having diarrhea again and was readmitted today. She has had only one stool within the last four hours. The stools mostly seem to be nocturnal. She has had no antibiotics recently, no one else is ill.

FINDINGS: The Pentax videosigmoidoscope was inserted without difficulty to 50 cm. Careful inspection of the mid and distal descending, sigmoid, and rectum revealed patchy erythema, minimal friability, and some mild edema. There was no discrete ulceration, no exudate. No biopsies were obtained. The patient tolerated the procedure well.

IMPRESSION: Mild patchy colitis that appears to be resolving, consistent with infectious colitis.

PLAN: The diarrhea is slowly resolving and probably will resolve spontaneously. We will check the stools but no treatment for now unless she continues to be symptomatic; if so, I would give her ciprofloxacin.

CPT Code(s): _____

ICD-10-CM Code(s): _____

Abstracting Questions

1. According to the CPT definition of a sigmoidoscopy, does the documentation in this report support the reporting of a sigmoidoscopy? _____

2. Does the designation as a flexible sigmoidoscopy affect assignment of the CPT code? _____
_____

3. Does the fact that "no biopsies" were taken affect CPT code selection? _____

4. What does SLE stand for? _____

5. Define the following terms from this case.

   a. Erythema _____

   b. Friability _____

   c. Edema _____

   d. Exudate _____

Practice Exercise 17-18: Hernia Repair

OPERATIVE REPORT

LOCATION: Outpatient, Hospital

PATIENT: Thad Mark

PREOPERATIVE DIAGNOSIS: Left inguinal hernia.

POSTOPERATIVE DIAGNOSIS: Left indirect inguinal hernia.

SURGEON: Loren White, MD

PROCEDURE PERFORMED: Left inguinal hernia repair with large Prolene hernia graft.

ANESTHESIA: General.

INDICATION: The patient is a 32-year-old gentleman with a symptomatic left groin hernia, who presents today for elective repair, understands surgery and the risk for bleeding, infection, possible damage to the spermatic cord, and possible postoperative fluid collections, and he wishes to proceed.

PROCEDURE: The patient was brought to the operating room, placed under general anesthesia, and prepped and draped sterilely with Betadine solution. A left groin incision was made with a #10 blade, and dissection was carried down through subcutaneous tissues using electrocautery. External oblique was identified and opened along its fibers down to the external ring. Spermatic cord was isolated and looped with a Penrose drain. Hernia sac and cord lipoma were dissected free from the cord. These were reduced. A large Prolene hernia system patch was then placed with the underlay patch going through the patulous internal ring and lying underneath the transversalis fascia. The overlay patch was then tacked superiorly to the conjoined tendon, inferiorly to the inguinal ligament and medially to the fascia overlying the pubic tubercle. We had cut a slit in the overlay patch so that the cord could exit through. The external oblique was then closed with a running 3–0 Vicryl. We anesthetized the wound with 30 cc of 0.5% Sensorcaine with epinephrine solution and closed the skin with subcuticular 4–0 undyed Vicryl. Steri-Strips and sterile Band-Aids were applied. All sponge and needle counts were correct. He tolerated this well and was taken to the recovery room in stable condition.

Pathology Report Later Indicated: Mesothelial-lined fibrovascular tissue with skeletal muscle, consistent with left inguinal hernia.

CPT Code(s): _____

ICD-10-CM Code(s): _____

Abstracting Questions

1. Was the repair performed open or via endoscope? _____

2. Would the location of the hernia affect CPT code selection? _____

3. Would age affect CPT code selection? _____

4. What three other factors would affect CPT code selection? _____

5. Would the mesh repair be reported separately? _____

6. What factors would affect the diagnosis coding? _____

Practice Exercise 17-19: Cholangiopancreatogram and Sphincterotomy

OPERATIVE REPORT

LOCATION: Outpatient, Hospital

PATIENT: Brenda Langford

PREOPERATIVE DIAGNOSIS: Severe abdominal pain and elevated liver enzymes.

POSTOPERATIVE DIAGNOSIS: Same.

SURGEON: Loren White, MD

PROCEDURES PERFORMED

1. Endoscopic retrograde cholangiopancreatogram.

2. Endoscopic retrograde pancreatic sphincterotomy with removal of sludge.

INDICATION: This is a 23-year-old white female who is admitted with severe abdominal pain and elevated liver enzymes. Her alkaline phosphatase was 120. Bilirubin 1.8. AST 42. ALT 282. Amylase normal at 18. Lipase normal at 1. The patient had an ultrasound that showed normal size ducts, but there was evidence for possible cholelithiasis. The patient's alkaline phosphatase has risen to 154 and bilirubin now to 4. AST down to 106. ALT down to 284. The patient continues to have pain.

PREOPERATIVE MEDICATION

1. Demerol 75 mg.

2. Versed 6 mg.

3. Atropine 0.4 mg IV.

FINDINGS: The Pentax video duodenoscope was inserted without difficulty into the oropharynx. The stomach was rapidly viewed, and no lesions were seen. The pylorus was intubated and the endoscope was advanced to the second duodenum. Immediately seen was a fairly normal-appearing ampulla. There was a slight amount of heme on the surface. The first duct cannulated was the pancreatic duct. The pancreatic head, body, and tail were normal in size and course. There were no filling defects. The next duct cannulated was the common bile duct. The common bile duct was normal in size. There were no filling defects initially seen, except perhaps one air bubble after sphincterotomy was performed. We did perform a pancreatic sphincterotomy because the patient had continued in pain and elevated/rising bilirubin. She was obese, and the fluoroscopic imaging was suboptimal because of this. The ducts were not dilated.

As mentioned, a 1-cm sphincterotomy was performed. We then inserted a 1-cm balloon and pulled the balloon through the opening four times and took occlusion cholangiograms each time. The first time we pulled the balloon through there was some sludge present, dark color material, but other subsequent films did not reveal any filling defects and no other sludge was pulled out. The patient tolerated the procedure well without sequelae.

IMPRESSION: Normal pancreatogram and normal cholangiogram without initially any stones. A 1-cm sphincterotomy was performed and sludge was removed.

PLAN: The patient will have her amylase and liver enzymes checked in the morning. She should be able to undergo an attempt at laparoscopic cholecystectomy in the morning.

CPT Code(s): _____

ICD-10-CM Code(s): _____

Abstracting Questions

1. Would the sphincterotomy be reported separately? _____

2. Was a definitive diagnosis determined? _____

Practice Exercise 17-20: Cholecystectomy

OPERATIVE REPORT

LOCATION: Outpatient, Hospital

PATIENT: Josette Fox

PREOPERATIVE DIAGNOSIS: Acute cholecystitis with choledocholithiasis.

POSTOPERATIVE DIAGNOSIS: Acute cholecystitis with choledocholithiasis.

SURGEON: Loren White, MD

PROCEDURE PERFORMED: Laparoscopic cholecystectomy.

ANESTHESIA: General.

INDICATION: This is a 29-year-old-female who was admitted with acute cholecystitis and ele-vated liver function tests. These levels continued to climb, and she underwent ERCP. They retrieved stones, and she presented today for elective laparoscopic cholecystectomy. She under-stands the risks for bleeding, infection, damage to the biliary system, and conversion to open procedure and she wishes to proceed.

PROCEDURE: The patient was brought to the operating room and placed under general anes-thesia. A Foley catheter and orogastric tubes were inserted. She was prepped and draped sterilely. A supraumbilical skin incision was made with a #11 blade and dissection was carried down through subcutaneous tissues bluntly. The midline fascia was grasped with a Kocher clamp and a 0 Vicryl suture was placed on either side of the midline fascia. A Veress needle was inserted in the abdominal cavity. Drop test confirmed placement within the peritoneal space. The abdomen was then insufflated with carbon dioxide. A 10-mm trocar port and laparoscope were introduced showing no damage to the underlying viscera. Under direct vision, 3 additional trocar ports were placed, 1 upper midline 10 mm and 2 right upper quadrant 5 mm. The gallbladder was grasped and elevated from its fossa, and the cystic duct and artery were dissected free, doubly clipped proximally and distally before dividing them with Hook scissors. The gallbladder was then shelled from its fossa using electrocautery. It was very inflamed and edematous. We then brought it up and out of the upper midline incision.

We irrigated the abdomen with saline until returns were clear. We took a good look at the liver bed, there was no evidence of bleeding and clips were in good position. We removed all trocar ports under direct vision with no evidence of bleeding and closed the supraumbilical port site fascial defect with a single interrupted 0 Vicryl suture. The skin at all port sites was closed with subcuticular 4–0 undyed Vicryl. Steri-Strips and sterile Band-Aids were applied.

All sponge and needle counts were correct. Prior to leaving the operating room, the wounds were anesthetized with a total of 30 cc of 0.5% Sensorcaine with epinephrine solution.

Pathology Report Later Indicated: Consistent with choledocholithiasis.

CPT Code(s): _____

ICD-10-CM Code(s): _____

Abstracting Questions

1. What was the approach for this procedure? _____

2. Does the location of the stone affect the diagnosis coding? _____

■ Urinary System Subsection (50010-53899)

Anatomical division:

- Kidney
- Ureter
- Bladder
- Urethra

Further divided by procedure, such as:

- Incision
- Excision
- Introduction
- Repair
- Laparoscopy
- Endoscopy

Kidney Subheading (50010-50593)

Endoscopy codes are used for procedures performed through a previously established stoma or incision

Caution: Codes may be unilateral or bilateral

Introduction Category (50382-50435)

Codes divided by renal pelvis catheter procedures or other introduction procedures

Renal pelvis catheters further divided; internally dwelling or externally accessible

Catheters for drainage and injections for radiography

Aspirations

Insertion of guidewires

Tube changes

Includes radiological supervision and interpretation

Ureter Subheading (50600-50980)

Caution: Codes may be unilateral or bilateral

Divided by type of procedure

- Incision
- Excision
- Introduction
- Repair
- Laparoscopy
- Endoscopy

Bladder Subheading (51020-52700)

Includes codes for

- Incision
- Removal
- Excision
- Introduction

- Urodynamics
- Repair
- Laparoscopy
- Endoscopy
  - Cystoscopy
  - Urethroscopy
  - Cystourethroscopy
- Transurethral surgery

Vesical neck and prostate

Many bundled codes

> *Example:* Urethral dilation is included with insertion of cystoscope

Read all descriptions carefully

Urodynamics (51725-51798)

Procedures relate to motion and flow of urine

Used to diagnose urine flow obstructions

Bundled: All instruments, equipment, fluids, gases, probes, catheters, technician's fees, medications, gloves, trays, tubing and other sterile supplies

Vesical Neck and Prostate (52400-52700)

Contains codes for transurethral resection of the prostate (TURP)

> *Example:* 52601 reports a complete transurethral electrosurgical resection of the prostate and includes vasectomy, meatotomy, cystourethroscopy, urethral calibration and/or dilation, internal urethrotomy, and control of any postoperative bleeding

Other approaches are reported with 55801-55845

> *Example:* 55801 reports removal of the prostate gland (prostatectomy) through an incision in the perineum and includes vasectomy, meatotomy, urethral calibration and/or dilation, internal urethrotomy, and control of any postoperative bleeding

■ Male Genital System Subsection (54000-55899)

- Penis (most codes)
- Testis
- Epididymis
- Tunica Vaginalis
- Scrotum
- Vas Deferens
- Spermatic Cord
- Seminal Vesicles
- Prostate

Biopsy Codes

Located in anatomical subheading to which the codes refer

> *Example:* Biopsy codes in subheadings

- Epididymis (Excision)
> *Example:* 54800, needle biopsy of epididymis

- Testis (Excision)

  Example: 54500, needle biopsy of testis

Penis (54000-54450)

Incision codes (54000-54015) differ from Integumentary System codes

- Penis incision codes assigned for deeper structures

Destruction (54050-54065)
Codes divided by

- Extent: Simple or extensive
- Method of destruction (e.g., chemical, cryosurgery)

Extensive destruction can be by any method

Excision (54100-54164)
Commonly used codes for biopsy and circumcision

Introduction (54200-54250)
Many procedures for corpora cavernosum (spongy body of penis)

- Injection procedures for Peyronie disease (toughening of corpora cavernosum)
- Treatments and tests for erectile dysfunction

Repair (54300-54440)
Many plastic repairs

Some repairs are staged (more than one procedure)

- Stage indicated in code description

■ Female Genital System Subsection (56405-58999)

Anatomical division: From vulva to ovaries

- Many bundled services

Vulva, Perineum, and Introitus (56405-56821)

Skene's gland reported with Urinary System, Incision or Excision codes

- Group of small mucous glands, lower end of urethra
- Paraurethral duct

Incision (56405-56442)
I&D of abscess of vulva, perineal area, or Bartholin's gland

Marsupialization (56440)
Cyst incised

Drained

Edges sutured to sides to keep cyst open, creating a pouchlike repair

Destruction (56501, 56515)
Lesions destroyed by variety of methods

- Destruction = Eradication, not to be confused with excision; excision is removal

Divided by whether destruction is simple or extensive

- Complexity based on physician's judgment
- Stated in medical record

Destruction has no pathology report

Excision (56605-56740)

Biopsy includes

- Local anesthetic
- Biopsy
- Simple closure
- Code based on number of lesions biopsied

Vulvectomy: Surgical Removal of Portion of Vulva (56620-56640)

Based on extent and size of area removed

Extent:

- Simple: Skin and superficial subcutaneous tissues
- Radical: Skin and deep subcutaneous tissues

Size:

- Partial: <80% vulvar area
- Complete: >80% vulvar area

Extent and size indicated in operative report

Repair (56800-56810)

Many plastic repairs

Read notes following category

- If repair procedure involves skin wound of genitalia, use Integumentary System code

Endoscopy (56820, 56821)

By means of a colposcopy with or without biopsy(ies)

Vagina (57000-57426)

Codes divided based on service (e.g., incision, excision)

Introduction (57150-57180)

Includes vaginal irrigation, insertion of devices, diaphragm, cervical caps

Report the inserted device separately

- 99070 or HCPCS National Level II code, such as A4261 (cervical cap)

Repair (57200-57335)

For nonobstetric repairs

- For obstetric repairs, report Maternity Care and Delivery codes

Manipulation (57400-57415)

Dilation: Speculum inserted into vagina and enlarged using dilator

Endoscopy/Laparoscopy (57420-57426)

Colposcopy codes based on purpose

- e.g., biopsy, diagnostic
- Includes code for laparoscopic approach for repair of paravaginal defect

Cervix Uteri (57452-57800)

Cervix uteri, narrow lower end of uterus

Services include excision, manipulation, repair

Excision (57500-57558)

Conization codes

- **Conization:** Removal of cone of tissue from cervix

LEEP (loop electrocautery excision procedure) technology can be used for conizations

Excision (58100-58294)

Dilation & curettage (D&C, 58120) of nonobstetric uterus

- After dilation, curette used to scrape uterus
- Coded according to circumstances: obstetrical or nonobstetrical

Do not report postpartum hemorrhage service with 58120

- Use 59160—Maternity and Delivery code

Many hysterectomy codes

- Based on approach (vaginal, abdominal), extent (uterus, fallopian tubes, etc.), and weight of uterus

Often secondary procedures performed with hysterectomy

Do not report secondary, related minor procedures separately

Only 58110 (endometrial biopsy), 58120 (dilation and curettage), and 58145 (myomectomy, vaginal approach) are performed on an outpatient basis

Corpus Uteri (58100-58579)

Many complex procedures

- Often very similar wording in code descriptions
- Requires careful reading

Introduction (58300-58356)

Common procedures

- e.g., insertion of an IUD

Report supply of device separately

Specialized services

- e.g., artificial insemination procedures

Used to report physician component of service

Component coding

- Necessary with catheter procedures for hysterosonography
- Notes following codes indicate radiology guidance component codes

Laparoscopy/Hysteroscopy (58541-58579)

Laparoscopic approach for:

- Removal of myomas
- Radical hysterectomy
- Supracervical and laparoscopic vaginal hysterectomies

Codes divided by tissue removed and weight of uterus

- Hysteroscopies divided on procedure performed (e.g., lysis of uterine adhesions, endometrial ablation)

Oviduct/Ovary (58600-58770)

Oviduct

Fallopian Tube

Incision category contains tubal ligations

- When it occurs during the same hospitalization but not at same session as delivery, ligation is reported separately

Laparoscopy (58660-58679)
Through abdominal wall

Codes in the laparoscopy section are divided by procedure performed (e.g., lysis of adhesions, removal adnexal structures)

Caution: If only diagnostic laparoscopy

- Do not use Female Genital System codes
- Use 49320, Digestive System

Many codes can be reported separately with appropriate modifiers

> *Example:* 58660, Laparoscopy, surgical, with lysis of adhesions, can be reported with any of the indented codes that follow 58660 (58661-58673)

Ovary (58800-58960)

Two categories only: Incision and Excision

- **Incision:** Primarily for drainage of cysts and abscesses
  - Divided by surgical approach
- **Excision:** Biopsy, wedge resection, and oophorectomy

In Vitro Fertilization (58970-58976)

Specialized codes usually used by physicians trained in fertilization procedures

- Codes divided by type of procedure and method used

■ Maternity Care and Delivery Subsection (59000-59899)

Divided by service, such as:

- Antepartum and Fetal Invasive Services
  Amniocentesis
  Fetal non-stress test
  Fetal monitoring during labor
- Type of delivery
  Vaginal delivery
  C-section
  Delivery after a previous C-section
- Abortion

Gestation

Fetal gestation: Approximately 266 days (40 weeks)

EDD: Estimated date of delivery

- 280 days from last menstrual period (LMP)

Trimesters
First, LMP to less than 14 weeks 0 days

Second, 14 weeks 0 days to less than 28 weeks 0 days

Third, 28 weeks 0 days until deliver

Excision (59100-59160)

Postpartum curettage: Removes remaining pieces of placenta or clotted blood (59160)

Nonobstetric curettage: 58120 (Corpus Uteri, Excision)

Introduction (59200)

Insertion of cervical dilator: Used to prepare cervix for an abortive procedure or delivery (for abortive procedures, see 59855)

Cervical ripening agents may be introduced to prepare cervix

- "Separate procedure" and not reported when part of more major procedure

Repair (59300-59350)

Only for repairs during pregnancy

Repairs done as a result of delivery or during pregnancy

Episiotomy or vaginal repair by other than attending physician

Suture closure (cerclage) of cervix or repair of uterus (hysterorrhaphy)

Abortion Services (59812-59857)

Spontaneous: Happens naturally (for a complete spontaneous abortion, report with a code from the E/M section [99201-99233])

Incomplete: Requires medical intervention

Missed: Fetus dies naturally during first 22 weeks' gestation

Septic: Abortion with infection

Medical intervention:

- Dilation and curettage or evacuation (suction removal)
- Intra-amniotic injections (saline or urea)
- Vaginal suppositories (prostaglandin)

PRACTICE EXERCISES

Practice Exercise 17-21: Kidney Biopsy

OPERATIVE REPORT

LOCATION: Outpatient, Hospital

PATIENT: Lilly Brown

PREOPERATIVE DIAGNOSIS: Acute renal failure, possible rejection, possible ischemic nephropathy.

POSTOPERATIVE DIAGNOSIS: Same.

SURGEON: George Orbitz, MD

PROCEDURE PERFORMED: Transplant kidney biopsy.

PROCEDURE: The transplanted kidney in the right iliac fossa was visualized with ultrasound. The previous arteriovenous malformation was noted in the lower pole. We avoided that area as much as we could. At least three core biopsies were obtained after prepping the area in the usual fashion and injecting 1% lidocaine. A post-biopsy ultrasound showed no evidence of hematoma or new AVM. The patient had some pain after the procedure and was sent to the post-procedure area. She will be getting some intravenous morphine.

Hemoglobin will be checked in 6 hours.

Pathology Report Later Indicated: Acute necrotizing glomerulitis.

CPT Code(s): _____

ICD-10-CM Code(s): _____

Abstracting Questions

1. Was the biopsy performed as an open procedure? _____

2. What further reference is found when you locate the main term "Glomerulitis" in the ICD-10-CM Index? _____

3. What is the meaning of AVM, and would it be reported? _____

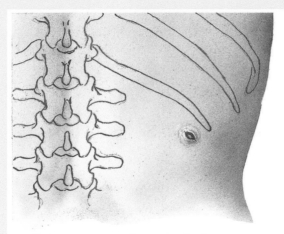

Small skin incision made in wheal at biopsy site

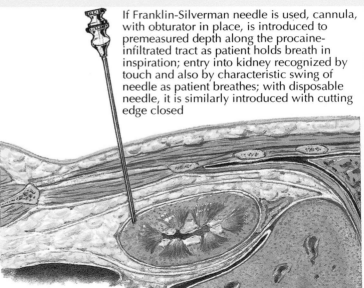

If Franklin-Silverman needle is used, cannula, with obturator in place, is introduced to premeasured depth along the procaine-infiltrated tract as patient holds breath in inspiration; entry into kidney recognized by touch and also by characteristic swing of needle as patient breathes; with disposable needle, it is similarly introduced with cutting edge closed

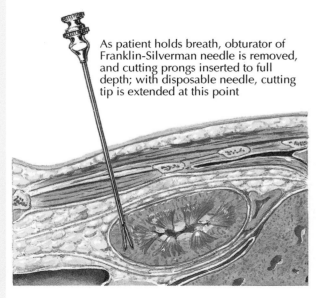

As patient holds breath, obturator of Franklin-Silverman needle is removed, and cutting prongs inserted to full depth; with disposable needle, cutting tip is extended at this point

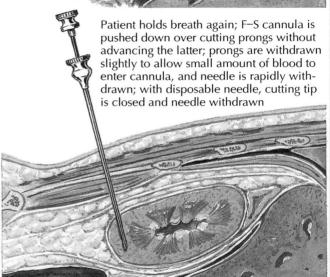

Patient holds breath again; F–S cannula is pushed down over cutting prongs without advancing the latter; prongs are withdrawn slightly to allow small amount of blood to enter cannula, and needle is rapidly withdrawn; with disposable needle, cutting tip is closed and needle withdrawn

Surgical biopsy

A 2-inch incision is made below outer end of 12th rib; musculature and fascia are penetrated by blunt dissection; lower pole of kidney identified by index finger of left hand which then guides needle into kidney parenchyma; biopsy specimen then taken in usual manner

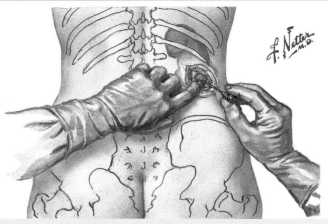

Practice Exercise 17-22: Kidney Biopsy

OPERATIVE REPORT

LOCATION: Outpatient, Hospital

PATIENT: Melissa Hart

SURGEON: George Orbitz, MD

PROCEDURE PERFORMED: Kidney biopsy.

REASON FOR PROCEDURE: Proteinuria.

After the procedure and potential complications were explained to the patient and consent was obtained, she was prepped for a right native kidney biopsy. The area was prepped with Betadine solution. Sterile drapes were then applied around the area in the usual fashion. One-percent lidocaine was used as a local anesthetic, which was infiltrated in the intended biopsy site. The patient's right kidney was directly visualized prior to the procedure using ultrasound. After the lidocaine was given, a small skin incision was made at the biopsy site. The intended biopsy needle track was also infiltrated with lidocaine using a spinal needle under direct ultrasonographic guidance. A biopsy of the lower pole of the right kidney was taken with an 18-gauge Tru-Cut needle. Four attempts were made to obtain three good core samples. Postbiopsy ultrasound with color flow did not show any hematomas.

The patient tolerated the procedure well. There was minimal bleeding. There were no acute complications. She was given a total of 2 mg of Versed, with 100 mcg of Fentanyl for sedation and analgesia.

Pathology Report Later Indicated: Membranous glomerulonephritis.

CPT Code(s): _____

ICD-10-CM Code(s): _____

Abstracting Questions

1. Was the biopsy of a transplanted kidney? _____

2. If the kidney was not native but transplanted, would that affect the diagnosis coding for this case? _____

3. What type of glomerulonephritis was identified? _____

Practice Exercise 17-23: Hysteroscopy

OPERATIVE REPORT

LOCATION: Outpatient, Hospital

PATIENT: Calley Olson

PREOPERATIVE DIAGNOSIS: Postmenopausal bleeding.

POSTOPERATIVE DIAGNOSIS: Endometrial polyp.

SURGEON: Andy Martinez, MD

OPERATIVE PROCEDURE: Diagnostic hysteroscopy with polypectomy and dilation and curettage.

PREAMBLE: The patient is a 42-year-old woman seen with complaints of postmenopausal bleeding. An attempt at endometrial biopsy in the office was, unfortunately, unsuccessful. The patient is therefore taken to the operating room for diagnostic hysteroscopy with D&C.

PROCEDURE NOTE: The patient was taken to the operating room and a general anesthetic was administered. The patient was then prepped and draped in the usual manner in the lithotomy position, and straight catheterization of the bladder was carried out. A weighted speculum was placed to allow for visualization of the cervix, which was grasped anteriorly using single-toothed tenaculum. The cervix was then dilated to allow for insertion of the diagnostic hysteroscope. Uterine cavity was entered, and there were two small endometrial polyps visible. Attempt was made to resect these with the hysteroscopic scissors, but unfortunately, this was unsuccessful. The hysteroscopic resecting loop, unfortunately, could not be made operational and could not be used.

Polyp forceps was therefore placed, and a small amount of the polypoid tissue was grasped for biopsy. A sharp curettage was also carried out with minimal products obtained.

The patient tolerated the procedure well and went to the recovery room in good condition. There were no complications. Estimated blood loss was minimal.

Pathology Report Later Indicated: Benign endometrial polyp.

CPT Code(s): _____

ICD-10-CM Code(s): _____

Abstracting Questions

1. What was the approach for this procedure? _____

2. Was this procedure diagnostic only? _____

3. What definitive procedures were performed? _____

4. How many codes are required to report the diagnostic hysteroscopy, biopsy, and curettage?
_____

5. Is there a definitive diagnosis to report or is the presenting problem reported? _____
_____

Practice Exercise 17-24: Amniocentesis

OPERATIVE REPORT

LOCATION: Outpatient, Hospital

PATIENT: Jennifer Barron

PREOPERATIVE DIAGNOSES

1. Intrauterine pregnancy at 32 weeks.

2. Insulin-dependent diabetes, type 2.

3. Diabetic nephropathy.

POSTOPERATIVE DIAGNOSIS: Same.

SURGEON: Andy Martinez, MD

PROCEDURE PERFORMED: Amniocentesis.

INDICATIONS: The patient is a 23-year-old with a complicated pregnancy who has been on bed rest because of diabetic nephropathy. Due to the fact that the fetus might be in a hostile environment, we believed that accelerated pulmonary maturity might be a possibility; therefore, at this time we elected to go with amniocentesis to help us manage her pregnancy. She had been fully informed of the risks and benefits of the procedure prior to proceeding.

DESCRIPTION OF PROCEDURE: The technologist did ultrasound scanning, and the placenta was posterior. We prepped the abdomen and draped it. We used a sterile covered ultrasound transducer with guide and located a pocket of fluid. The 20-gauge needle was inserted. As we got into the uterus the baby moved into the area, therefore the needle was immediately withdrawn; the fetus was palpated a little bit, and we stimulated the baby and it moved out of the area. We then repositioned the transducer and were able to drop into the pocket of amniotic fluid and withdrew 20 cc of clear yellow amniotic fluid. The fluid was sent for maturity studies. The patient tolerated the procedure without difficulty.

CPT Code(s): _____

ICD-10-CM Code(s): _____

Abstracting Questions

1. Was the procedure diagnostic or therapeutic? _____

2. Would the ultrasound guidance be included in the procedure, or would it be separately reported? _____

3. Would the pregnancy affect the primary diagnosis code selection? _____

4. In ICD-10-CM, what does the sixth character "3" in the O24 code represent? _____
_____

5. Would the diabetes and nephropathy be reported? _____

6. Would the diabetic code assignment be affected by the nephropathy? _____

Practice Exercise 17-25: Cystoscopy

OPERATIVE REPORT

LOCATION: Outpatient, Hospital

PATIENT: Eunice Nehring

SURGEON: Ira Avila, MD

The patient's maximal flow was 63.5 and average flow 37.5. Voided volume is 686 with residual urine of 150 cc. The CMG, EMG, and IRP show a lot of artifactual activity, but she was leaking throughout the procedure. Her first desire to void was 37 cc. Normal desire to void was 96 cc. Maximal capacity, however, was 161 cc. However, the information does not easily match the flow study where she had a much larger capacity with residual urine. The leak was noted very early on in the study and leaking continued throughout the study. The baseline shows a lot of artifacts but nothing that I can truly call uninhibited contractions of the bladder.

The patient had a cystoscopy performed today. She was prepared and draped in a sterile fashion. Following this, an endoscope was introduced through the urethra into the bladder. There is actually fairly good coaptation of the urethra at the bladder neck. Ureteral orifices were normal in size, shape, and position and well-developed interureteric ridge. There was no evidence of stone or tumor in the bladder. No trabeculation was present. There appeared to be a very mild subacute cystitis, but this was likely due to the fact that the patient had just had her urodynamic studies performed. The bladder was filled several times and emptied several times and re-examined. Examination of the mucosa revealed no evidence of any interstitial cystitis. With the bladder fairly well filled, I had the patient cough and bear down and she does have a lot of loss of urine from that position. This is relieved to some extent by pressure lateral to the urethra at the level of the bladder neck.

IMPRESSION:

1. Urinary incontinence with a predominant element of urinary stress incontinence.

2. Probable intrinsic sphincteric deficiency.

3. Elevated residual urine.

4. Some inconsistencies in urodynamic testing.

RECOMMENDATION: I gave the patient a prescription for Cipro following the procedure but she did not want to get that filled since she has lots of antibiotics she tells me at home, and she does have Augmentin and I suspect that is okay for her to take. I would recommend that at the time that she has her cystocele and rectocele repair and hysterectomy, consideration be given to also placing a sling at the bladder neck to see if this could overcome her urinary incontinence. I told her about the elevated residual urine and discussed with her timed voiding and double voiding to try and get that bladder to empty better. The patient, if she has her operative procedure, is at a bit of a risk for urinary retention postoperatively, and I talked to her about the fact that if she has those procedures done, she may require intermittent self-catheterization for a while until it all balances out.

CPT Code(s): _____

ICD-10-CM Code(s): _____

Abstracting Questions

1. Was this a diagnostic or surgical procedure? _____

2. Would you report a diagnosis code for the incontinence? _____

■ Endocrine System Subsection (60000-60699)

Nine glands in endocrine system; only four included in subsection

1. Thyroid
2. Parathyroid
3. Thymus
4. Adrenal

Pituitary and Pineal
See Nervous System subsection

Pancreas
Digestive System

Ovaries and Testes
Respective genital systems

Divided into two subheadings

- Thyroid Gland
- Parathyroid, Thymus, Adrenal Glands, Pancreas and Carotid Body

Carotid Body
Refers to area adjacent to the bifurcation of the carotid artery

Can be site of tumors

Thyroid Gland, Excision Category (60100-60281)

Code descriptions often refer to

- Lobectomy (partial or subtotal): Something less than total
- Thyroidectomy (total): All

Thyroid, 1 gland with 2 lobes

■ Nervous System Subsection (61000-64999)

Divided anatomically:

- Skull, Meninges, and Brain
- Spine and Spinal Cord
- Extracranial Nerves, Peripheral Nerves, and Autonomic Nervous System

Skull, Meninges, and Brain Subheading (61000-62258)

Category Examples:
Injection, Drainage, or Aspiration

Twist Drills, Burr Hole(s), or Trephination

Conditions that Require Openings into Brain to

- Relieve pressure
- Insert monitoring devices
- Place tubing
- Inject contrast material

Craniectomy or Craniotomy Category (61304-61576)

Craniectomy involves removal of portion of skull, at operative site, performed emergently to prevent herniation of brain into the brainstem

Craniotomy—bone flap is replaced after surgery

Codes divided by site and condition for which procedure is performed

Performed only on an inpatient basis

Surgery of Skull Base Category (61580-61619)

Skull base: Area at base of cranium

- Lesion removal from this area very complex

Surgery of Skull Base Terminology

Approach procedure used to gain exposure of lesion

Definitive procedure is what is done to lesion

Repair/reconstruction procedure reported separately only if extensive repair

Approach procedure and definitive procedure coded separately

Example: Removal of an intradural lesion using middle cranial fossa approach

- 61590 approach procedure, middle cranial fossa, and
- 61608 definitive procedure of intradural resection of lesion

Most of these procedures are performed only on an inpatient basis

Cerebrospinal Fluid (CSF) Shunt Category (62180-62258)

Performed to drain fluid

Codes describe, e.g.,

- Placement of devices
- Reprogramming
- Replacement
- Removal of shunting devices

Most performed only on an inpatient basis

Spine and Spinal Cord (62263-63746)

Codes divided by condition and approach

Often used are

- Unilateral or bilateral procedures (-50)
- Radiologic supervision and fluoroscopic guidance coded separately

Includes codes for

- Myelography injections (62302-62305)
  - Spinal anesthetic or steroid injections 62310-62319
  - Intrathecal or epidural catheter placement/implantation 62350-62355

Extracranial Nerves, Peripheral Nerves, and Autonomic Nervous System (64400-64999)

Introduction/Injection of Anesthetic Agent (Nerve Block), Diagnostic or Therapeutic Category (64400-64530)

Includes codes for

- Nerve blocks 64486-64489, 64505-64530
  - Bundled when used as anesthesia for procedure

- Paravertebral facet joint injections 64490-64495, diagnostic or therapeutic

Epidural injections 64479-64484

- Used to provide pain relief
- As compared to an epidural catheter placement used for anesthetic purposes

Eye and Ocular Adnexa Subsection (65091-68899)

Terminology extremely important

- Code descriptions often vary only slightly

Understanding of eye anatomy is necessary for proper coding in this subsection

Codes divided anatomically, e.g.,

- Eyeball
- Anterior segment
- Posterior segment
- Ocular adnexa
- Conjunctiva

Some codes specifically for previous surgery

Example: Insertion of ocular implant, secondary 65130

Much bundling:

Example: Subheading Posterior Segment, Prophylaxis category notes indicate:

- "The following descriptors (67141, 67145) are intended to include all sessions in a defined treatment period."

Cataracts

Method used depends on type of cataract and surgeon preference

Nuclear cataract: Most common, center of lens (nucleus), due to aging process

Cortical cataract: Forms in cortex of lens and extends outward; frequent in patients with diabetes

Subcapsular cataract: Forms at back of lens, increased rate in diabetics, those who take steroid medications, certain genetic factors and eye trauma

Lens Removal (66830-66986)

- Extracapsular cataract extraction (ECCE)

Patient retains posterior outer shell of the lens

Soft cortex and rest of shell is removed in multiple pieces

Posterior shell helps prevent vitreous prolapse

- Intracapsular cataract extraction (ICCE) is total removal

Removes lens and capsule in one piece as in

Incision is large

- Phacoemulsification

Small incision into eye and introduction of probe

High-frequency waves fragment cataract (extracapsular); then suctioned out

Lens placed through same small incision

Eyelids (67700-67999)

Blepharotomy (67700)

- Incision into eyelid for drainage of abscess

Blepharoplasty

- Repair of eyelid
- Codes in Integumentary System (15820-15823) report removal of excess skin
- Codes in Eye and Ocular Adnexa (67916, 67917, 67923, 67924) report muscle repairs and slings

These codes strictly for ectropion and entropion

Selection of code depends on technique used to repair eyelid

- Blepharoplasty coded with specific techniques (67901-67908)

Auditory System Subsection (69000-69979)

Codes divided by

- External Ear (69000-69399)
- Middle Ear (69420-69799)
- Inner Ear (69801-69949)
- Temporal Bone, Middle Fossa Approach (69420-69979)

Understanding of ear anatomy is necessary for proper coding in this subsection

External, middle, and inner ear further divided by procedure, such as

- Incision
- Excision
- Removal
- Repair

Myringotomy and tympanostomy

- Eustachian tube connects middle ear to back of throat for drainage
- Fluid collects in middle ear when tube does not function properly
- Prevents air from entering middle ear and pressure builds
- Surgical intervention

  Myringotomy (incision into tympanic membrane)

  Tympanostomy (placement of PE [pressure equalization] tube)

Operating Microscope Subsection (+69990)

Employed with procedures using microsurgical techniques

Code in addition to primary procedure performed

Do not report separately when primary procedure description includes microsurgical techniques

Example: 15758, Free fascial flap with microvascular anastomosis

Note that following 15758 is the statement:

"(Do not report code 69990 in addition to code 15758)," indicating to the coder not to report the use of operating microscope separately

Do not code 69990 when magnifying loupes are used

PRACTICE EXERCISES

Practice Exercise 17-26: Blepharoplasty

OPERATIVE REPORT

LOCATION: Outpatient, Hospital

PATIENT: Anna Penn

PREOPERATIVE DIAGNOSES

1. Upper lid entropion, each eye.

2. History of herpes simplex keratitis, left eye.

3. Diabetes mellitus type I.

POSTOPERATIVE DIAGNOSES: Same.

SURGEON: Rita Wimer, MD

PROCEDURE: Wedge resection with mini-blepharoplasty, upper lids, OU (both eyes).

ANESTHESIA: MAC (Monitored Anesthesia Care).

INDICATION: This 45-year-old white female has had recurrent eye pain and irritation of her eye secondary to upper lid entropion, both eyes. She was counseled as to the repair, risk for infection, recurrence, and exposure.

DESCRIPTION OF PROCEDURE: After the patient was prepped and draped in the usual sterile fashion for ophthalmic surgery, the amount of skin to be resected was determined by the open eye/close eye method. This was marked with a sterile marking pen and infiltrated with 2% Xylocaine with 0.75% Marcaine and bicarbonate. A #15 Bard-Parker blade then made a free hand dissection, and a 2-mm strip of orbicularis was removed. Epinephrine-soaked sponges were then applied for 10 minutes under cool water compresses, and the cautery was used. It was determined that no fat was prolapsing and that the fat pads were left undisturbed. The wound was then closed with multiple interrupted 6–0 nylon sutures, and Maxitrol ointment, Telfa, and two half-eye pads were applied. There were no complications.

Pathology Report Later Indicated: Benign tissue.

CPT Code(s): _____

ICD-10-CM Code(s): _____

Abstracting Questions

1. Does the wedge resection method affect code selection? _____

2. What type of modifiers would you assign for the services provided in this case? _____
_____

3. Does the unspecified type of entropion affect diagnosis code selection? _____

4. Would the diabetes be reported? _____

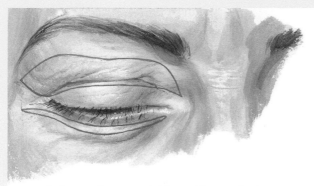

A. Areas of proposed skin excision marked out by methylene blue

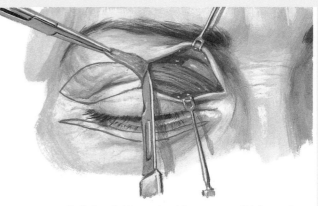

B. Strip of skin excised from upper lid; fat pad shining through orbital fascia and orbicularis oculi muscle

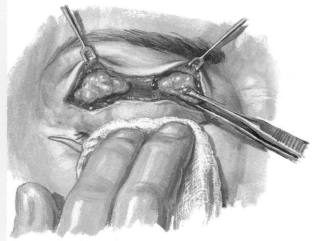

C. Orbital fascia opened in two places (medially and laterally). Pressure on eyeball causes fat pads to bulge. They are teased out meticulously

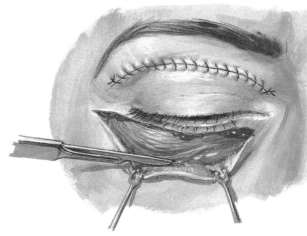

D. Upper lid incision sutured with no. 6–zero silk continuous stitches. Orbicularis oculi fibers are being separated from skin

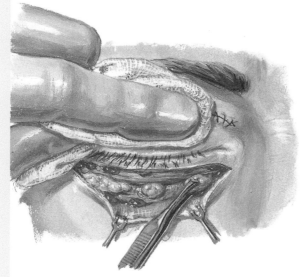

E. Orbital fascia opened; fat pads bulge due to digital pressure and are teased out meticulously

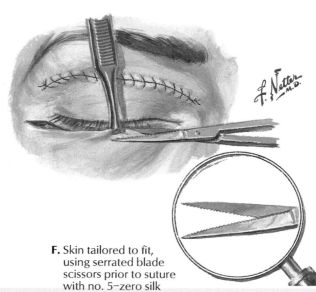

F. Skin tailored to fit, using serrated blade scissors prior to suture with no. 5–zero silk

Practice Exercise 17-27: Discectomy

OPERATIVE REPORT

LOCATION: Outpatient, Hospital

PATIENT: Neil Wills

PREOPERATIVE DIAGNOSIS: Left L5-S1 herniated disc.

POSTOPERATIVE DIAGNOSIS: Same.

SURGEON: John Hodgson, MD

PROCEDURE: Left L5-S1 discectomy.

INDICATIONS: This is a 37-year-old male who presented with left lower extremity pain. He had motor, sensory, and reflex findings all consistent with a left S1 radiculopathy. He had a large midline and, slightly to the left, a herniated L5-S1 disc. He failed to respond to conservative treatment. After discussion of the options and risks, he elected surgery.

PROCEDURE AS FOLLOWS: The patient was taken to the operating room and underwent induction of general endotracheal anesthesia in the supine position. He was then flipped over to the prone position on the operating room table. The lumbosacral area was sterilely prepped and draped. The C-arm was draped and moved into position. A K-wire was placed one fingerbreadth to the left of the L5-S1 interspace. This was confirmed with the C-arm. I then used a sequential series of dilators and eventually placed a 5-cm-long, 18-mm-diameter tubular retractor. This was verified again to be over the L5-S1 interspace with the C-arm. I then removed the redundant muscle with a Kerrison rongeur. I incised the ligamentum of flavum with a #15 blade and removed it with various sizes of Kerrison rongeurs. I retracted the common dural sac and the left S1 nerve root medially. There was a very significant bulge compressing the left S1 nerve root. I incised this and removed two large pieces of extruded disc. I then went into the disc space, which was narrow, and removed additional pieces of disc. At the end of the decompression, I could pass a nerve hook underneath the common dural sac across the midline, toward the right side, and I did not feel any further compression. I could also pass a nerve hook along the exiting S1 nerve root and did not feel any compression. At no time was there a dural tear or spinal fluid leak. I was content that the neural elements were nicely decompressed. I irrigated with copious amounts of saline. Surgicel was placed over the exposed dura. The tubular retractor was withdrawn. The subcutaneous tissue was closed with interrupted 2–0 Vicryl. The skin was closed with a running 3–0 Vicryl subcuticular stitch. Benzoin and $^1/_4$-inch Steri-Strips and a sterile dressing were placed. The patient tolerated the procedure well without apparent complications. Sponge, instrument, and needle counts were correct. He was taken to the recovery room in stable condition.

Pathology Report Later Indicated: Benign disc fragments.

CPT Code(s): _____

ICD-10-CM Code(s): _____

Abstracting Questions

1. When reporting the CPT code for the service in this case, is the location of the disc(s) a factor?
   _____

2. Does the number of discs involved affect code assignment? _____

3. What is the direction in the Index of the ICD-10-CM when you reference the terms "Hernia, disc"? _____

Practice Exercise 17-28: Ventricular Puncture

OPERATIVE REPORT

LOCATION: Outpatient, Hospital

PATIENT: Sam Dillard

PREOPERATIVE DIAGNOSIS: Increased intracerebral pressure.

POSTOPERATIVE DIAGNOSIS: Same.

SURGEON: John Hodgson, MD

OPERATIVE PROCEDURE: Percutaneous aspiration of ventricular reservoir.

COMPLICATIONS: None.

INDICATIONS: This is a 19-year-old male with a high-grade glioma of the posterior fossa. He has shunt-dependent hydrocephalus due to the neoplasm. He comes to my office complaining of nausea, vomiting, lethargy, and headache. After obtaining consent from the parents, I went ahead and tapped the valve.

PROCEDURE: The patient was placed in the lateral supine position with the right side up. His neck and head was supported with a pillow. I prepped the site of the shunt reservoir with Betadine. I then took a 23-gauge needle attached to a 60-cc syringe and aspirated approximately 55 cc of xanthochromic CSF that had some particulate matter in it. I then withdrew the needle. I sent the fluid for total protein, glucose, cell count with differential, Gram stain culture, and Vancomycin level. The patient tolerated the procedure well. The needle was withdrawn. There were no complications.

Pathology Report Later Indicated: Normal cerebral spinal fluid.

CPT Code(s): _____

ICD-10-CM Code(s): _____

Abstracting Questions

1. Does the needle placement for the percutaneous aspiration of the ventricular reservoir (ventricular puncture) affect the CPT code assignment? _____

2. Was there an injection as well as aspiration in this case? _____

3. What was the underlying condition? _____

4. Would a secondary diagnosis be reported? _____

Practice Exercise 17-29: Insertion of Intrathecal Catheter and Pump

OPERATIVE REPORT

LOCATION: Outpatient, Hospital

PATIENT: Josh Ring

PREOPERATIVE DIAGNOSES

1. Osteoporosis.

2. Multiple compression fractures of the spine, status post multilevel kyphoplasty.

3. Lumbar spinal stenosis without neurogenic claudication.

4. Degenerative disc disease of the lumbar spine.

5. Alzheimer's disease.

6. Benign prostatic hypertrophy.

POSTOPERATIVE DIAGNOSES: Same.

SURGEON: John Hodgson, MD

PROCEDURE PERFORMED: Insertion of permanent intrathecal catheter and SynchroMed pump.

ANESTHESIA: General.

ESTIMATED BLOOD LOSS: Minimal.

PROCEDURE: The patient was brought to the operating room. General endotracheal anesthesia was instituted. He was placed in left lateral position. Parts were prepped and draped. Fluoroscopy guidance was obtained. Skin and subcutaneous tissue at the site of back incision, site of needle insertion, and right lower quadrant incision and tunneling tract were infiltrated with local anesthetic, 0.25% Sensorcaine with epinephrine; total amount used was 25 cc. I attempted to do the spinal tap at L5-S1, L4-L5 level under fluoroscopy guidance. I was unable to do that. I made the spinal tap at L3-4 level in one attempt without any difficulty. CSF was clear. There was free flow. Under fluoroscopy guidance, I inserted intraspinal catheter to T9 level. Stylet was removed. The flow was excellent. Under fluoroscopy guidance, I withdrew the intraspinal needle 1 cm making sure the intraspinal catheter did not get dislodged.

I made an incision, 3 inches long, in the right lower quadrant and carried that into the subcutaneous tissue. I made a pocket over abdominal wall fascia by blunt and sharp dissection. Hemostasis was achieved. This pocket was packed with antibiotic solution–soaked lap pad.

I made an incision in the back 2 inches long vertical along the intraspinal needle. I carried that incision into the subcutaneous tissue and made a pocket over the back muscle fascia by blunt and sharp dissection to accommodate the anchoring device. I placed 2–0 silk pursestring suture times two around the intraspinal needle. Intraspinal needle was removed under fluoroscopy guidance making sure the intraspinal catheter did not get dislodged. Pursestring sutures were tightened around the intraspinal catheter. This was done to prevent CSF leak around the intraspinal catheter. After tightening the pursestring sutures, I made sure the CSF flow was adequate through the catheter. Then I inserted anchoring device on the intraspinal catheter; the anchor was secured to back muscle fascia with 2–0 silk suture times two. I passed a tunneler from right lower quadrant incision into the back incision in one pass, then brought the intraspinal catheter through the right lower quadrant incision. Excess portion of the catheter was trimmed. Implanted catheter length is 64 cm with volume of 0.141 ml. Pump was made ready by the scrub nurse and Medtronics clinical specialist. It was filled with Bupivacaine and Dilaudid solution. I connected the connecting tube to the intraspinal catheter. Connection was secured with 2–0 silk tie. This connection was connected to the pump, and this connection was secured with 0 silk tie.

Lap pad in the pump pocket was removed. Hemostasis was checked. Pump pocket was irrigated with antibiotic solution. The pump was placed in its pocket, making sure the filling port is anterior. The pump was secured to abdominal wall fascia with 0 silk suture at each anchoring site, one on the inferior side and one on the lateral side of the pump.

Both incisions were checked for hemostasis. They were irrigated with antibiotic solution. They were closed in two layers, 0 Vicryl interrupted for subcutaneous tissue, 3–0 Monocryl for subcuticular. Incisions were clean. Dermabond was applied. Pump was programmed to deliver Bupivacaine 5 mg and Dilaudid 500 mcg per day.

Pathology Report Later Indicated: Normal cerebral spinal fluid.

CPT Code(s): _____

ICD-10-CM Code(s): _____

Abstracting Questions

1. Was the intrathecal (CSF) catheter placement performed during a laminectomy? _____
   _____

2. Does the placement of the intrathecal catheter include insertion of the pump? _____
   _____

3. Was the type of pump inserted programmable? _____

4. Does the type of pump inserted affect the CPT code selection? _____

5. What was the primary diagnosis and secondary diagnoses (there were two secondary diagnoses) for the insertion of the pump? _____

Practice Exercise 17-30: Carpal Tunnel Release

OPERATIVE REPORT

LOCATION: Outpatient, Hospital

PATIENT: Henry Judge

PREOPERATIVE DIAGNOSIS: Left carpal tunnel syndrome.

POSTOPERATIVE DIAGNOSIS: Left carpal tunnel syndrome.

SURGEON: Johns Hodgson, MD

PROCEDURE PERFORMED: Left carpal tunnel release.

COMPLICATIONS: None.

INDICATION: This is a 58-year-old male with left carpal tunnel syndrome. He failed to respond to conservative treatment. After a discussion of the options and risks, he elected surgery.

PROCEDURE: The patient was taken to the operating room. He underwent IV sedation. The planned incision was infiltrated with local anesthetic and then an incision was made beginning at the base of the proximal phalanx in line between the 3rd and 4th metacarpals and extending to but not across the wrist crease. I cut the subcutaneous tissue and then sectioned the transverse carpal ligament. I initially exposed the median nerve and completed a proximal transection of the ligament and undermined the wrist crease. I then completed a distal transection of the ligament. The nerve was purplish colored. I was able to see more pink healthy-appearing nerve both at the proximal and distal ends of the decompression. I was content the nerve was adequately decompressed. I irrigated with copious amounts of saline. Subcutaneous tissue was closed with interrupted 2–0 Vicryl. The skin was closed with running 3–0 nylon stitches. A bulky dressing was placed. The patient tolerated the procedure well without apparent complications. Sponge, instrument, and needle counts were correct. He was moving his hand well after the surgery.

CPT Code(s): _____

ICD-10-CM Code(s): _____

Abstracting Questions

1. Was this procedure open or endoscopic (through a scope)? _____

2. Does the nerve involved affect the CPT code assigned for the service? _____

3. Define neuroplasty. _____

4. Where is the "carpal tunnel" located? _____

CHAPTER 18: HCPCS CODING

Developed by Centers for Medicare and Medicaid Services (CMS)
- Formerly HCFA

HCPCS developed in 1983

CPT did not contain all codes necessary for Medicare services reporting.

One of Two Levels of Codes

1. Level I, CPT
2. Level II, HCPCS, also known as national codes

Phased out Level III, Local Codes

Developed by Medicare and other carriers for use at local level

Varied by locale

Discontinued October 2002 due to HIPAA code set regulations

- Some codes incorporated into HCPCS Level I and Level II

Level II, National Codes

Codes for wide variety of providers

- Physicians
- Hospital outpatient facilities
- Orthodontists

Codes for wide variety of services

- Specific drugs
- Durable medical equipment (DME)
- Ambulance services

Format

Begins with letter, followed by four digits

> *Example:* E0605, vaporizer, room type

Each letter represents group codes

> *Example:* "J" codes used to report drugs, J0585, Botox, per unit

Temporary Codes

Certain letters indicate temporary codes

> *Example:* K0552, Supplies for external drug infusion pump, syringe type cartridge, sterile

- K codes are temporary codes

Code book published every year, but codes are added and deleted throughout the year and providers are notified through carrier bulletins

HCPCS National Level II Index

Directs coder to specific codes

Do not code directly from index

Reference main portion of text before assigning code

Alphabetical order

▪ Ambulance Modifiers

Origin and destination used in combination

- First letter: Origin
- Second letter: Destination

  Example:

  - -R = Residence
  - -H = Hospital
  - -RH origin (first letter), residence, and destination (second letter), hospital

▪ PET Modifiers

Positron Emission Tomography: Noninvasive Imaging Procedure
Assesses metabolic organ activity

▪ Table of Drugs

Listed by generic name, not brand name

Often used when reporting immunizations or injections

> On the CCS examination, you will be assigning ICD-10-CM, ICD-10-PCS, CPT and HCPCS codes to both inpatient and outpatient (ASC) services.

UNIT 4

ICD-10-CM/PCS Coding

ICD-9-CM versions of Units 4-5 and the Practice Examinations can be found in the Student Evolve Resources.

Some of the CPT code descriptions for physician services include physician extender services. Physician extenders, such as nurse practitioners, physician assistants, and nurse anesthetists, etc., provide medical services typically performed by a physician. Within this educational material the term "physician" may include "and other qualified health care professionals" depending on the code. Refer to the official CPT® code descriptions and guidelines to determine codes that are appropriate to report services provided by non-physician practitioners.

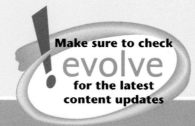

Make sure to check
evolve
for the latest
content updates

CHAPTER 19: ICD-10-CM/PCS OVERVIEW

■ Introduction

Morbidity (illness)

Mortality (death)

CM = Clinical Modification

PCS = Procedural Coding System

Provides continuity of data

World Health Organization's ICD-10 used globally

The United States develops ICD-10-CM and ICD-10-PCS version

On January 16, 2009, HHS published a final rule adopting ICD-10-CM and ICD-10-PCS

- Effective implementation date: October 1, 2015

Uses of ICD-10-CM

Facilitate payment of health services

Evaluate patients' use of health services

Fiscal entities track health care costs

Research

- Health care quality
- Future needs
- Newer cancer center built if patient use warrants
- Predict health care trends
- Plan for future health care needs

ICD-10-CM on Insurance Forms (Figure 19-1)

Diagnoses establish medical necessity

Services and diagnoses must correlate

■ Format

Diseases, Tabular List

Diseases, Alphabetic Index

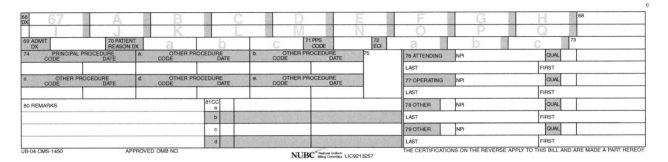

Figure **19-1** Blocks 66-81 of UB04/837I.

Diseases, Tabular List

Contains alphanumeric codes with descriptions

A00-Z99 diagnosis codes describe condition

21 chapters

Diseases, Alphabetic Index

Appears first in book

Refers coder to alphanumeric code in Volume 1

Never code directly from Index!

Placeholder

Character "X" is used as a placeholder for future expansion

Example: T36-T50 range of codes, "X" is placeholder

- T36.4X2A: Poisoning by, tetracyclines, intentional self-harm, initial encounter

7th Character

Certain categories have 7th character

Example: T36-T50 range of codes, "A" is 7th character to report initial encounter

- T36.4X2A: Poisoning by, tetracyclines, intentional self-harm, initial encounter

Abbreviations

Symbols, abbreviations, punctuation, and notations

NEC: Not elsewhere classifiable

- No more-specific code exists
- Means "other specified"

NOS: Not otherwise specified

- Unspecified in documentation

Punctuation

[ ] Brackets

Tabular:

- Enclose synonyms, alternative wording, or explanatory phrases
- Helpful, additional information
- Can affect code
- Located in Tabular List A00-Z99

Index: Brackets enclose manifestation codes

( ) Parentheses

Located in Tabular List and Index

- Contain nonessential modifiers
- Take them or leave them

Does not affect code

: Colon

Located in Tabular

Completes statement with one or more modifiers

Bold type

Codes and code titles in Tabular

Italicized Type
Located in Tabular

see

Located in Index

see also, *see* condition, *see also* condition, *omit code*

Includes, Excludes, Use Additional Code
Includes: Conditions included in code

Excludes1: Condition not coded here

Excludes2: Not included here; not part of condition being coded but may be used as an additional code, when condition documented

Use additional code: Assignment of other code(s) as necessary

And/With
And: Means "and/or"

With: One condition with (in addition to) another condition; "associated with" or "due to"

Code, if Applicable, any Causal Condition First
May be principal or first-listed diagnosis if no causal condition applicable or known

- If the causal condition is known, then a code for that condition should be sequenced as the principal or first-listed code diagnosis

■ Alphabetic Index

Nonessential modifiers: Have no effect on code selection

- Enclosed in parentheses
- Clarify diagnosis

  Example: Ileus (bowel) (colon) (inhibitory) (intestine) K56.7

Terms
Main terms (bold typeface)

Subterms

- Indented two spaces to right
- Not bold

Cross References in the Index
Directs you: *see, see also*

- "*see*" directs you to specific term, must be reference

  Example: Pelade—*see* Alopecia, areata
- "*see also*" directs you to another term for more information, may also be reference

  Example: Pneumopericarditis—*see also* Pericarditis
- "*see* condition" directs you to specific information about assignment of the code

  Example: Vesicourethrorectal—*see* condition
- "*see also* condition" directs you to specific information about assignment of the code

  Example: Abdomen, abdominal—*see also* condition

Notes
Define terms

Give further coding instructions

Example: Tabular H00-H59

- Note: Use an external cause code following the code for the eye condition, if applicable, to identify the cause of the eye condition

Eponyms

Disease or syndromes named for person

Example: Goldberg-Maxwell syndrome E34.51

Etiology and Manifestation of Disease

Etiology = cause of disease

Manifestation = symptom

Combination codes = etiology and manifestation in one code

Example: E11.341 Type 2 diabetes mellitus with severe nonproliferative diabetic retinopathy with macular edema

Index to Diseases

Largest part

First step in coding, locate main term in Index by condition, sign, symptom, or disease—not body area

Subterms indented two spaces to right

May have more than one subterm

Table of Neoplasms

Table of Neoplasms (illustrated in Figure 19-2)

- Located after the Z Index entries

Table of Drugs and Chemicals

Located after the Index of Diseases

Contains classification of drugs and substances to identify poisoning, adverse effects, and underdosing

- Adverse effect occurs when substance is taken correctly but patient has a negative reaction to substance

	Malignant Primary	Malignant Secondary	Ca in situ	Benign	Uncertain	Unspecified Behavior
bile or biliary (tract)	C24.9	C78.89	D01.5	D13.5	D37.6	D49.0
canaliculi (biliferi) (intrahepatic)	C22.1	C78.7	D01.5	D13.4	D37.6	D49.0
cands, interlobular	C22.1	C78.89	D01.5	D13.4	D37.6	D49.0
duct or passage (common) (cystic) (extrahepatic)	C24.0	C78.89	D01.5	D13.5	D37.6	D49.0
interlobular	C22.1	C78.89	D01.5	D13.4	D37.6	D49.0
intrahepatic	C22.1	C78.7	D01.5	D13.4	D37.6	D49.0
and extrahepatic	C24.8	C78.89	D01.5	D13.5	D37.6	D49.0

Figure **19-2** Table of Neoplasms.

Condition code for drug found under "Adverse Effect" column

- Poisoning occurs when substance is incorrectly taken

  Examples: Amoxicillin prescribed for bronchitis causes rash (adverse effect); or rather than one tablet of prescribed amoxicillin, patient takes 4 tablets and nausea results (poisoning)

Drug name placed alphabetically on left under heading "Substance" (Figure 19-3)

First column: "Poisoning Accidental (Unintentional)" lists code for substance involved if not related to an adverse effect

External cause codes identify how poisoning occurred (V, W, X, Y codes)

Table Headings

Poisoning, Accidental (Unintentional)

Poisoning, Intentional Self-Harm

Poisoning, Assault

Poisoning, Undetermined

Adverse Effect

Underdosing (never a primary or first-listed code)

V, W, X, Y Codes

External Causes of Injuries and Poisonings

Provides additional information about the nature of the injury/poisoning, locality, activity and status codes

Never principal (inpatient) or first-listed/primary (outpatient) diagnosis

Separate Index to External Causes

Located after Table of Drugs and Chemicals

		External Cause (T-Code)				
Substance	Poisoning, Accidental (Unintentional)	Poisoning, Intentional Self-Harm	Poisoning, Assault	Poisoning, Undetermined	Adverse Effect	Underdosing
Acetylsulfamethoxypyridazine	T37.0X1	T37.0X2	T37.0X3	T37.0X4	T37.0X5	T37.0X6
Achromycin	T36.4X1	T36.4X2	T36.4X3	T36.4X4	T36.4X5	T36.4X6
ophthalmic preparation	T49.5X1	T49.5X2	T49.5X3	T49.5X4	T49.5X5	T49.5X6
topical NEC	T49.0X1	T49.0X2	T49.0X3	T49.0X4	T49.0X5	T49.0X6
Aciclovir	T37.5X1	T37.5X2	T37.5X3	T37.5X4	T37.5X5	T37.5X6
Acid (corrosive) NEC	T54.2X1	T54.2X2	T54.2X3	T54.2X4	–	–
Acidifying agent NEC	T50.901	T50.902	T50.903	T50.904	T50.905	T50.906
Acipimox	T46.6X1	T46.6X2	T46.6X3	T46.6X4	T46.6X5	T46.6X6
Acitretin	T50.991	T50.992	T50.993	T50.994	T50.995	T50.996
Aclarubicin	T45.1X1	T45.1X2	T45.1X3	T45.1X4	T45.1X5	T45.1X6
Aclatonium napadisilate	T48.1X1	T48.1X2	T48.1X3	T48.1X4	T48.1X5	T48.1X6
Aconite (wild)	T46.991	T46.992	T46.993	T46.994	T46.995	T46.996

Figure **19-3** Table of Drugs and Chemicals.

- Alphabetical listing with main terms in bold
- Subterms indented 2 spaces to right under main term

A Word of Caution about the Alphabetic Index
Some words in Index do not appear in Tabular—saves space

Exact word may not be in code description in Tabular

- Usually found in Alphabetic Index
- Must locate term in Index and then locate in Tabular
- Additional coding instructions found in Tabular

▪ Tabular List

Major Division
Classification of Diseases and Injuries

- 21 Chapters

Classification of Diseases and Injuries
Main portion of ICD-10-CM

Codes from A00-Z99

Most chapters are body systems

Example:
- Digestive System
- Respiratory System

Divisions of Classification of Diseases and Injuries
Blocks: A group of related conditions

Category: Represents single disease/condition

Subcategory: More specific to etiology, anatomical site and severity

7th character requirement

Available for select codes in Chapters 13, 15, 18, 19, 20

Assign to highest level of specificity, based on documentation

- If 4th to 7th characters exist, do not report a code with fewer characters

---

Remember: ICD-10-CM and ICD-10-PCS are required for the CCS certification examination.

CHAPTER 20: USING ICD-10-CM

ICD-10-CM OGCR developed by Cooperating Parties
- American Hospital Association (AHA)
- American Health Information Management Association (AHIMA)
- Centers for Medicare and Medicaid Services (CMS)
- National Center for Health Statistics (NCHS)

▪ Official Guidelines

Appendix A of this text contains Evolve Resources to link to the ICD-10-CM OGCR

You must know and follow Guidelines when assigning diagnoses codes

- All certification examinations adhere to the OGCR

  In ICD-10-CM, the chapter instructions take precedence over the OGCR
- As you review this ICD-10-CM material, locate the information in the OGCR
- In this way, you will become familiar with the location of OGCR content to be able to quickly reference the OGCR during the examination
- Some Guidelines specific to place of service: inpatient/outpatient

Guidelines for Following Labels

You have to be able to code inpatient and outpatient facility services on the CCS certification examination

"(I)" indicates inpatient setting guidelines

"(O)" indicates outpatient setting guidelines

"(I/O)" guidelines apply to both inpatient and outpatient settings

■ Steps to Diagnosis Coding (I/O)

Identify MAIN term(s) in diagnosis

Locate MAIN term(s) in Index

Review subterms

Follow cross-reference instructions (e.g., *see, see also*)

Verify code(s) in Tabular

Remember (I/O)

Read Tabular notes

Code to highest specificity

NEVER CODE FROM INDEX!

A dot/dash (./-) after a code means additional character(s) required

OGCR Section I.B.2. Level of Detail in Coding (I/O)

Assign diagnosis to highest level of specificity

Do NOT use 3-character code if there is 4-character code

Do NOT use 4-character code if there is 5, 6, 7 character available

OGCR Section I.A.9. Other (NEC) and Unspecified (NOS) (I/O)

NEC = Not elsewhere classifiable

- More specific code does NOT exist

NOS = Not otherwise specified (means "unspecified")

- Available information NOT specific enough
- Use ONLY if more specific code NOT available

OGCR Section I.B.8. Acute and Chronic Conditions (I/O)

Exists alone or together

May be separate or combination codes

If two codes, code acute first

> *Example:* Acute (K85.9) and chronic (K86.1) pancreatitis

Combination code: Both acute and chronic conditions in one code

> *Example:* K80.46 Calculus of bile duct with acute and chronic cholecystitis without obstruction

OGCR Section I.B.9. Combination Code (I/O)

Always use combination code if one exists

Example: Rubella encephalitis B06.01

OGCR Section I.B.7. Multiple Coding for Single Condition

Etiology (cause)

Manifestation (symptom)

- Slanted brackets *[ ]*

  Example: Disease, heart, amyloid E85.4 *[I43]*

OGCR Section II.H. Uncertain Diagnosis (I)

If diagnosis at time of discharge states

- Probable
- Suspected
- Likely
- Questionable
- Possible
- Rule Out

Code condition as if condition existed until proven otherwise

Example: "Cough and fever, probably pneumonia" (I/O)

- Inpatient: Code pneumonia, do NOT code cough and fever (I)
- Outpatient: Code cough and fever, do NOT code pneumonia (O)

OGCR Section I.B.11. Impending or Threatened Condition (I)

Code any condition described at time of discharge as impending or threatened

- Did occur: Code as confirmed diagnosis
- Did NOT occur: Code as impending or threatened (MAIN terms)

OGCR Section I.B.13. Laterality (I/O)

Laterality may be right, left, bilateral, or unspecified

- M93.271 Osteochondritis dissecans, right ankle and joints of right foot
- M93.272 Osteochondritis dissecans, left ankle and joints of left foot
- If no bilateral code is available and condition is bilateral, assign separate codes for left and right

OGCR Section I.B.14. Documentation for BMI, Non-pressure Ulcers, and Pressure Ulcer Stages

Code assignment based on medical documentation

May be health care provider other than physician, such as nurse

- Associated diagnosis must be documented by physician

BMI is assigned as secondary diagnosis only

Selection of Principal Diagnosis (I)

Condition established after study (tests)

Responsible for patient admission

Selection of Primary/First-Listed Diagnosis (O)

Condition for encounter

Documented

Responsible for services provided

Also list coexisting condition(s) or comorbidity(ies)

Diagnosis and Services (I/O)

Diagnosis and procedure MUST correlate

Medical necessity established

No correlation = No reimbursement

OGCR Section II.A. Symptoms, Signs, and Ill-Defined Conditions (I)

Inpatient coders do NOT use when definitive or possible diagnosis has been established

Can be the provisional diagnosis if a more specific diagnosis is not available

Chapter 18 of ICD-10-CM, Symptoms, Signs, and Abnormal Clinical and Laboratory Finds, Not Elsewhere Classified (R00-R99), contains many but not all codes for symptoms

OGCR Section I.A.7. Codes in Brackets (I/O)

Never sequence as first-listed diagnosis

Always sequence in order listed in Index

> *Example:* Chorioretinitis, in (due to) histoplasmosis B39.9 *[H32]*
>
> - Code first histoplasmosis (B39.9), then chorioretinitis (H32)

OGCR Section II.B. Two or More Interrelated Conditions (I/O)

When two or more interrelated conditions exist and either could be the principal or first-listed diagnosis, either is sequenced first

> *Example:* Patient with mitral valve stenosis and coronary artery disease (two interrelated conditions)

- Either can be principal diagnosis and sequenced first
- Resource intensiveness affects choice

OGCR Section II.C. Two or More Equal Diagnoses (I/O)

Either can be sequenced first

> *Example:* Diagnosis of viral gastroenteritis and dehydration

OGCR Section II.D. Two or More Comparative or Contrasting Conditions (I)

"Either/or" diagnoses coded as confirmed

If determination CANNOT be made, either can be sequenced first

- Pneumonia or lung cancer
- Lung cancer or pneumonia

OGCR Section II.E. Symptom(s) Followed by Contrasting/Comparative Diagnoses (I)

Symptom code sequenced first

- Followed by other diagnoses

OGCR Section I.C.21.c.6. Observation and Evaluation for Suspected Conditions Not Found (I/O)

Z03.6-Z03.89 Assigned as principal diagnosis for:

- Admissions for evaluation

- Following an accident that would ordinarily result in health problem, BUT there is none

  Example: Car accident, driver hits head, no apparent injury, admit to R/O head trauma

OGCR Section II.F. Original Treatment Plan Not Carried Out (I)
Principal diagnosis becomes

- Condition that after study was reason for admission

Treatment does NOT have to be carried out for condition

  Example: Patient admitted for elective surgery, develops pneumonia; surgery canceled

- Code reason for surgery first
- Code "Surgical or other procedure NOT carried out because of other contraindication" Z53.09
- Also code pneumonia

Sequela (Late Effects) (I/O)

Location in the OGCR: Section I.B.10.

Late effect residual of (remaining from) previous illness/injury

- e.g., Burn that leaves scar

Residual coded first (scar)

Cause (burn) coded second

Late effect codes are not in a separate chapter; rather, throughout Tabular

Reference the term "Late, effect(s)" in the Index; you are directed to "*see* Sequelae"

There is no time limit on developing a residual

There may be more than one residual

  Example: Patient has a stroke (I63.9) and develops paralysis on right dominant side (hemiparesis, I69.351) and loss of ability to communicate (aphasia, I69.320)

CHAPTER 21: ICD-10-CM CHAPTERS 1-10

Chapter 1, Certain Infectious and Parasitic Diseases (I/O)

Divided based on etiology (cause of disease)

Many combination codes

  Example: B37.0 candidiasis stomatitis infection of mouth, which reports both the organism and condition with one code

Multiple Codes (I/O)
Sequencing must be considered.

- UTI due to Escherichia coli
  - N39.0 (UTI) etiology
  - B96.2- (*E. coli*) organism (in this order)

OGCR Section I.C.1.a. Human Immunodeficiency Virus (I/O)
Code HIV or HIV-related illness ONLY if stated as confirmed in diagnostic statement

- B20 HIV or HIV-related illness
- Z21 Asymptomatic HIV status
- R75 Inconclusive HIV serology

Previously Diagnosed HIV-Related Illness (I/O)

Code prior diagnosis HIV-related disease B20 (HIV)

NEVER assign these patients to:

- Z21 (Asymptomatic) or
- R75 (Nonspecific serologic evidence of HIV)

HIV Sequencing (I)

If admitted for HIV-related illness (e.g., pneumonia due to *Pneumocystis carinii*)

- Code B20 (HIV)
- Followed by current illness (B59, Pneumonia due to *Pneumocystis carinii*)

If admitted for other than HIV-related illness (unilateral inguinal hernia)

- Code reason for admittance K40.90 (Unilateral inguinal hernia NOS)
- Then B20 (HIV)

Sequencing (O)

- Sequence first reason most responsible for encounter
- Followed by secondary diagnosis that affects encounter or patient care

HIV and Pregnancy (I/O)

This is an exception to HIV sequencing

During pregnancy, childbirth, or puerperium, code:

- O98.7--(Other specified infections and parasitic diseases)
- Followed by B20 (HIV)

Asymptomatic HIV during pregnancy, childbirth, or puerperium

- O98.7--(Other specified infections and parasitic diseases)
- Z21 (Asymptomatic HIV infection status)
- Reporting asymptomatic HIV varies by state
  - Check the state's reporting laws

Inconclusive Laboratory Test for HIV (I/O)

R75 (Inconclusive serologic test for HIV)

- Reporting inconclusive laboratory HIV tests varies by state
  - Check the state's reporting laws
- Typically used in infants of mothers who are HIV positive

HIV Screening (I/O)

Code Z11.4 (Screening for human immunodeficiency virus [HIV])

- Patient in high-risk group for HIV
- Z72.89 (Other problems related to lifestyle)

Patients returning for HIV screening results = Z71.7 (HIV counseling)

Caution (I/O)

Incorrectly applying these HIV coding rules can cause patient hardship

Insurance claims for patients with HIV usually need patient's written agreement to disclosure

OGCR Section I.C.1.d. Septicemia, Severe Sepsis, and Septic Shock

Sepsis: Assign systemic infection code as first-listed diagnosis when sepsis is present

- Assign a sepsis code as secondary when sepsis develops during encounter

Septicemia/SIRS: Usually an A41.9 septicemia code and a R65.- SIRS code (in this order)

- Code the organ system dysfunction by the SIRS (e.g., J96.9- respiratory failure followed by R65.2-)

Septic Shock: Organ dysfunction associated with severe sepsis

- Code underlying systemic infection (e.g., A41.9) followed by the combination code for severe sepsis with septic shock (R65.21)

■ Chapter 2, Neoplasms (I/O)

Two steps for coding neoplasms

- Incorrectly applying these neoplasm codes can also cause patient hardship
    1. Index: Locate histologic type of neoplasm (e.g., Sarcoma, melanotic—*see* Melanoma); review all instructions
    2. Locate code identified (usually in Neoplasm Table in Index) by body site

Neoplasm Table divided into columns:

- Malignant (Primary)
- Malignant (Secondary)
- Ca in situ
- Benign
- Uncertain
- Unspecified Behavior

Example: Pathology report confirmed diagnosis stated in operative report of primary malignant neoplasm of the bladder neck

- ICD-10-CM, Neoplasm Table, bladder, neck, under Malignant, Primary column, C67.5
- Reference in the Tabular to ensure accurate assignment

Coded as primary site unless specified as secondary site (metastasis)

Bone	Meninges	Brain
Peritoneum	Diaphragm	Pleura
Heart	Retroperitoneum	Liver
Lymph nodes	Spinal cord	Mediastinum

OGCR Section I.C.2. Neoplasms (I/O)
Treatment directed at neoplasm: Neoplasm is principal/first-listed diagnosis

- Except for chemotherapy, immunotherapy, or radiotherapy:
    - Therapy (treatment), listed first (Z51.-)
    - Neoplasm, listed second

Chemotherapy: Z51.11

Radiotherapy: Z51.0

Immunotherapy: Z51.12

First-Listed Diagnosis, Neoplasms (I/O)
Surgical removal of neoplasm and subsequent chemotherapy or radiotherapy

- Code neoplasm as principal/first-listed diagnosis

Surgery to determine extent of malignancy (staging)

- Code neoplasm as principal/first-listed diagnosis

History and Secondary Metastasis of Neoplasms (I/O)
Report Z85.-, Personal history of malignant neoplasm, if:

- Neoplasm was previously destroyed, AND
- No longer being treated

If patient receives treatment for secondary neoplasm (metastasis)

- Secondary neoplasm is principal/first-listed diagnosis
- Even though primary is known

Admission for Neoplasms (I)

Admission for symptoms of primary or secondary neoplasm

- Neoplasm principal diagnosis

Do NOT code symptoms or signs

Anemia and Complications with/of Neoplasm (I/O)

Patient treated for anemia due to neoplasm or dehydration due to neoplasm or therapy, code in this order:

- Anemia or dehydration
- Neoplasm

Code for antineoplasm drug adverse effect (T code)

Patient admitted to repair complication of surgery for an intestinal neoplasm

- Complication, principal/first-listed diagnosis
- Complication is reason for encounter
- Neoplasm, secondary diagnosis

Report T code first if anemia is an adverse effect of chemotherapy

Z Codes and Neoplasms (I/O)

Patient receiving chemotherapy or radiotherapy post-op removal of neoplasm code:

- Therapy
- Active neoplasm

Do NOT report H/O (history of) neoplasm

■ Chapter 3, Diseases of the Blood and Blood-Forming Organs and Certain Disorders Involving the Immune Mechanism (I/O)

Includes anemia, blood disorders, coagulation defects

Often used code: Anemia

Many different types of anemia:
- Hereditary hemolytic (D58.9)
- Iron deficiency (D50.9)
- Acquired hemolytic (D59.9)
- Aplastic (D61.9)
- Other specified (D64.8-)
- Unspecified (D64.9)

Multiple coding often necessary

Identify underlying disease condition

■ Chapter 4, Endocrine, Nutritional, and Metabolic Diseases (I/O)

Disorders of Other Endocrine Glands (I/O)

Diabetes Mellitus (E10 or E11) coded frequently

- Combination codes include type of DM, body system affected, and complications

Example:

- E11.39 reports Type 2 diabetes mellitus with other diabetic ophthalmic complications (etiology)
- Often requires two codes
  - Z79.4 used in addition to diabetes code to report long-term use of insulin

  Temporary insulin use not coded to Z79.4; only long-term

If type not indicated, report type 2

Type 1 diabetic is always insulin-dependent

Patient with type 2 diabetes may be insulin-dependent

Other Metabolic and Immunity Disorders Section (I/O)

Disorders such as gout and dehydration

Disorders often have many names

- E05.00 Toxic diffuse goiter, also known as
  - Basedow's disease
  - Graves' disease
  - Hyperthyroidism with goiter

Chapter 5, Mental, Behavioral, and Neurodevelopmental Disorders (I/O)

Includes codes for:

- Personality disorders
- Stress disorders
- Neuroses
- Psychoses
- Sexual dysfunction, etc.

Pain disorders related to psychological factors

- Assign F45.42 for psychological factors related to pain and code also a G89.- code (acute or chronic pain)

Mental and behavioral disorders due to psychoactive substance use

- In remission, F10-F19
- Psychoactive substance use, abuse, dependence, one code assigned based on hierarchy (see OGCR, Section I.C.5.b.2.)

Chapter 6, Diseases of Nervous System (I/O)

Central Nervous System

Peripheral Nervous System

Pain—Category G89

Acute or chronic pain not elsewhere classified due to:

- Acute pain due to trauma G89.11
- Acute post-thoracotomy pain G89.12
- Central pain syndrome G89.0
- Other acute postoperative pain G89.18
- Neoplasm related pain (acute) (chronic) G89.3
- Chronic pain due to trauma G89.21

- Chronic post-thoracotomy pain G89.22
- Other chronic postprocedural pain G89.28
- Chronic pain syndrome G89.4

Principal/Primary diagnosis

- Pain management is reason for encounter/admission

Chapter 7, Diseases of Eye and Adnexa (I/O)

Does not contain all the eye and adnexa codes

Example: Traumatic injury to eye and orbit of eye, S05.-

Hordeolum, infection of sebaceous gland of eyelid (stye)

Reported on location and type

Example: Externum, report H00.01- or internum, report H00.02-

Chalazion, infection of eyelid that forms mass

Reported based on location

Entropion = turning inward of eyelid (H02.0--)

Ectropion = turning outward of eyelid (H02.1--)

Lacrimal System, category H04

Reported based on right, left, bilateral, unspecified

Chapter 8, Diseases of Ear and Mastoid Process (I/O)

Excludes2 indicates other categories for reporting other ear conditions

Examples: Endocrine, nutritional and metabolic disease (E00-E90)

H60-H95 reports diseases of:

- External ear
- Middle ear
- Inner ear
- Mastoid
- Other
- Surgical complications NEC

Chapter 9, Diseases of Circulatory System (I/O)

OGCR Section I.C.9.a. Hypertension (I/O)

Assign hypertension (arterial, benign, essential, malignant, primary, systemic) to I10

OGCR Section I.C.9.a.1. Hypertension with Heart Disease (I/O)

Category I11

- Certain heart conditions when stated "due to hypertension" or implied ("hypertensive")
- Any condition in I50.- or I51.4-I51.9 due to hypertension
- Use additional code to specify type of heart failure (I50.-)

OGCR Section I.C.9.a.2. Hypertensive Chronic Kidney Disease (I/O)

Cause-and-effect relationship assumed in chronic kidney failure with hypertension

Category I12 Hypertensive chronic kidney disease

- Includes any condition in N18.- due to chronic kidney disease

Use additional code to identify stage of chronic kidney disease N18.1-N18.9

OGCR Section I.C.9.a.3. Hypertensive Heart and Chronic Kidney Disease (I/O)

Assign category I13 when both hypertensive chronic kidney disease and hypertensive heart disease stated in diagnosis

Assume cause-and-effect relationship between hypertension and chronic kidney disease

Includes any condition in I11.- with any condition in I12.- cardiorenal disease; cardiovascular renal disease

- Use additional code from category I50 to identify type of heart failure
- Use additional code to identify stage of chronic kidney disease (N18.1-N18.9)

OGCR Section I.C.9.a.4. Hypertensive Cerebrovascular Disease (I/O)

Use additional code to identify presence of hypertension (I10-I15)

Code:

- Cerebrovascular disease (I60-I69)
- Type of hypertension (I10-I15)

OGCR Section I.C.9.a.5. Hypertensive Retinopathy (I/O)

Code:

- Hypertensive retinopathy (H35.0)
- Type of hypertension (I10-I15)

The sequencing is based on the reason for the encounter.

OGCR Section I.C.9.a.6. Hypertension, Secondary (I/O)

Hypertension caused by an underlying condition

Code:

- Underlying condition
- Type of hypertension (I15)

OGCR Section I.C.9.a.7. Hypertension, Transient (I/O)

Transient hypertension: Temporary elevation of BP

Do NOT assign I10-I15, Hypertensive disease

- Hypertension diagnosis NOT established
- Assign either:
  - R03.0, Elevated blood pressure
  - O13.-, Gestational hypertension without significant proteinuria (pregnancy induced)
  - O14.-, Pre-eclampsia, for transient hypertension of pregnancy with significant proteinuria

OGCR Section I.C.9.a.8. Hypertension, Controlled (I/O)

Hypertension controlled by therapy

- Assign appropriate code from categories I10-I15

OGCR Section I.C.9.a.9. Hypertension, Uncontrolled (I/O)

Untreated hypertension

Uncontrolled hypertension

Assign appropriate code from categories I10-I15

■ Chapter 10, Diseases of Respiratory System (I/O)

Watch for "Use additional code to identify infectious organism"

- Some codes include the specific organism and do not need an additional code
- Respiratory Failure Sequencing

If the respiratory failure is due to an acute condition (such as MI [myocardial infarction]) or acute exacerbation of a chronic condition (such as COPD [chronic obstructive pulmonary disease]), sequence the acute condition first

Example: MI (acute condition) and respiratory failure

- Sequence MI (I21.3) first and respiratory failure (J96.00) second

If the respiratory failure (acute condition) is due to a chronic nonrespiratory condition (such as myasthenia gravis), sequence the respiratory failure first

Example: Acute respiratory failure (acute) and myasthenia gravis (chronic)

- Sequence acute respiratory failure (J96.00) first and myasthenia gravis (G70.00) second

Acute Respiratory Infection Section (I/O)

Frequently assigned codes, such as:

- Common cold (J00, acute nasopharyngitis)
- Sore throat (J02, acute pharyngitis)
- Acute tonsillitis (J03)
- Acute bronchitis (J20-J21), chronic bronchitis (J41-J42)
- Acute upper respiratory infection (J06.9)
- Influenza (J09-J10)
- Pneumonia (J12-J18)

Read OGCR Section I.C.10.a., or Chapter 10 for specifics on coding COPD and asthma

CHAPTER 22: ICD-10-CM CHAPTERS 11-14

■ Chapter 11, Diseases of Digestive System (I/O)

Mouth to anus and accessory organs

Extensive subcategories

Cholelithiasis (K80)

Commonly assigned codes

- Ulcers (K25-K28)
  - Gastric (K25)
  - Duodenal (K26)
  - Peptic (K27)
  - Gastrojejunal (K28)
- Hernias (K40-K46)

■ Chapter 12, Diseases of Skin and Subcutaneous Tissue (I/O)

Skin

Epidermis

Dermis

Subcutaneous tissue

Infectious skin/Subcutaneous tissue

Scar tissue

Accessory Organs

Sweat glands

Sebaceous glands

Nails

Hair and hair follicles

Other

> *Example:* Cellulitis of right finger due to *Staphylococcus aureus*, report:
>
> - Cellulitis L03.011
> - *Staphylococcus aureus* B95.61

■ Chapter 13, Diseases of Musculoskeletal System and Connective Tissue (I/O)

Bone

Bursa

Cartilage

Fascia

Ligaments

Muscle

Synovia

Tendons

Sections (I/O)

Infectious arthropathies (joint disease)

Inflammatory polyarthropathies

Osteoarthritis

Other joint disorders

Dentofacial anomalies

Systemic connective tissue disorders

Deforming dorsopathies

Spondylopathies

Other dorsopathies

Disorders of muscle

Disorders of synovium and tendons

Other soft tissue disorders

Disorders of bone density and structure

Other osteopathies

Chondropathies

Other disorders of the musculoskeletal system and connective tissue

Intraoperative and postprocedural complications and disorders of musculoskeletal system, not elsewhere classified

Biomechanical lesions, not elsewhere classified

■ Chapter 14, Diseases of Genitourinary System (I/O)

Commonly assigned codes categories:

- Urinary tract infection (N39.0)
- Inflammatory diseases of prostate (N41.-)
- Inflammatory diseases of female pelvic organs (N70-N77)

Stages of chronic kidney disease

- Stage 1: Blood flow through kidney increases, kidney enlarges (N18.1)
- Stage 2: (mild) Small amounts of blood protein (albumin) leak into urine (microalbuminuria) (N18.2)
- Stage 3: (moderate) Albumin and other protein losses increase. Patient may develop high blood pressure and kidney loses ability to filter waste (N18.3)
- Stage 4: (severe) Large amounts of urine pass through kidney: blood pressure increases (N18.4)
- Stage 5: Ability to filter waste nearly stops (N18.5)
- End-stage renal failure (N18.6)

When documentation indicates chronic renal disease (CKD) and ESRD, report ESRD

- Unspecified (N19)

Status post kidney transplant, assign Z94.0

- Patient may still have CKD

CHAPTER 23: ICD-10-CM CHAPTERS 15-21

■ Chapter 15, Pregnancy, Childbirth, and the Puerperium (I/O)

Used only on the **maternal** record

Admission for pregnancy, complication

- Obstetric complication = first-listed diagnosis

Chapter 15 codes take precedence over codes from other chapters unless the documentation indicates the condition being treated is not affecting the management of the pregnancy

The majority of codes in Chapter 15 have a final character indicating the trimester of pregnancy

7 characters are required on specified codes in Chapter 15

OGCR Section I.C.15.a. General Rules (I/O)

Not all encounters are pregnancy-related

Example: Pregnant woman, broken ankle; report:

- Broken ankle
- Z33.1 Pregnant state incidental

Must be documented in medical record that condition being treated is not affecting pregnancy

- If NOT documented, assume condition is affecting pregnancy

Trimesters

Trimesters are counted from the first day of the last menstrual period

- 1st trimester: Less than 14 weeks 0 days
- 2nd trimester: 14 weeks 0 days to less than 28 weeks 0 days
- 3rd trimester: 28 weeks 0 days until delivery

OGCR Section I.C.15.a.2. Complications of Pregnancy, Childbirth, and the Puerperium (I/O)

Chapter 15 codes (O00-O9A)

- Assigned only to mother's medical record
- Not assigned to newborn medical record

Episodes when no delivery occurs

- Principal diagnosis should correspond to the principal complication of the pregnancy which necessitated the encounter.

OGCR Section I.C.15.b.4., When a delivery occurs

OGCR Section I.C.15.b.5., Outcome of delivery code (Z37) when delivered

OGCR Section I.C.15.b.3., Selection of Principal Diagnosis when no delivery occurs—Obstetric (I)

OGCR Section I.C.15.b.1.-2. Selection of Principal or First-listed Diagnosis (O)

Routine prenatal visits, no complications:

- Z34, Supervision, normal pregnancy, or

Prenatal outpatient visits for high-risk pregnancies

- O09, Supervision of high-risk pregnancy

OGCR Section I.C.15.n.1.-3. Normal Delivery, Code O80 (I)

Normal delivery includes:

- Vaginal delivery
- Minimal or no assistance
- With or without episiotomy
- No fetal manipulation or instrumentation
- Full-term, single, liveborn infant

No complications, principal diagnosis = O80

With complications = NOT O80 (normal delivery)

- Only outcome for O80 is normal delivery

Z37.0 (Single liveborn) only outcome of delivery code appropriate for use with O80

Delivery Procedure Codes (I)

If delivered prior to admission:

- In ambulance
- At home
- In ED

Do NOT code delivery

Code any postpartum repairs

Postpartum Period (I/O)

After delivery and continues for 6 weeks

Peripartum Period (I/O)

Defined as the last month of pregnancy to five months postpartum

Abortions (I/O)

No identifiable fetus

500 grams or less

Less than 22 weeks' gestation

Codes O00-O08

Abortions with Liveborn Fetus (I/O)

Attempted abortion results in liveborn fetus

- Category O60 (Early onset of delivery) appropriately

Assign Z37 (Outcome of delivery)

Attempted abortion code also assigned

■ Chapter 16, Certain Conditions Originating in the Perinatal Period (I/O)

Birth through 28 days following birth

Conditions Originating in Perinatal Period P00-P96

- Perinatal period through 28th day following birth
- Codes can be used after 28th day, if documented that condition originated during perinatal period

Chapter 16 codes are for use on the maternal record

Assign Z38.– as first-listed diagnosis according to type of birth

Use of Codes Z00 (I/O)

Z00.11 Newborn health examination

Infant 28 days or less

Excludes1 health check for child over 28 days old (Z00.12-)

Use of Codes Z37 (I)

Liveborn infant(s) according to place and type of birth

Example:

- Z37.0 Single liveborn
- Z37.2 Liveborn twins

Inpatient: Principal diagnosis

NOTE: Z37 assigned ONLY once, hospital record where baby delivered

Coding Additional Diagnosis (I)

Code conditions that require

- Treatment
- Further investigation
- Additional resource

Prolonged length of stay (LOS)

Implications for future care

Insignificant conditions, signs, symptoms

- Resolve with no treatment
- Need no code
- EVEN IF documented

Prematurity and Fetal Growth Retardation (I)

Codes from categories

- P05 (Slow fetal growth and fetal malnutrition) and
- P07 (Disorders relating to short gestation and low birthweight NEC)

Not assigned solely on birthweight or gestational age

Use physician's assessment of maturity

Use additional code for weeks of gestation (P07.30, P07.31, P07.32)

Chapter 17, Congenital Malformations, Deformations and Chromosomal Abnormalities

When a malformation/deformation/or chromosomal abnormality does not have a unique code assignment, assign additional code(s) for any manifestations that may be present.

Codes from Chapter 17 may be used throughout the life of the patient. If a congenital malformation or deformity has been corrected, a personal history code should be used to identify the history of the malformation or deformity.

Chapter 18, Symptoms, Signs, and Abnormal Clinical and Laboratory Findings, Not Elsewhere Classified

Do NOT code a sign or symptom if

- Definitive diagnosis made (symptoms are part of disease)

Used only if no specific diagnosis made or symptoms are not linked to the diagnosis

One category requires 7 characters (Coma, R40.2-)

Chapter 19, Injury, Poisoning and Certain Other Consequences of External Causes

Block Examples (I/O)

- S00-S09 Injuries to the head
- S10-S19 Injuries to the neck
- S20-S29 Injuries to the thorax
- S30-S39 Injuries to the abdomen, lower back, lumbar spine, pelvis and external genitals
- S40-S49 Injuries to the shoulder and upper arm
- S50-S59 Injuries to the elbow and forearm
- S60-S69 Injuries to the wrist, hand, and fingers
- S70-S79 Injuries to the hip and thigh
- S80-S89 Injuries to the knee and lower leg
- S90-S99 Injuries to the ankle and foot

When Coding Injuries:

- Assign separate codes for each injury unless a combination code is provided, in which case the combination code is assigned.
- Multiple injury codes are provided in ICD-10-CM but should not be assigned unless information for a more specific code is not available
- Traumatic injury codes (S00-T14.9) are not assigned for normal, healing surgical wounds or to identify complications of surgical wounds
- Most categories in Chapter 19 have 7th character extensions that are required for each applicable code.

  Most categories in this chapter have three extensions (with the exception of fractures):

    A, initial encounter

    D, subsequent encounter

    S, sequela

External Cause Codes: Index and Tabular

V, W, X, Y code Index located following the Table of Drugs and Chemicals

Directly before the Tabular

Not in the Index to Disease and Injuries

Codes V, W, X, Y are located in Chapter 20 in the Tabular

▪ Chapter 20, External Causes of Morbidity (I/O)

The only external cause codes assigned on the CCS examination are those for adverse effects of correct medication correctly given and correctly taken

Provide supplemental information

Identify

- Cause of an injury or poisoning
- Intent (unintentional or intentional)
- Place it occurred
- Activity

Chapter 20 General Code Guidelines (V01-Y99)

Use with any code in Volume 1 in the range of A00.0-T88.9, Z00-Z99

7th character required on most codes to describe the initial encounter, subsequent encounter, or sequela (late effect)

Assign as many external cause codes as necessary

Certain external cause codes are combination codes

Initial encounter

- Use external cause code, if applicable

Table of Drugs and Chemicals (I/O)

Follows the Neoplasm Table in Index

Alphabetic listing with codes

Do NOT code directly from Table

Always reference Tabular

Late Effects of External Cause (I/O)

Should be used with late effect of a previous injury/poisoning

Should NOT be used with related current injury code

Report using the external cause code with the 7th character extension "S" for Sequela

These codes should be used with any report of a late effect or sequela resulting from a previous injury

Signs and Symptoms and Definitive Diagnosis (I/O)

Do NOT code a sign/symptom if definitive diagnosis made

- Symptoms are part of disease

Use only if no specific diagnosis is made

Burns/Corrosions Classified (I/O)

According to extent of body surface involved

Burn site NOT specified

Additional data required

Burn—heat

Corrosion—chemical

Category (I/O)

Category T31.- = % body surface involved and

% body surface involved in 3rd-degree burns

Rule of Nines applies

> Burn Example: 3rd-degree burn of abdomen (10%) and 2nd-degree burn of left thigh (5%) by hot water, initial encounter

- T21.32XA Burn, abdomen, 3rd degree
- T24.212A Burn, thigh, left, 2nd degree
- T31.11 15% total burn area and 10% 3rd degree
- X12.XXXA Burn by hot liquid

Debridement of Wound, Infection, or Burn (I)

Excisional debridement

- Cut away
- Performed by physician or other health care provider

Nonexcisional procedure

- Shaved or scraped
- Performed by physician or nonphysician

Coding for Multiple Injuries (I/O)

Separate code for each injury

Most serious injury first

Vessel and Nerve Damage (I/O)

Code primary injury first

- Use additional code if nerve damage minor

Primary injury = Nerve damage

- Code nerve damage first

Multiple Fractures (I/O)

Same coding principles as multiple injuries

Code multiple fractures by site

Sequenced by severity

Fractures (I/O)

Not indicated as closed or open = closed

Same bone fractured AND dislocated:

- Code fracture ONLY (highest level of injury)
  - Laterality

■ Chapter 21, Factors Influencing Health Status and Contact with Health Services

Z Codes

Located after Y99.9 in Tabular

Main terms: Contraception, counseling, dialysis, status, examination

Uses of Z Codes (I/O)

Not sick BUT receives health care (e.g., vaccination)

Services for known disease/injury (e.g., chemotherapy)

A circumstance/problem that influences patient's health BUT NOT current illness/injury

Example: Organ transplant status

Example: Birth status and outcome of delivery (newborn)

Special Note about "History of" (I/O)

Index to Disease, MAIN term "History"

Entries between "family" and "visual loss Z82.1" = "family history of"

Entries after "family" and after "visual loss Z86.69" = "personal history of"

Draw a line in the Index of your ICD-10-CM coding manual to indicate end of "family history" entries and beginning of "personal history" entries

History Z Codes

Section I.C.21. of the OGCR contains specific guidelines that identify how Z codes can be listed (first, first/additional, additional only)

Categories in Tabular

Z85	Personal history of malignant neoplasm
Z86.59	Personal history of mental and behavioral disorder
Z87.89	Personal history of other specified conditions

Except: Z87.39 Personal history of arthritis, and Z87.79 Personal history of congenital malformations. These conditions are life-long so are not true history codes

Z88	Allergy status to medicinal agents
Z91.89	Other personal risk factors presenting hazards to health
Z80	Family history of primary malignant neoplasm
Z82.8	Family history of certain other disabilities and chronic diseases
Z84.89	Family history of other specified conditions

CHAPTER 24: OUTPATIENT CODING

■ OGCR Section IV, Diagnostic Coding and Reporting Guidelines for Outpatient Services (O)

Hospital-based outpatient services = OPPS

Part of ICD-10-CM OGCR, Section IV

Guideline A

Use term first-listed diagnosis for outpatient settings

Outpatient surgery: If procedure is not performed due to contraindications, report the reason for the surgery as first-listed diagnosis

Observation stay: Report medical condition as first-listed diagnosis

Patient admitted for outpatient surgery develops complications requiring admission to observation, report reason for admission, followed by codes for complications

Guideline B

Use codes A00.0-T88.9, Z00-Z99 to report diagnosis, symptoms, conditions, problems, complaints, or other reason(s) for visit

Guideline C

Accurate reporting of ICD-10-CM diagnosis codes, documentation should include patient's condition, specific diagnosis(es), symptoms, problems, or reason for encounter

Guideline D

Codes that describe symptoms and signs (rather than diagnoses) are acceptable for outpatient coding

Guideline E

Encounters for circumstances other than a disease or injury are reported with Z00-Z99

Guideline F

Level of detail in coding ICD-10-CM: code to highest number of characters available

Guideline G

First-listed diagnosis is the diagnosis, condition, problem, or other reason for encounter/visit

Guideline H

Uncertain diagnoses are not reported in outpatient settings

Report the condition that is the reason for the encounter, such as symptoms, signs, abnormal test results

Guideline I

Chronic diseases are treated on an ongoing basis

Report the disease each time the disease is treated or managed

Guideline J

Code all documented conditions that coexist

Do not code conditions that were previously treated and no longer exist

Guideline K

Patients receiving diagnostic services only, the first-listed code is the diagnosis, condition, problem or other reason for encounter that is chiefly responsible for services

Routine laboratory/radiology tests

- When no signs, symptoms, or diagnoses are available, report Z01.89
- When test is to evaluate sign, symptom, or diagnosis, report both the V code and a code to report the reason for the test

  Report any confirmed or definitive diagnosis(es) documented in the test result interpretation

  - Do not code signs and symptoms as additional diagnoses

Guideline L

Patients receiving therapeutic services only, sequence first the diagnosis, condition, problem or reason for encounter chiefly responsible for service

- Report other diagnosis(es), such as chronic conditions, as secondary diagnosis(es)

Guideline M

Patients receiving preoperative evaluations only

- Report a code from subcategory Z01.81 as first-listed diagnosis
- Report condition that prompted surgery as secondary diagnosis
- Code also any findings related to preoperative evaluation

Guideline N

Ambulatory surgery: Report the diagnosis for which the surgery was performed

Report the postoperative diagnosis if different from preoperative diagnosis

Guideline O

See OGCR, Section I.C.15

Routine prenatal visits, no complications:

- Z34, Supervision, normal first pregnancy

Prenatal outpatient visits for high-risk pregnancies

- O09, Supervision of high-risk pregnancy

Guideline P

Encounters for general medical examinations, with or without abnormal findings, report Z00.0-

If examination results in abnormal finding, report as first-listed diagnosis a code for general medical examination with abnormal findings

   - Secondary code to report the abnormal finding

Guideline Q

Encounters for routine health screening, see OGCR, Section I.C.21.

CHAPTER 25: ICD-10-PCS, REPORTING INPATIENT PROCEDURES

Appendix A of this text contains Evolve Resources to link to ICD-10-PCS OGCR

90% of codes refer to surgical procedures

10% refer to diagnostic and therapeutic procedures

- Codes assigned by hospitals to report facility services provided to inpatients
- Procedures done in physician's office or outpatient ASC are coded using CPT/HCPCS codes
- Surgeon uses CPT to report services to inpatients

GEMs file maps ICD-9-CM, Volume 3 to ICD-10-PCS (illustrated in Figure 25-1)

> **Example**:
> ICD-9-CM Volume 3 code 00.01 maps to 6A750Z4 or 6A751Z4

■ Table of Contents

Contains the Sections of the ICD-10-PCS coding system

Appendix A of the manual contains the definitions used within the system

■ Alphabetic Index

Index terms in bold

- Subterms not in bold

Alphabetical arrangement as illustrated in Figure 25-2

Cross-reference feature is "*see*"

> **Example**: Inferior tarsal plate
> *see* Eyelid, Lower, Right
> *see* Eyelid, Lower, Left

Never code directly from Index.

```
0001  6A750Z4 10000 ⎫
0001  6A751Z4 10000 ⎬
0002  6A750Z5 10000
0002  6A751Z5 10000
0003  6A750Z6 10000
0003  6A751Z6 10000
0009  6A750Z7 10000
0009  6A750ZZ 10000
0009  6A751Z7 10000
0009  6A751ZZ 10000
0009  6A930ZZ 10000
0009  6A931ZZ 10000
```

Figure **25-1** ICD-9-CM Volume 3 mapping to ICD-10-PCS.

A

Abdominal aortic plexus *see* Nerve, Abdominal Sympathetic
Abdominal esophagus *see* Esophagus, Lower
Abdominohysterectomy
  see Excision, Uterus 0UB9
  see Resection, Uterus 0UT9
Abdominoplasty
  see Alteration, Wall, Abdominal 0W0F
  see Repair, Wall, Abdominal 0WQF
  see Supplement, Wall, Abdominal 0WUF
Abductor hallucis muscle
  see Muscle, Foot, Right
  see Muscle, Foot, Left

Figure **25-2** ICD-10-PCS Tables.

■ Tabular List

Tables of Sections

Usually subdivided by:

- Body System
- Operation
- Body Part
- Approach
- Device
- Qualifier

Tables of Characters to Be Assigned (Illustrated in Figure 25-3)
All PCS codes have 7 characters.

Figure 25-4 illustrates a PCS coding grid.

Example of a code from the grid: 00160J6

0 = Medical and Surgical section	First = section of medical service
0 = Central Nervous System	Second = body system
1 = Bypass	Third = type of operation
6 = Cerebral Ventricle	Fourth = body part
0 = Open	Fifth = approach
J = Synthetic Substitute	Six = device
6 = Peritoneal Cavity	Seventh = qualifier

■ Index

Use Index to locate code by means of alphabetic lookup

Index based on root operation terms with subentries based on:

- Body System
- Body Part
- Operation
- Device

SECTIONS

0	Medical and Surgical
1	Obstetrics
2	Placement
3	Administration
4	Measurement and Monitoring
5	Extracorporeal Assistance and Performance
6	Extracorporeal Therapies
7	Osteopathic
8	Other Procedures
9	Chiropractic
B	Imaging
C	Nuclear Medicine
D	Radiation Therapy
F	Physical Rehabilitation and Diagnostic Audiology
G	Mental Health
H	Substance Abuse Treatment

Figure **25-3** Sections of ICD-10-PCS.

Section: **0 MEDICAL AND SURGICAL**
BODY SYSTEM: **0 CENTRAL NERVOUS SYSTEM**
OPERATION: 1 BYPASS: Altering the route of passage of the contents of a tubular body part

Body Part	Approach	Device	Qualifier
6 Cerebral Ventricle	0 Open 3 Percutaneous	7 Autologous Tissue Substitute J Synthetic Substitute K Nonautologous Tissue Substitute	0 Nasopharynx 1 Mastoid Sinus 2 Atrium 3 Blood Vessel 4 Pleural Cavity 5 Intestine 6 Peritoneal Cavity 7 Urinary Tract 8 Bone Marrow B Cerebral Cisterns
U Spinal Canal	0 Open 3 Percutaneous	7 Autologous Tissue Substitute J Synthetic Substitute K Nonautologous Tissue Substitute	4 Pleural Cavity 6 Peritoneal Cavity 7 Urinary Tract 9 Fallopian Tube

Figure **25-4** ICD-10-PCS Table.

■ Guidelines

ICD-10-PCS has separate Official Guidelines for Coding and Reporting

www.cms.gov/Medicare/Coding/ICD10/Downloads/pcs-2015-guidelines.pdf   or   http://evolve.elsevier.com/Buck.facilityexam

▪ Bundling

Included in all surgical procedures

- Opening and closing of surgical site
- Approach, except where approach differs from code description

  Example: Microscopic approach used instead of described approach

- Do not unbundle and code these separately
- If closure takes place during separate surgical procedure, closure can be coded separately

Coding Challenge

ICD-9-CM versions of Units 4-5 and the Practice Examinations can be found in the Student Evolve Resources.

Some of the CPT code descriptions for physician services include physician extender services. Physician extenders, such as nurse practitioners, physician assistants, and nurse anesthetists, etc., provide medical services typically performed by a physician. Within this educational material the term "physician" may include "and other qualified health care professionals" depending on the code. Refer to the official CPT® code descriptions and guidelines to determine codes that are appropriate to report services provided by non-physician practitioners.

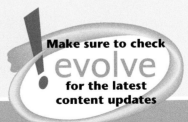

Make sure to check
evolve
for the latest
content updates

CHAPTER 26: EXAMINATIONS

You have three opportunities to practice taking an examination:

- Pre-Examination (before study)
- Post-Examination (after study)
- Final Examination (at the end of your complete program of study)

You should have the following manuals:

- 2016 ICD-10-CM, *(International Classification of Diseases, 10th Revision, Clinical Modification)*
- 2016 ICD-10-PCS *(International Classification of Disease, 10th Revision, Procedure Coding System)*
- 2016 HCPCS (Healthcare Common Procedure Coding System)
- On the certification examination, HCPCS questions are on the theory portion of the examination, not on the practical portion of the examination
- 2016 CPT *(Current Procedural Terminology)*

No other reference material, other than a medical dictionary, is allowed for any of the examinations.

- For the Pre-, Post-, and Final Examinations, you will need a computer that has Internet access and the four coding references listed above (ICD-10-CM, ICD-10-PCS, HCPCS, CPT).
- Each organization's certification examination has different scoring requirements, but as you take these examinations, you should strive for 80% to 90% on the Post-Examination and 65% as a minimum on the Final Examination.

  ICD-9-CM versions of the Pre-/Post- and Final Examinations can be found in the Student Evolve Resources.

NOTE: To enable the learner to calculate an examination score, minimums have been identified as "passing" within this text; however, this may or may not be the percentage identified by the certifying organization as a "passing" grade. It is your responsibility to review all certification information published by the certifying organization.

Guidelines

The number of spaces provided on Part II of the Exam represent the exact number of correct codes.

Do not assign E codes, M codes, or modifiers.

The Final Examination has more difficult questions and cases than the Pre-/Post-Examination to ensure that you have had adequate practice with the more complex coding cases.

The Practice Examinations are divided into two sections.

Part I: Multiple Choice Section—This section includes 97 single-response multiple-choice questions to be completed without reference material.

Part II: Fill in the Blank Section (Case Studies)—This section includes 8 case studies to be completed with the use of coding manuals.

Pre-Examination and Post-Examination

The Pre-Examination contains 105 questions and is located on the companion Evolve website. The purpose of the Pre-Examination is only to assess your beginning level of knowledge and skill—your starting place. Based on your scores, you can tailor your study to target your weakest areas and increase your scores. Take this examination before you begin your studies.

The multiple choice questions (Part I) are located on Evolve and answered on the computer screen. The cases for Part II are provided as you click through each case. Read the case and assign all necessary service and diagnosis codes. These codes are then entered into the blocks on the computer. The electronic program on Evolve will calculate your score and retain this information for later use.

Immediately on completion of your study, you should complete the Post-Examination. After you are finished, the electronic program will automatically compare your Pre-Examination scores with your Post-Examination scores, and will store the results for when you take the Final Examination. By comparing the results of the Pre-Examination and the Post-Examination, the electronic program illustrates the improvements you have achieved.

Rationales for each question are available for review after you complete the Post-Examination. Study the questions for which you did not choose the right response. Did you misread the question, did you not know the material well enough to answer correctly, or did you run out of time? Knowing why you missed a question is an important step to improving your skill level.

Ideally, you should complete each examination in one sitting (4 hours, or 240 minutes); if time does not allow, spread the examination times over several periods. There are no time extensions in an actual examination setting, and learning how to judge the amount of time you spend on each question is an important part of this learning experience to prepare you for the real certification examination.

Final Examination

If you scored well on all areas of the Post-Examination (80%-90%), you are ready to move on to the Final Examination, which is also on the companion Evolve website. The real certification examination is computer-based. Once you have completed the Final Examination, the software will compare all your scores to illustrate your improvement.

If you did not attain a minimum score on each section, you should develop a plan to restudy those particular areas where the examination indicates you are having difficulties. There are rationales for each question in the Final Examination, and you should review that information as well as material in the text. You can take any of the practice examinations again after your additional study.

Grading of the Examination

The grading for the Pre-/Post-Examination includes 146 possible points as follows:
- Part I contains 97 total questions
  - Each correct answer is worth 1 point
  - Possible points on Part I are 97
  - One point will be deducted for each unnecessary or missing code
  - Strive for a minimum score of 65%, or 63 correct answers, to consider Part I successful
- Part II contains 8 coding cases
  - Each correct code is worth 1 point
  - Possible points to award on Part II are 49
  - One point will be deducted for each unnecessary or missing code
  - Strive for a minimum score of 65%, or 31 points, to consider Part II successful

The grading for the Final Examination based on 144 points is as follows:

- Part I contains 97 total questions
  - Each correct answer is worth 1 point
  - Possible points on Part I are 97
  - Strive for a minimum score of 65%, or 63 correct answers, to consider Part I successful
- Part II contains 8 coding cases
  - Each correct answer is worth 1 point
  - Possible points on Part II are 47
  - One point will be deducted for each unnecessary or missing code
  - Strive for a minimum score of 65%, or 30 points, to consider Part II successful

Let's look at how this is calculated by reviewing the examination results of a student who received the following scores on her final examination:

Awarded

Part I, 69 questions correct:	$69 \times 1 = +69$
69 correct/97 possible	Parts I, **71%**
Part II, 34 correct codes and units:	$34 \times 1 = +34$
Part II, 4 unnecessary or missing codes and units:	$4 \times -1 = -4$ $(+34 - 4 = +30)$
30 points/47 possible	Part II, **65%**

This student carefully reviewed the incorrect codes to determine her areas of weakness and then developed a plan to study those areas that had presented her with difficulties.

Figure Credits

7-3   From Kumar V, Abbas AK, Aster JC: *Robbins and Cotran Pathologic Basis of Disease*, ed 9, Philadelphia, 2015, Saunders.

8-7   From Damjanov I: *Pathology for the Health Professions*, ed 4, St. Louis, 2012, Saunders.

8-8   From Kissane JM, editor: *Anderson's Pathology*, ed 9, St. Louis, 1990, Mosby.

11-2   From Canale ST, Beaty JH, *Campbell's Operative Orthopaedics*, ed 11, Philadelphia, 2008, Mosby.

11-3   From Patton KT, Thibodeau GA: *Anatomy & Physiology*, ed 8, St. Louis, 2013, Mosby.

13-2   From Yanoff M, Duker J, eds: *Ophthalmology*, ed 4, St. Louis, 2014, Saunders.

14-1   From *Federal Register*, January 23, 2015, Vol. 80, No. 15, Notices.

14-3   Final changes to the ASC Payment System and CY 2015 Payment Rates, January 2015, www.cms.gov/ASCpayment/ascm/list.asp.

14-6   From www.cms.gov/icd10manual/fullcode_cms/p0002.html.

14-7   From www.cms.gov/icd10manual/fullcode_cms/p0018.html.

14-8   From www.cms.gov/icd10manual/fullcode_cms/p0003.html

14-9   From www.cms.gov/icd10manual/fullcode_cms/p0038.html.

14-10   Modified from www.cms.gov/icd10manual/fullcode_cms/p0048.html.

14-11   From www.cms.gov/icd10manual/fullcode_cms/p0004.html.

19-1   Courtesy U.S. Department of Health and Human Services, Centers for Medicare and Medicaid Services.

19-2   Modified from Buck, CJ: 2016 *ICD-10-CM Hospital Professional Edition*, St. Louis, 2016, Saunders.

19-3   Modified from Buck, CJ: 2016 *ICD-10-CM Hospital Professional Edition*, St. Louis, 2016 Saunders.

25-1   Courtesy U.S. Department of Health and Human Services, Centers for Disease Control and Prevention.

25-2   Modified from Buck, CJ: 2016 *ICD-10-CM Hospital Professional Edition*, St. Louis, 2016, Saunders.

25-3   Modified from Buck, CJ: 2016 *ICD-10-CM Hospital Professional Edition*, St. Louis, 2016, Saunders.

25-4   Modified from Buck, CJ: 2016 *ICD-10-CM Hospital Professional Edition*, St. Louis, 2016, Saunders.

Resources

The most current coding guidelines and code system updates are posted to the Evolve website at **http://evolve.elsevier.com/Buck/facilityexam**.

Once registered for your free Evolve resources, go to the *Course Documents* section to reference the following:

Exam Review

Mobile Quick Quizzes

ICD-9-CM Content

Unit 4—ICD-9-CM Coding
Unit 5—Coding Challenge

Resources

Coding Updates, Tips, and Links
GEMs Files
ICD-10-CM Official Guidelines for Coding and Reporting
ICD-9-CM Official Guidelines for Coding and Reporting
1995 Guidelines for E/M Services
1997 Documentation Guidelines for Evaluation and Management Services
CPT Updates
ICD-10-CM Updates
ICD-9-CM Updates
HCPCS Updates
Study Tips
Weblinks
Content Updates—Student

Some of the CPT code descriptions for physician services include physician extender services. Physician extenders, such as nurse practitioners, physician assistants, and nurse anesthetists, etc., provide medical services typically performed by a physician. Within this educational material the term "physician" may include "and other qualified health care professionals" depending on the code. Refer to the official CPT® code descriptions and guidelines to determine codes that are appropriate to report services provided by non-physician practitioners.

Answers

Unit 1 Quiz Answers

■ Chapter 1—Integumentary System

Anatomy and Terminology Quiz		Pathophysiology Quiz	
1. c	6. c	1. c	6. c
2. d	7. d	2. c	7. d
3. a	8. b	3. a	8. b
4. b	9. c	4. d	9. d
5. d	10. c	5. b	10. a

■ Chapter 2—Musculoskeletal System

Anatomy and Terminology Quiz		Pathophysiology Quiz	
1. b	6. d	1. d	6. d
2. c	7. b	2. c	7. a
3. a	8. d	3. b	8. c
4. c	9. a	4. a	9. b
5. a	10. c	5. d	10. d

■ Chapter 3—Respiratory System

Anatomy and Terminology Quiz		Pathophysiology Quiz	
1. b	6. c	1. b	6. a
2. d	7. c	2. a	7. c
3. c	8. b	3. d	8. b
4. a	9. d	4. d	9. a
5. a	10. d	5. d	10. c

■ Chapter 4—Cardiovascular System

Anatomy and Terminology Quiz		Pathophysiology Quiz	
1. d	6. b	1. b	6. a
2. a	7. d	2. c	7. c
3. c	8. a	3. c	8. c
4. a	9. d	4. c	9. a
5. d	10. d	5. d	10. d

Chapter 5—Female Genital System and Pregnancy

Anatomy and Terminology Quiz		Pathophysiology Quiz	
1. d	6. a	1. b	6. a
2. a	7. b	2. d	7. a
3. a	8. b	3. a	8. c
4. b	9. c	4. c	9. b
5. c	10. d	5. b	10. c

Chapter 6—Male Genital System

Anatomy and Terminology Quiz		Pathophysiology Quiz	
1. c	6. a	1. a	6. b
2. a	7. a	2. b	7. d
3. d	8. d	3. d	8. b
4. b	9. d	4. a	9. a
5. a	10. b	5. c	10. b

Chapter 7—Urinary System

Anatomy and Terminology Quiz		Pathophysiology Quiz	
1. c	6. d	1. c	6. c
2. d	7. c	2. d	7. a or c
3. a	8. b	3. d	8. c
4. c	9. d	4. c	9. b
5. b	10. a	5. b	10. c

Chapter 8—Digestive System

Anatomy and Terminology Quiz		Pathophysiology Quiz	
1. b	6. b	1. c	6. c
2. d	7. a	2. a	7. a
3. d	8. c	3. d	8. c
4. b	9. a	4. b	9. a
5. c	10. b	5. a	10. a

Chapter 9—Mediastinum and Diaphragm

Anatomy and Terminology Quiz	
1. a	6. b
2. b	7. a
3. d	8. b
4. c	9. a
5. c	10. d

Chapter 10—Hemic and Lymphatic System

Anatomy and Terminology Quiz		Pathophysiology Quiz	
1. b	6. c	1. c	6. b
2. d	7. a	2. a	7. a
3. a	8. d	3. b	8. a
4. d	9. b	4. d	9. c
5. c	10. d	5. b	10. b

■ Chapter 11—Endocrine System

Anatomy and Terminology Quiz		Pathophysiology Quiz	
1. c	6. a	1. a	6. b
2. d	7. d	2. b	7. a
3. b	8. a	3. c	8. d
4. a	9. b	4. a	9. a
5. d	10. d	5. d	10. c

■ Chapter 12—Nervous System

Anatomy and Terminology Quiz		Pathophysiology Quiz	
1. b	6. c	1. a	6. b
2. a	7. a	2. c	7. a
3. a	8. d	3. b	8. b
4. b	9. b	4. d	9. b
5. b	10. a	5. a	10. c

■ Chapter 13—Senses

Anatomy and Terminology Quiz		Pathophysiology Quiz	
1. d	6. b	1. d	6. a
2. d	7. c	2. b	7. a
3. a	8. b	3. c	8. a
4. a	9. d	4. a	9. b
5. a	10. a	5. b	10. b

Unit 2 Quiz Answers

■ Chapter 14—Reimbursement Issues

Reimbursement Quiz

1. b	6. b
2. d	7. a
3. d	8. b
4. b	9. b
5. d	10. b

Unit 3 Practice Exercise Answers and Rationales

■ Chapter 16—Evaluation and Management (E/M) Section

Practice Exercise 16-1

Professional Services: 99282 (Evaluation and Management, Emergency Department)

ICD-10-CM: S13.4XXA (Sprain, neck, cervical spine), **V49.9XXA** (External Cause Index Accident, transport, car occupant)

Facility Services: 99282 (Level 2, Point 6)

ICD-10-CM: S13.4XXA (Sprain, neck, cervical spine), **V49.9XXA** (External Cause Index Accident, transport, car occupant)

Rationale: The highest level was Level 2, Point 6, Simple trauma not requiring x-ray.

The diagnosis is stated in the assessment as acute neck strain (S13.4XXA). The neck pain is not reported because a more definitive diagnosis is the neck strain. The injury was due to a motor vehicle collision (MVC) in which the patient was a passenger. Code V49.9XXA reports occupant, either a driver or passenger, of a car in unspecified accident. The seventh character "A" indicates this is the first encounter for this injury.

Practice Exercise 16-2

Professional Services: 99283 (Evaluation and Management, Emergency Department)

ICD-10-CM: M54.5 (Pain, low back), **K59.00** (Constipation, unspecified)

Facility Services: 99283 (Level 3, Point 3)

ICD-10-CM: M54.5 (Pain, low back), **K59.00** (Constipation, unspecified)

Rationale: The highest level for the facility was Level 3, Point 3, X-ray, one area.

The diagnosis is stated in the assessment area of the report as mechanical back pain. Code M54.9 would not be reported because the exact area of pain is indicated in the report (M54.5). The patient is also experiencing right-sided abdominal pain, but the report states in the assessment area that the pain is secondary to constipation. The constipation (K59.00) is reported, not the abdominal pain.

Practice Exercise 16-3

Professional Services: 99285 (Evaluation and Management, Emergency Department)

ICD-10-CM: R07.9 (Pain, chest [central]), **D64.9** (Anemia)

Facility Services: This is an inpatient stay. The entire record would need to be reviewed before coding. We will not be assigning codes on inpatients. The facility charges for the emergency department visit would be included on the inpatient billing.

ICD-10-CM: R07.9 (Pain, chest [central]), **D64.9** (Anemia)

Rationale: The highest level was Level 5, Point 8, Admission to hospital.

The diagnosis is stated in the Assessment section of the report as chest pain (R07.9) and no more definitive diagnosis or reason for the chest pain was given. The patient also was found to be slightly anemic on laboratory results. The type of anemia is not specified, thus D64.9, unspecified anemia, would be reported. This case will now be referred to a cardiologist to identify the reason for the chest pain.

Practice Exercise 16-4

Professional Services: 99283 (Evaluation and Management, Emergency Department)

ICD-10-CM: S90.122A (Contusion, toe[s] [lesser]), **S90.222A** (Contusion, toe[s] [lesser], with damage to nail), **W20.8XXA** (External Cause Index, Struck by, object, falling)

Facility Services: 99283 (Level 3, Point 3)

ICD-10-CM: S91.205A (Wound, open, toe[s], lesser, left, with damage to nail), **S90.122A** (Contusion, toe[s] [lesser]), **S90.222A** (Contusion, toe[s] [lesser], with damage to nail), **W20.8XXA** (External Cause Index, Struck by, object, falling)

Rationale: The highest level was Level 3, Point 3, X-ray of one area (left foot, emphasis on the distal third and fourth toes).

The diagnosis is stated in the Assessment as injury to the toes with a partial nail avulsion. The x-ray is negative for gross bony abnormalities (no fracture seen), thus a contusion of the toe is reported for the third left toe (S90.122A) and contusion with partial nail avulsion for the left fourth toe (S90.222A). The report states possible fracture of the nail; therefore, injury of the nail S90.222A is not reported for professional services. The Index for Avulsion, toenail, indicates "*see* Wound, open, toe(s)" (S90.222A) for the left fourth toe. This injury was due to an external cause, thus an external cause code would be assigned. Code W20.8XXA reports the injury was a result of a TV falling on the patient's foot, with a seventh character "A" indicating this is the initial encounter.

Practice Exercise 16-5

Professional Services: 99283 (Evaluation and Management, Emergency Department)

ICD-10-CM: R10.32 (Pain, abdomen, lower, left quadrant), **R19.7** (Diarrhea)

Facility Services: 99383 (Level 3, Points 3 and 10)

ICD-10-CM: R10.32 (Pain, abdomen, lower, left quadrant), **R19.7** (Diarrhea)

Rationale: The highest level was Level 3 because of the x-ray (Point 3). In this report, no assessment is given listing the diagnoses.

The diagnosis of lower left quadrant (LLQ) abdominal pain would be correct to report. To assign an ICD-10-CM code, reference the Index terms "Pain, abdominal" and "lower," followed by "left quadrant" (R10.32). Code R19.7 (diarrhea) would also be reported.

■ Chapter 17—Surgery Section

Practice Exercise 17-1

Facility: 14060 (Tissue Transfer, Adjacent, Skin)

ICD-10-CM: C44.311 (Neoplasm, nose, skin, basal cell carcinoma, Malignant Primary)

Rationale: The CPT index under Skin Graft and Flap, subheading Tissue Transfer directs you to codes 14000-14350. The CPT Guidelines for Adjacent Tissue Transfer and Rearrangement are used for excision of the lesion and the adjacent tissue transfer. Excision of the lesion is not reported separately. The adjacent tissue rearrangement for this lesion is of the nose and less than 10 sq cm, reported with 14060.

To locate the diagnosis for the neoplasm, you would refer to the Neoplasm Table in the ICD Index. Basal cell carcinoma is the most common type of malignant skin cancer. This lesion is reported as a malignant primary lesion of the skin of the nose (C44.311).

Practice Exercise 17-2

Facility: 13101 (Repair, Skin, Wound, Complex, Trunk, 2.6 cm-7.5 cm) and **+13102** (each additional 5 cm or less)

ICD-10-CM: L98.499 (Ulcer, skin, specified site)

Rationale: This was a complex repair. By definition in CPT, it includes debridement (removal of clot and debridement of necrotic tissue), layered closure, stents, and Jackson-Pratt drain. It also includes creation of the defect. The total repair was noted as 8-cm in diameter, reported with 13101 and add-on code 13102, for each additional 5 cm.

The diagnosis must support the service provided. This patient has a chronic ulcer of the ischium, which is part of the hip area. Code L98.499 reports chronic ulcer of "other specified area."

Practice Exercise 17-3

Facility: 11043 (Debridement, Muscle)

ICD-10-CM: L89.894 (Ulcer, pressure [area], Stage 4, specified site NEC)

Rationale: The "Procedure" statement indicates this debridement went down to the muscle but included fascia. It did not state that it extended into the muscle. However, on reading the body of the report, the surgeon states that there was sharp debridement of necrotic tissue, which "included some tendinous tissues" and "was down into some **muscle** in a couple of spots." Further on the surgeon states, "We debrided all the necrotic tissue." Based on this, 11042 would not be the correct code because that code is for a more superficial debridement. Rather, 11043 correctly reports this service because the code description states, "muscle." Code 11043 stated the service is debridement for the first 20 sq cm or less. This report stated 4-5 cm in length by 3 cm. Use the smallest measurements to calculate the sq cm, which in this case would be $4 \times 3 = 12$ sq cm.

Another name for a pressure ulcer is decubitus ulcer (L89.894). When reporting decubitus ulcers, the area affected by the pressure needs to be known. In this case, the area affected is the patient's leg. The necrosis is part of the ulcer when the skin around the edges of the ulcer dies.

The report states that necrotic tissue was debrided down to the muscle and tendon. The sixth character "4" indicates a stage IV ulcer, which includes muscle in the description.

Practice Exercise 17-4

Facility: 15120 (Skin Graft and Flap, Split Graft)

ICD-10-CM: L97.511 (Ulcer, lower limb, foot, right, with, skin breakdown only), **L97.311** (Ulcer, lower limb, ankle, right, with, skin breakdown only)

Rationale: This is a repair of ulcers with a split-thickness graft to the right foot and the right ankle. The specific code for the foot is 15120 for the first 100 sq cm. The graft required for the lateral foot was 35 sq cm (7 cm × 5 cm). The graft required for the anterior ankle was 6 sq cm (2 cm × 3 cm). Since both locations are reported with code 15120, the graft required is added together for a total of 41 sq cm. The code is for up to 100 sq cm, so it is reported only one time.

These ulcers are both of the right lower extremity, but the diagnoses for the specific area of each would be reported separately. In this case, the ulcers are located on the right foot (L97.511) and another on the ankle (L97.311). The ICD-10-CM codes designate the location with the fourth characters, the right side with the fifth characters, and the extent of ulcer with the sixth characters. Skin breakdown only is selected for extent based on the repair being split thickness skin graft, not any deeper levels.

Practice Exercise 17-5

Facility: 11401 (Excision, Skin, Lesion, Benign)

ICD-10-CM: D22.5 (Nevus, skin, chest wall)

Rationale: When reporting the removal of lesions from the skin, one approach is to begin your search by referencing the CPT index under "Excision." The status of the lesion as benign or malignant determines the specific code that will be assigned. The size of the lesion is the other determining factor. This lesion was reported as 5 mm, with the widest margins being 5 mm on distal margin and 2 mm on the lateral margins. As noted in CPT under Excision—Benign Lesions, the largest diameter plus the narrowest margin is measured (5 mm + 2 mm + 2 mm). This is a total of 9 mm excised. Codes are reported as cm, so this would convert to 0.9 cm. Code 11401 is for excised diameter 0.6 to 1.0 cm.

There are many indicators that indicate the lesion was of the skin. The surgeon calls the lesion a "nevus," it is visible to the eye; the closure of the defect was superficial. The lesion is located on the skin of the chest wall. In the Index of the ICD-10-CM, reference Nevus, skin, chest wall, D22.5. The pathology indicated benign tissue, reported with code D22.5.

Practice Exercise 17-6

Facility: 25606-LT (Fracture, Radius, Percutaneous Fixation)

ICD-10-CM: S52.572A (Fracture, traumatic, radius, lower end, intraarticular NEC)

Rationale: This patient has a distal intra-articular radial fracture. A closed reduction is performed via traction and fixated percutaneously with the application of an external fixation device (25606). Modifier -LT is added to indicate left arm. CPT code 25600 would not be the correct code to assign due to the skeletal fixation that was applied.

To assign a diagnosis code to the fracture, you need to identify the location of the fracture and whether the fracture was open or closed. When referencing the distal radius fracture in the ICD-10-CM Index, the coder is directed to report a code for the lower end of the radius, intraarticular (S52.572A). Note that for the ICD-10-CM code, the code identifies the intra-articular location of the fracture, the left arm, the closed nature of the fracture, and the initial encounter, indicated with a seventh character "A".

Practice Exercise 17-7

Facility: 29877-78-LT (Arthroscopy, Surgical, Knee), **29874-78-LT** (Arthroscopy, Surgical, Knee)

ICD-10-CM: T85.622S (Complication, suture, permanent [wire] NEC, mechanical, displacement), **M12.862** (Arthropathy, specified form NEC, knee)

Rationale: This patient is 6 weeks post repair of a femoral condyle fracture. The patient now returns to the operating room for an arthroscopy. The Procedure Performed section states synovectomy, but the body of the report does not state that the synovium was removed. This procedure would be coded as a debridement. The arthroscopic debridement was performed on the suprapatellar area, medial gutter, and femoral notch, reported with 29877. The removal of the piece of retained metal, a staple in this case, would be reported with 29874. Each of the procedures would be reported separately. Modifier -LT is appended to each code to indicate left knee and modifier -78 reports a return to the operating room for a complication in the global period.

The diagnosis is an internal staple that has come loose. This would be considered a mechanical complication of a nonabsorbable surgical material (T85.622S). There is no code specific to scar tissue; therefore, M12.862 is assigned to indicate arthropathy of the knee joint. The ICD-10-CM code T85.622S reports a complication of a surgical procedure, permanent suture, in this case a loose staple. When referencing the Index for Complication, mechanical, you are instructed to "*see* Complication," by site or type. In this case, the type is surgical material, nonabsorbable; again the instructions are to "*see* Complication, suture, permanent," T85.89. It is important that the coder verifies the code in the Tabular to ensure that the most specific code available is reported. The seventh character "S" indicates sequelae.

Practice Exercise 17-8

Facility: 29888-RT (Arthroscopy, Surgical, Knee)

ICD-10-CM: M23.611 (Derangement, knee, ligament, anterior cruciate)

Rationale: This report states a reconstruction of the anterior cruciate ligament (ACL). When you reference "Reconstruction, Knee, Ligament" in the CPT, you are directed to code range 27427-27429. In the main section of the CPT, the code descriptions state these codes are for open procedures, and the procedure in this report was performed by means of an arthroscope. Before coding orthopedic procedures, you must know how the procedure was performed, as this often determines the code choice. The correct code for this procedure is found in the index by referencing "Arthroscopy, Surgical, Knee," which directs the coder to range 29871-29889. Careful review of the range indicates the correct code is 29888. The harvesting of the graft is included in this code and is not to be reported separately. Modifier -RT is added to the code to indicate right. The preoperative diagnosis indicates that this procedure is "staged" reconstruction after medial meniscus repair. If this procedure is within the global period of the initial procedure, modifier -58 would be appended. This is not documented; therefore it is not applied in this case.

For the diagnosis, the meniscal tear injury would not be reported because this was already repaired in a prior procedure. For ICD-10-CM code M23.611 reports the derangement of the right anterior cruciate ligament, with the sixth character of "1" indicating right knee.

Practice Exercise 17-9

Facility: 29866-RT (Knee, Arthroscopy, Surgical)

ICD-10-CM: M17.11 (Osteoarthritis, primary, knee)

Rationale: A mosaicplasty is a repair of the knee when some piecing together and grafting is performed. This was accomplished by use of an arthroscope, through ports in the skin. In the CPT index, under "Arthroscopy, Surgical" is "Cartilage Autograft," and the coder is directed to 29866. Never code from the index. When referencing the code in the main portion of the CPT, you will see that the information in parentheses indicates that the code "(includes harvesting of the autografts)"; therefore, the harvesting would not be reported separately. Also note that parenthetical information, "(eg, mosaicplasty)," indicates that this is the correct code.

This patient has an internal derangement of the knee, but the location was not specified; thus M23.91 would be assigned, as the code description indicates "unspecified." Note "Derangement" is a specific heading in ICD. The fifth character "1" indicates the right knee.

The patient also has arthritis of the femoral condyle (the articulation surface of the knee), which is arthritis of the lower femur and includes the knee joint and is reported with M17.11. The ICD-10-CM Index indicates "Arthritis, degenerative—*see* Osteoarthritis." Osteoarthritis, primary, knee, M17.11, the primary diagnosis for this surgery. This is the definitive diagnosis for the mosaicplasty; therefore, the knee derangement (M23.91) is not reported.

Practice Exercise 17-10

Facility: 29805-RT (Arthroscopy, Diagnostic, Shoulder), **23430-RT** (Tenodesis, Biceps Tendon, Shoulder)

ICD-10-CM: S46.111A (Injury, muscle, biceps, long head, strain), **X58.XXXA** (External Cause Index, Injury [accidental] NOS)

Rationale: Both the diagnostic arthroscopy and the open procedure would be reported. Note that the preoperative and postoperative diagnoses for this report are different. When coding, use the postoperative findings. In this case, the patient was found to have a tear of the tendon in the shoulder/biceps area. A scope was used and would be coded as a diagnostic procedure (29805). Some insurance carriers will not pay for a diagnostic scope when it leads to an open procedure. Coders need to check with their local carriers. The open tenodesis procedure would be correctly reported with 23430, with modifier -RT to indicate right shoulder. The open procedure is more work-intensive than the arthroscopy and is reported first.

The Index entry in the ICD-10-CM for "Tear, tendon" directs the coder to "*see* Strain." Under "Strain, muscle (tendon)," the coder is directed to "*see* Injury, muscle, by site, strain." Code S46.111A reports the injury to the long head of the right bicep tendon. The seventh character "A" denotes the service was an initial encounter. The biceps long head tendon attaches to the glenoid cavity. This was transected near its attachment, which was then moved and attached to the biceptal groove in the upper humerus.

At the beginning of the note, the coder is directed to assign an external cause code to indicate how injury occurred. There is no indication in the documentation of the mechanism of the injury, so Injury NOS is reported (X58.XXXA). Note, typically, external cause codes are only reported at the initial contact for an injury, not after work up (patient seen and arthrogram performed) and surgery is being performed. The seventh character "A" reports the initial encounter.

Practice Exercise 17-11

Facility: 38221 (Bone Marrow, Needle Biopsy)

ICD-10-CM: D61.9 (Anemia, aplastic), **C85.90** (Lymphoma [malignant])

Rationale: This is a needle biopsy of bone marrow and reported with 38221. The aspiration is included in 38221 and not reported separately.

The patient has aplastic anemia (D61.9) and lymphoma (C85.90).

Practice Exercise 17-12

Facility: 31628-RT (Bronchoscopy, Biopsy), **31632-RT** (Bronchoscopy, Biopsy), **31623-RT** (Bronchoscopy, Brushing, Protected Brushing), **31624-RT** (Bronchoscopy, Alveolar Lavage)

ICD-10-CM: R91.8 (Infiltrate, pulmonary)

Rationale: "Bronchoscopy" is stated under the Procedure Performed section of the report. You would need to read the body of the report to see what procedures were performed once the lung was entered–in this case brushings (31623), washings, and exploration bilaterally, which are included in the base procedure and are not reported separately with code 31622, and bronchoalveolar lavage, reported with 31624. Also, transbronchial biopsies were taken of two separate lobes of the right lung; thus code 31628 would be assigned for one lobe and the add-on code 31632 would be the biopsy of the additional lobe of the right lung. The modifier

-RT would be assigned to indicate the procedure was performed on the right lung. The left lung was also evaluated and determined to be normal, which could be reported with 31622, diagnostic bronchoscopy; however, this code is designated as a "separate procedure," meaning that when a diagnostic bronchoscopy is performed during a surgical bronchoscopy, it is not separately reported. The evaluation of the left lung, because it was normal and nothing more was done, is included in the rest of the procedures and not separately reported.

The diagnosis to report would be the pulmonary infiltrates (R91.8).

Practice Exercise 17-13
Facility: 94060 (Pulmonology, Diagnostic, Spirometry), **94729** (Pulmonology, Diagnostic, Carbon Monoxide Diffusion Capacity)

ICD-10-CM: R06.02 (Shortness, breath), **R06.2** (Wheezing), **R09.02** (Hypoxia)

Rationale: This is a pulmonary function study to measure the patient's respiratory function (94060). The patient was tested for CO diffusing capacity (94729), and bronchodilation responsiveness, which is included in 94060.

The report states the diagnosis of shortness of breath (R06.02), wheezes (R06.2), and hypoxia (R09.02).

Practice Exercise 17-14
Facility: 32551 (Thoracostomy, Tube), **75989** (Ultrasound, Drainage, Abscess)

ICD-10-CM: J90 (Effusion, pleura)

Rationale: This patient has fluid in the right lung that is hindering the lung to expand and contract properly for normal breathing. Code 32551 is for placement of the chest tube to drain the effusion. The ultrasound guidance is used during the procedure and reported with 75989.

The pleural effusion (J90) would be reported as the diagnosis. A chest tube is inserted to drain fluid out of the pleural space to restore adequate airflow.

Practice Exercise 17-15
Facility: 36558 (Insertion, Catheter, Venous)

ICD-10-CM: N17.9 (Failure, renal, acute)

Rationale: A variety of CPT codes are used for the insertion of central lines depending on the purpose of the line, whether the catheter is tunneled under the clavicle bone or not tunneled, and the age of the patient. In this case, the catheter was a central venous catheter inserted for the purpose of hemodialysis and was tunneled into place and the patient is "age 5 years or older," reported with 36558.

This patient is in acute renal failure (N17.9) and requires dialysis. The venous catheter will be used in cleansing this patient's blood.

Practice Exercise 17-16
Facility: 45385 (Colonoscopy, Removal, Polyp), **45384-59** (Colonoscopy, Removal, Polyp)

ICD-10-CM: D12.5 (Neoplasm, intestine, large, colon, sigmoid, Benign), **K57.30** (Diverticulosis, large intestine)

Rationale: This patient has benign polyps of the descending and sigmoid colon. A flexible colonoscopy is performed to better visualize the polyps. Code 45385 is the correct code for the colonoscopy with removal of the polyp by snare technique. Code 45384 is the correct code for removal of polyps by hot biopsy forceps. Modifier -59 is appended to indicate a distinctive procedural service. Even though the polyps were biopsied, they were actually totally removed and then sent for pathology examination. This is sometimes called an excisional biopsy. The entire lesion is excised. These procedures are removals rather than biopsies.

The benign polyps of the descending and sigmoid colon are reported with D12.5. This patient also has diverticula of the descending and sigmoid colon. Diverticula are pouches in the walls of the colon that can get inflamed and/or infected if not treated. Treatment is often diet modification. Diverticula of the colon is reported with K57.30.

Practice Exercise 17-17
Facility: 45330 (Sigmoidoscopy, Exploration)

ICD-10-CM: A09 (Enteritis, infectious NOS), **R50.9** (Fever)

Rationale: This is a diagnostic examination of the sigmoid colon (sigmoidoscopy). Take care not to report a colonoscopy, which is an exploration of the entire colon. Also, do not report a surgical procedure when only a diagnostic procedure was performed.

The diagnosis for this procedure is diarrhea, but the result of the procedure determined the cause of the diarrhea was infectious colitis, A09. The ICD-10-CM Index for "Colitis" refers the coder to "*see* Enteritis, infectious." The fever (R50.9) is reported because the report indicated that the infectious colitis may not be the cause of the fever.

Practice Exercise 17-18
Facility: 49505-LT (Hernia, Repair, Inguinal, Initial, Child 5 Years or Older)

ICD-10-CM: K40.90 (Hernia, inguinal [indirect])

Rationale: A hernia is a protrusion of an organ or part of an organ through the wall of the cavity that contains it. In this case, it is an inguinal hernia that is indirect (a herniation of the sac that contains the intestine protruding through the internal inguinal ring and often descending into the scrotum). This type of hernia is the most common of all hernias and is usually caused by overexertion; for example, lifting something too heavy. When reporting hernia procedures, you need to know the age of the patient, whether the repair is initial or recurrent, and whether the hernia is reducible, incarcerated, or strangulated. In this case, 49505 would be the correct code because this is the initial repair of a reducible hernia. Because there is a right and a left inguinal canal, the -LT modifier is added to indicate the left side was repaired. The mesh implantation (Prolene hernia system patch) is included in the hernia repair code and is not reported separately.

For the diagnosis this report states the hernia was inguinal and unilateral, but the report does not specify whether the hernia was recurrent (K40.90).

Practice Exercise 17-19
Facility: 43262 (Bile Duct, Endoscopy, Sphincterotomy)

ICD-10-CM: R10.9 (Pain, abdominal, unspecified), **R74.8** (Abnormal, serum level [of], enzymes, specified NEC)

Rationale: When coding the sphincterotomy, you would need to know whether the procedure was performed endoscopically. Endoscopic retrograde cholangiopancreatography is also known as ERCP. The pancreatic duct was cannulated and a sphincterotomy was performed, and there is a specific procedure code for this procedure when performed with ERCP (43262).

This patient is experiencing abdominal pain, but the area of pain is not specified (R10.9). For the elevated liver enzymes, there is no specific code that directly reports the enzymes of the liver, thus R74.8 would be assigned because it reports "other serum enzymes." Note when locating abnormal test result in ICD-10-CM Index the main term is "Abnormal."

Practice Exercise 17-20
Facility: 47562 (Laparoscopy, Biliary Tract, Cholecystectomy)

ICD-10-CM: K80.42 (Calculus, bile duct, with cholecystistis [with cholangitis], acute)

Rationale: When reporting a cholecystectomy, you need to know whether the procedure was performed laparoscopically or via open incision. In this case, the procedure is correctly reported with 47562 to report a laparoscopic procedure.

When referencing the main term "Choledocholithiasis" in the ICD-10-CM Index, the coder is directed to "*see* Calculus, bile duct." From the entry "Calculus, bile duct," reference the entry "with cholecystitis, acute." The code reported would be K80.42. There are additional options for "with obstruction," and in this case there was not documentation of obstruction.

Practice Exercise 17-21
Facility: 50200-RT (Biopsy, Kidney), **76942** (Ultrasound, Guidance, Needle Biopsy)

ICD-10-CM: N05.8 (Glomerulonephritis, necrotic, necrotizing, NEC), **Z94.0** (Transplant, kidney)

Rationale: This is a biopsy of a transplanted kidney. To assign the procedure code you would consider this kidney as the patient's own. You need to know the method used to obtain the biopsy. In this case, a needle biopsy was performed. You would not assign 50205 because this reports an open biopsy and the biopsy in this report was performed closed with a needle (50200). Modifier -RT indicates that the biopsy was performed on the right kidney. 76942 reports the ultrasound guidance for the needle biopsy.

The diagnosis is acute necrotizing glomerulitis (N05.8), as substantiated by the pathology report. An additional code is reported to indicate status post kidney transplant, Z94.0.

Practice Exercise 17-22
Facility: 50200-RT (Biopsy, Kidney), **76942** (Ultrasound, Guidance, Needle Biopsy)

ICD-10-CM: N05.2 (Glomerulonephritis, membranous NEC)

Rationale: The title of this report states simply "Kidney Biopsy." This is an example of why it is important not to code from the Procedure Performed section of the report. Rather, the coder must read the body of the report to know whether the biopsy is performed as an open or closed procedure. The operative report states a needle was used for the biopsy. Code 50200 is the correct code for the needle kidney biopsy. Modifier -RT indicates that the biopsy was performed on the right kidney. 76942 reports the ultrasound guidance for the needle biopsy.

The pathology report indicated membranous glomerulonephritis (N05.2). In the Reason for Procedure section of the report, it states the procedure is being performed due to proteinuria. Proteinuria (R80.9) is a symptom of membranous glomerulonephritis and is therefore not reported separately. The physician should be queried to ensure the proteinuria is a symptom of the patient's membranous glomerulonephritis.

Practice Exercise 17-23
Facility: 58558 (Hysteroscopy, Surgical, with Biopsy)

ICD-10-CM: N84.0 (Polyp, endometrium)

Rationale: This report states that three procedures were performed: hysteroscopy, polypectomy, and dilation and curettage (D&C). The report states that the polyps could not be fully removed; thus only a portion was removed for biopsy. Code 58558 reports the scoping procedure of the uterus with the biopsy and includes the diagnostic D&C. The 58558 code states with **or** without polypectomy. The fact that the surgeon was unable to perform the procedure does not affect reporting this code.

The patient is having postmenopausal bleeding. During the procedure two polyps of the endometrium were found, which was the cause of this bleeding based on the Postoperative Diagnosis section of the report. The most definitive diagnosis would be reported, N84.0, endometrial polyp, not the postmenopausal bleeding, N95.0.

Practice Exercise 17-24
Facility: 59000 (Amniocentesis, Diagnostic), **76946** (Ultrasound, Guidance, Amniocentesis)

ICD-10-CM: Z36 (Screening, antenatal, of mother), **O24.113** (Pregnancy, complicated by, diabetes, pre-existing, type 2), **E11.21** (Diabetes, type 2, with nephropathy), **Z79.4**

(Long-term [current] drug therapy [use of] insulin), **Z3A.32** (Pregnancy, weeks of gestation, weeks, 32)

Rationale: This is a diagnostic amniocentesis, 59000. The technologist performed the ultrasound scanning, reported with code 76946.

The patient has diabetic nephropathy, type 2, that is complicating her pregnancy. She is now on bed rest, and an amniocentesis is to be performed to check the maturity of the fetus's lungs (Z36). The pregnancy is complicated by pre-existing type 2 diabetes and is reported with O24.113, with a sixth character "3" that denotes the third trimester of pregnancy. Code E11.21 reports both the type 2 diabetes and the nephropathy. The reports also indicates long-term insulin use, reported with Z79.4. The gestation of the fetus is reported with Z3A.32.

Practice Exercise 17-25
Facility: 52000 (Bladder, Endoscopy)

ICD-10-CM: N39.3 (Incontinence, urine, stress [female])

Rationale: This was a cystoscopy performed for diagnostic purposes only and reported with 52000.

The code for urinary incontinence (R32) would not be reported because this report specifies that this patient's condition is predominately stress incontinence (N39.3). The diagnosis of intrinsic sphincteric deficiency would not be reported because it is stated as a probable diagnosis. All other findings are part of the urinary incontinence.

Practice Exercise 17-26
Facility: 67923-E1, 67923-E3 (Repair, Eyelid, Entropion, Excision Tarsal Wedge)

ICD-10-CM: H02.001 (Entropion [eyelid], right, upper), **H02.004** (Entropion [eyelid], left, upper)

Rationale: This is a mini-blepharoplasty of the eyelids, which is a reconstruction of an inversion of the edge of the upper eyelid. This repair involved dissection of deep structures, as indicated by the removal of a 2-mm strip of the orbicularis muscle. The procedure is reported with 67923, with modifier -E1 to indicate the upper left eyelid and 67923 listed again with modifier -E3 to indicate the upper right eyelid. The coder may also have considered 15823; however, this code describes a more superficial procedure that involves dissection of the skin only.

The diagnoses for unspecified type of entropion is reported twice, first for right upper eyelid (H02.001) and second for left upper eyelid (H02.004).

Practice Exercise 17-27
Facility: 63030-LT (Hemilaminectomy)

ICD-10-CM: M51.27 (Displacement, intervertebral disc, lumbosacral region)

Rationale: When you reference "Discectomy" in the index of the CPT, you are directed to code range 63075-63078. Checking these codes in the main portion of the CPT, you will see that these codes are not performed on the lumbar spine and are accomplished from an anterior (front) approach. This surgery was performed on the lumbar disc and used a posterior (back) approach. The patient's lumbar nerve is compressed and a part of the lamina and some muscle is removed to free up space (decompress) for the lumbar nerve. This procedure is a laminotomy, which includes the partial removal of the lamina. This procedure is also known as a hemilaminectomy. If the entire lamina had been removed, that would be a laminectomy. When you reference "Hemilaminectomy" in the index of the CPT, you are directed to the correct code range, 63020-63044. Code 63030 describes the surgery performed on the lumbar spine specifically performed for a herniated disc. In reading the operative report, decompression of the nerve root at S1 was performed. The decompression would be included in the code 63030 because it was at the same level as the discectomy. If the nerve decompression was performed in a different level from where the excision of the disc is taking place, this procedure would be reported separately. Modifier -LT indicates that the procedure was performed on the left side only.

In the Index of the ICD-10-CM under "Hernia, disc, intervertebral" the coder is directed to "*see* Displacement, intervertebral disc." The ICD-10-CM code for displacement of a disc in the lumbar region is reported with M51.26; the displacement in the lumbosacral region is reported with M51.27. In this case, the herniated disc was in the lumbosacral region (M51.27).

Practice Exercise 17-28

Facility: 61020 (Ventricular, Puncture)

ICD-10-CM: C71.6 (Neoplasm, cerebellum, Malignant Primary), **G91.4** (Hydrocephalus, in, neoplastic disease NEC)

Rationale: This patient has increased intracranial pressure. The reason for increased intracranial pressure is an increase in the severity of the hydrocephalus (fluid on the brain) due to a neoplasm of the brain. The surgeon is relieving pressure by percutaneous aspiration of fluid from the ventricular shunt reservoir. (Ventricle is an area of the heart, as well as the brain.) In the index of the CPT, reference "Ventricular Puncture" and you are directed to two ranges of codes. Referencing the first listed codes (61020-61021) in the main portion of the CPT, you will note that these punctures take place through a previously established access, such as a burr hole or catheter. The body of this report describes the aspiration was accomplished by tapping an existing shunt.

Although you did not need to check further for codes because 61020 described the service provided, the next range of codes from the index of the CPT was 61105-61120. In the code description for 61105-61108, a twist drill is used. A twist drill is manually operated. Because the procedure in the report was performed percutaneously, this range of codes was not correct to report the service. The next code is 61120 and describes the creation of a burr hole. A burr hole is created by means of an electronic drill.

The report indicates that the patient had a "high-grade glioma of the posterior fossa." This is a malignant neoplasm of the cerebellum (posterior fossa) and is reported with C71.6. The report also states the patient had hydrocephalus, reported with G91.4. The intracranial pressure is not reported separately because in the Index of the ICD-10-CM, under the main term "Pressure" and subterms "increased, intracranial, due to, hydrocephalus," the coder is directed to "*see* Hydrocephalus." There is a subterm under hydrocephalus stating "in neoplastic disease, NEC," which is appropriate in this case, reported with code G91.4, hydrocephalus in diseases classified elsewhere. The coder is directed to "*code first the underlying disease, such as … neoplastic disease.*" The presenting symptoms of nausea, vomiting, lethargy, and headache are not reported separately because they are due to the worsening hydrocephalus (increased intracranial pressure).

Practice Exercise 17-29

Facility: 62350 (Insertion, Catheter, Spinal Cord), **62362** (Insertion, Infusion Pump, Spinal Cord)

ICD-10-CM: M81.0 (Osteoporosis), **M48.06** (Stenosis, spinal, lumbar region), **M51.36** (Degeneration, intervertebral disc, lumbar region)

Rationale: This procedure was done for pain management. This patient had an intrathecal catheter placed within the spinal canal. The catheter (62350) is tunneled under the skin into the subcutaneous tissues. A pump was implanted in a pocket that was formed in the abdominal wall fascia. The pump was then attached to this catheter that will enable the delivery of the pain medication. The insertion of the infusion pump (62362) is reported separately from the insertion of the spinal catheter.

This patient has osteoporosis, but the type is not specified; therefore, the code for generalized osteoporosis would be assigned (M81.0). The multiple compression fractures of the spine would not be reported because these have already been repaired by kyphoplasty, so the fractures no longer exist. When reporting the stenosis of the spine, the location of the stenosis is important to know. In this case, the location is the lumbar spine, reported with M48.06. The patient also has degeneration of the lumbar spine, reported with M51.36. The codes for the Alzheimer's disease and benign prostatic hypertrophy (BPH) would not be reported because they do not pertain to the reason for the procedure, although it is not incorrect to report these conditions.

Facility: 64721-LT (Release, Carpal Tunnel)

ICD-10-CM: G56.02 (Syndrome, carpal tunnel)

Rationale: After all other treatment options were tried and did not relieve the pain for this patient, decompression or release of the left medial nerve was performed (64721). Once the nerve has been released (freed up), the pressure is gone and with that the pain. Modifier -LT is appended to the procedure code to indicate the left side.

One way to locate the diagnosis code (G56.02) in the Index of the ICD-10-CM is to reference "Syndrome." Another location would be "Carpal tunnel syndrome." Note that the fifth character "2" designates the left side.

Medical Terminology

ablation	removal or destruction by cutting, chemicals, or electrocautery
abortion	termination of pregnancy
absence	without
actinotherapy	treatment of acne using ultraviolet rays
adenoidectomy	removal of adenoids
adipose	fatty
adrenals	glands, located at the top of the kidneys, that produce steroid hormones
albinism	lack of color pigment
allograft	homograft, same species graft
alopecia	condition in which hair falls out
amniocentesis	percutaneous aspiration of amniotic fluid
amniotic sac	sac containing the fetus and amniotic fluid
A-mode	one-dimensional ultrasonic display reflecting the time it takes a sound wave to reach a structure and reflect back; maps the structure's outline
anastomosis	surgical connection of two tubular structures, such as two pieces of the intestine
aneurysm	abnormal dilation of vessels, usually an artery
angina	sudden pain
angiography	radiography of the blood vessels
angioplasty	procedure in a vessel to dilate the vessel opening
anhidrosis	deficiency of sweat
anomaloscope	instrument used to test color vision
anoscopy	procedure that uses a scope to examine the anus
antepartum	before childbirth
anterior (ventral)	in front of
anterior segment	those parts of the eye in the front of and including the lens (cornea, iris, ciliary body, aqueous humor)
anteroposterior	from front to back
antigen	a substance that produces a specific response

aortography	radiographic recording of the aorta
apex cardiography	recording of the movement of the chest wall over the end of the heart
aphakia	absence of the lens of the eye
apicectomy	excision of a portion of the temporal bone
apnea	cessation of breathing
arthrocentesis	injection and/or aspiration of joint
arthrodesis	surgical immobilization of joint
arthrography	radiography of joint
arthroplasty	reshaping or reconstruction of joint
arthroscopy	use of scope to view inside joint
arthrotomy	incision into a joint
articular	pertains to joint
asphyxia	lack of oxygen
aspiration	use of a needle and a syringe to withdraw fluid
assignment	Medicare's payment for the service, which participating physicians agree to accept as payment in full
asthma	shortage of breath caused by contraction of bronchi
astigmatism	condition in which the refractive surfaces of the eye are unequal
atelectasis	incomplete expansion of lung, collapse
atherectomy	removal of plaque by percutaneous method
atrophy	wasting away
audiometry	hearing test
aural atresia	congenital absence of the external auditory canal
auscultation	listening to sounds within the body
autograft	from patient's own body
avulsion	ripping or tearing away of part either surgically or accidentally
axillary nodes	lymph nodes located in the armpit
bacilli	plural of bacillus, a rod-shaped bacterium
barium enema	radiographic contrast medium
beneficiary	person who benefits from health or life insurance
bifocal	two focuses in eyeglasses, one usually for close work and the other for improvement of distance vision
bilaminate skin	skin substitute usually made of silicone-covered nylon mesh
bilateral	occurring on two sides
biliary	refers to gallbladder, bile, or bile duct
bilobectomy	surgical removal of two lobes of a lung
biofeedback	process of giving a person self-information
biometry	application of a statistical measure to a biologic fact

biopsy	removal of a small piece of living tissue for diagnostic purposes
block	frozen piece of a sample
brachytherapy	therapy using radioactive sources that are placed inside the body
bronchiole	smaller division of bronchial tree
bronchography	radiographic recording of the lungs
bronchoplasty	surgical repair of the bronchi
bronchoscopy	inspection of the bronchial tree using a bronchoscope
B-scan	two-dimensional display of tissues and organs
bulbocavernosus	muscle that constricts the vagina in a female and the urethra in a male
bulbourethral	gland with duct leading to the urethra
bundle of His	muscular cardiac fibers that provide the heart rhythm to the ventricles; blockage of this rhythm produces heart block
bundled codes	one code that represents a package of services
bunion	hallux valgus, abnormal increase in size of metatarsal head that results in displacement of the great toe
burr	drill used to create an entry into the cranium
bursa	fluid-filled sac that absorbs friction
bursitis	inflammation of bursa (joint sac)
bypass	to go around
calcaneal	pertaining to the heel bone
calculus	concretion of mineral salts, also called a stone
calycoplasty	surgical reconstruction of a recess of the renal pelvis
calyx	recess of the renal pelvis
cancellous	lattice-type structure, usually of bone
cardiopulmonary	refers to the heart and lungs
cardiopulmonary bypass	blood bypasses the heart through a heart-lung machine
cardioversion	electrical shock to the heart to restore normal rhythm
carotid body	located on each side of the common carotid artery, often a site of tumor
cartilage	connective tissue
cataract	opaque covering on or in the lens
catheter	tube placed into the body to put fluid in or take fluid out
caudal	same as inferior; away from the head, or the lower part of the body
causalgia	burning pain
cauterization	destruction of tissue by the use of cautery
cavernosa	connection between the cavity of the penis and a vein
cavernosography	radiographic recording of a cavity, e.g., the pulmonary cavity or the main part of the penis
cavernosometry	measurement of the pressure in a cavity, e.g., the penis

central nervous system	brain and spinal cord
cervical	pertaining to the neck or to the cervix of the uterus
cervix uteri	rounded, cone-shaped neck of the uterus
cesarean	surgical opening through abdominal wall for delivery
cholangiography	radiographic recording of the bile ducts
cholangiopancreatography	radiographic recording of the biliary system or pancreas
cholecystectomy	surgical removal of the gallbladder
cholecystoenterostomy	creation of a connection between the gallbladder and intestine
cholecystography	radiographic recording of the gallbladder
cholesteatoma	tumor that forms in middle ear
chondral	referring to the cartilage
chordee	condition resulting in the penis being bent downward
chorionic villus sampling	CVS, biopsy of the outermost part of the placenta
circumflex	a coronary artery that circles the heart
Cloquet's node	also called a gland; it is the highest of the deep groin lymph nodes
closed fracture repair	not surgically opened with/without manipulation and with/without traction
closed treatment	fracture site that is not surgically opened and visualized
coccyx	caudal extremity of vertebral column
collagen	protein substance of skin
Colles' fracture	fracture at lower end of radius that displaces the bone posteriorly
colonoscopy	fiberscopic examination of the entire colon that may include part of the terminal ileum
colostomy	artificial opening between the colon and the abdominal wall
component	part
computed axial tomography	CAT or CT, procedure by which selected planes of tissue are pinpointed through computer enhancement, and images may be reconstructed by analysis of variance in absorption of the tissue
conjunctiva	the lining of the eyelids and the covering of anterior sclera
contraction	drawn together
contralateral	opposite side
cordectomy	surgical removal of the vocal cord(s)
cordocentesis	procedure to obtain a fetal blood sample; also called a percutaneous umbilical blood sampling
corneosclera	cornea and sclera of the eye
corpectomy	removal of vertebrae
corpora cavernosa	the two cavities of the penis
corpus uteri	uterus
crackle	abnormal sound when breathing (heard on auscultation)

craniectomy	permanent, partial removal of skull
craniotomy	opening of the skull
cranium	that part of the skeleton that encloses the brain
curettage	scraping of a cavity using a spoon-shaped instrument
curette	spoon-shaped instrument used to scrape a cavity
cutdown	incision into a vessel for placement of a catheter
cyanosis	bluish discoloration
cystocele	herniation of the bladder into the vagina
cystography	radiographic recording of the urinary bladder
cystolithectomy	removal of a calculus (stone) from the urinary bladder
cystolithotomy	cystolithectomy
cystometrogram	CMG, measurement of the pressures and capacity of the urinary bladder
cystoplasty	surgical reconstruction of the bladder
cystorrhaphy	suture of the bladder
cystoscopy	use of a scope to view the bladder
cystostomy	surgical creation of an opening into the bladder
cystotomy	incision into the bladder
cystourethroplasty	surgical reconstruction of the bladder and urethra
cystourethroscopy	use of a scope to view the bladder and urethra
dacryocystography	radiographic recording of the lacrimal sac or tear duct sac
dacryostenosis	narrowing of the lacrimal duct
debridement	cleansing of or removal of dead tissue from a wound
deductible	amount the patient is liable for before the payer begins to pay for covered services
delayed flap	pedicle of skin with blood supply that is separated from origin over time
delivery	childbirth
dermabrasion	planing of the skin by means of sander, brush, or sandpaper
dermatologist	physician who treats conditions of the skin
dermatoplasty	surgical repair of skin
dialysis	filtration of blood
dilation	expansion
discectomy	removal of a vertebral disc
discography	radiographic recording of an intervertebral joint
dislocation	placement in a location other than the original location
distal	farther from the point of attachment or origin
diverticulum	protrusion in the wall of an organ
Doppler	ultrasonic measure of blood movement
dosimetry	scientific calculation of radiation emitted from various radioactive sources

drainage	free flow or withdrawal of fluids from a wound or cavity
duodenography	radiographic recording of the duodenum or first part of the small intestine
dysphagia	difficulty swallowing
dysphonia	speech impairment
dyspnea	shortness of breath, difficult breathing
dysuria	painful urination
echocardiography	radiographic recording of the heart or heart walls or surrounding tissues
echoencephalography	ultrasound of the brain
echography	ultrasound procedure in which sound waves are bounced off an internal organ and the resulting image is recorded
ectopic	pregnancy outside the uterus (i.e., in the fallopian tube)
edema	swelling due to abnormal fluid collection in the tissue spaces
elective surgery	nonemergency procedure
electrocardiogram	ECG, written record of the electrical action of the heart
electrocautery	cauterization by means of heated instrument
electrocochleography	test to measure the eighth cranial nerve (hearing test)
electrode	lead attached to a generator that carries the electrical current from the generator to the atria or ventricles
electroencephalogram	EEG, written record of the electrical action of the brain
electromyogram	EMG, written record of the electrical activity of the skeletal muscles
electronic claim submission	claims prepared and submitted via a computer
electronic signature	identification system of a computer
electro-oculogram	EOG, written record of the electrical activity of the eye
electrophysiology	study of the electrical system of the heart, including the study of arrhythmias
embolectomy	removal of blockage (embolism) from vessel
emphysema	air accumulated in organ or tissue
encephalography	radiographic recording of the subarachnoid space and ventricles of the brain
endarterectomy	incision into an artery to remove the inner lining so as to eliminate disease or blockage
endomyocardial	pertaining to the inner and middle layers of the heart
endopyelotomy	procedure involving the bladder and ureters, including the insertion of a stent into the renal pelvis
endoscopy	inspection of body organs or cavities using a lighted scope that may be inserted through an existing opening or through a small incision
enterolysis	releasing of adhesions of intestine
enucleation	removal of an organ or organs from a body cavity
epicardial	over the heart
epidermolysis	loosening of the epidermis

epidermomycosis	superficial fungal infection
epididymectomy	surgical removal of the epididymis
epididymis	tube located at the top of the testes that stores sperm
epididymography	radiographic recording of the epididymis
epididymovasostomy	creation of a new connection between the vas deferens and epididymis
epiglottidectomy	excision of the covering of the larynx
episclera	connective covering of the sclera
epistaxis	nosebleed
epithelium	surface covering of internal and external organs of the body
erythema	redness of skin
escharotomy	surgical incision into necrotic (dead) tissue
eventration	protrusion of the bowel through an opening in the abdomen
evisceration	pulling the viscera outside of the body through an incision
evocative	tests that are administered to evoke a predetermined response
exenteration	removal of an organ all in one piece
exophthalmos	protrusion of the eyeball
exostosis	bony growth
exstrophy	condition in which an organ is turned inside out
extracorporeal	occurring outside of the body
false aneurysm	sac of clotted blood that has completely destroyed the vessel and is being contained by the tissue that surrounds the vessel
fasciectomy	removal of a band of fibrous tissue
Federal Register	official publication of all "Presidential Documents," "Rules and Regulations," "Proposed Rules," and "Notices"; government-instituted national changes are published in the *Federal Register*
fee schedule	services and payment allowed for each service
femoral	pertaining to the bone from the pelvis to knee
fenestration	creation of a new opening in the inner wall of the middle ear
fissure	cleft or groove
fistula	abnormal opening from one area to another area or to the outside of the body
fluoroscopy	procedure for viewing the interior of the body using x-rays and projecting the image onto a television screen
fracture	break in a bone
free full-thickness graft	graft of epidermis and dermis that is completely removed from donor area
fulguration	use of electrical current to destroy tissue
fundoplasty	repair of the bottom of the bladder
furuncle	nodule in the skin caused by *Staphylococci* entering through hair follicle
ganglion	knot

gastrointestinal	pertaining to the stomach and intestine
gastroplasty	operation on the stomach for repair or reconfiguration
gastrostomy	artificial opening between the stomach and the abdominal wall
gatekeeper	a physician who manages a patient's access to health care
glaucoma	eye diseases that are characterized by an increase of intraocular pressure
globe	eyeball
glottis	true vocal cords
gonioscopy	use of a scope to examine the angles of the eye
Group Practice Model	an organization of physicians who contract with a Health Maintenance Organization to provide services to the enrollees of the HMO
grouper	computer used to input the principal diagnosis and other critical information about a patient and then provide the correct DRG code
Health Maintenance Organization	HMO, a healthcare delivery system in which an enrollee is assigned a primary care physician who manages all the healthcare needs of the enrollee
hematoma	mass of blood that forms outside the vessel
hemodialysis	cleansing of the blood outside of the body
hemolysis	breakdown of red blood cells
hemoptysis	bloody sputum
hepatography	radiographic recording of the liver
hernia	organ or tissue protruding through the wall or cavity that usually contains it
histology	study of structure of tissue and cells
homograft	allograft, same species graft
hormone	chemical substance produced by the body's endocrine glands
hydrocele	sac of fluid
hyperopia	farsightedness, eyeball is too short from front to back
hypogastric	lowest middle abdominal area
hyposensitization	decreased sensitivity
hypothermia	low body temperature; sometimes induced during surgical procedures
hypoxemia	low level of oxygen in the blood
hypoxia	low level of oxygen in the tissue
hysterectomy	surgical removal of the uterus
hysterorrhaphy	suturing of the uterus
hysterosalpingography	radiographic recording of the uterine cavity and fallopian tubes
hysteroscopy	visualization of the canal and cavity of the uterus using a scope placed through the vagina
ichthyosis	skin disorder characterized by scaling
ileostomy	artificial opening between the ileum and the abdominal wall
ilium	portion of hip

imbrication	overlapping
immunotherapy	therapy to increase immunity
implantable defibrillator	surgically placed device that directs an electrical shock to the heart to restore rhythm
incarcerated	regarding hernias, a constricted, irreducible hernia that may cause obstruction of an intestine
incise	to cut into
Individual Practice Association	IPA, an organization of physicians who provide services for a set fee; Health Maintenance Organizations often contract with the IPA for services to their enrollees
inferior	away from the head or the lower part of the body; also known as caudalingual
inguinofemoral	referring to the groin and thigh
inofemoral	referring to the groin and thigh
internal/external fixation	application of pins, wires, and/or screws placed externally or internally to immobilize a body part
intracardiac	inside the heart
intramural	within the organ wall
intramuscular	into a muscle
intrauterine	inside the uterus
intravenous	into a vein
intravenous pyelography	IVP, radiographic recording of the urinary system
introitus	opening or entrance to the vagina from the uterus
intubation	insertion of a tube
intussusception	slipping of one part of the intestine into another part
invasive	entering the body, breaking skin
iontophoresis	introduction of ions into the body
ischemia	deficient blood supply due to obstruction of the circulatory system
island pedicle flap	contains a single artery and vein that remain attached to origin temporarily or permanently
isthmus	connection of two regions or structures
isthmus, thyroid	tissue connection between right and left thyroid lobes
isthmusectomy	surgical removal of the isthmus
jaundice	a condition in which excessive bilirubin causes the skin and whites of the eyes to appear yellowish
jejunostomy	artificial opening between the jejunum and the abdominal wall
joint	the place at which two bones attach
jugular nodes	lymph nodes located next to the large vein in the neck
keloid	a fibrous growth that forms at the site of a scar
keratomalacia	softening of the cornea associated with a deficiency of vitamin A

keratoplasty	surgical repair of the cornea
ketones	compounds that are carbon-based by-products of fatty acid metabolism; excess ketone bodies in urine may indicate diabetes mellitus
kidney	organs that filter blood and balance the levels of water, salt, and minerals in the blood
kidney stones	formations of minerals and salt that may form in the urine
Kock pouch	surgical creation of a urinary bladder from a segment of the ileum
kyphosis	humpback
labyrinth	inner connecting cavities, such as the internal ear
labyrinthitis	inner ear inflammation
lacrimal	related to tears
lamina	flat plate
laminectomy	surgical excision of the lamina
laparoscopy	exploration of the abdomen and pelvic cavities using a scope placed through a small incision in the abdominal wall
laryngeal web	congenital abnormality of connective tissue between the vocal cords
laryngectomy	surgical removal of the larynx
laryngography	radiographic recording of the larynx
laryngoplasty	surgical repair of the larynx
laryngoscope	fiberoptic scope used to view the inside of the larynx
laryngoscopy	direct visualization and examination of the interior of larynx with a laryngoscope
laryngotomy	incision into the larynx
lateral	away from the midline of the body (to the side)
lavage	washing out
leukoderma	depigmentation of skin
leukoplakia	white patch on mucous membrane
ligament	fibrous band of tissue that connects cartilage or bone
ligation	binding or tying off, as in constricting the blood flow of a vessel or binding fallopian tubes for sterilization
lipocyte	fat cell
lipoma	fatty tumor
lithotomy	incision into an organ or a duct for the purpose of removing a stone
lithotripsy	crushing of a stone by sound waves or force
lobectomy	surgical excision of lobe of the lung
lordosis	anterior curve of spine
lumbodynia	pain in the lumbar area
lunate	one of the wrist (carpal) bones
lymph node	station along the lymphatic system

lymphadenectomy	excision of a lymph node or nodes
lymphadenitis	inflammation of a lymph node
lymphangiography	radiographic recording of the lymphatic vessels and nodes
lymphangiotomy	incision into a lymphatic vessel
lysis	releasing
magnetic resonance imaging	MRI, procedure that uses nonionizing radiation to view the body in a cross-sectional view
Major Diagnostic Categories	MDC, the division of all principal diagnoses into 25 mutually exclusive principal diagnosis areas within the DRG system
mammography	radiographic recording of the breasts
Managed Care Organization	MCO, a group that is responsible for the health care services offered to an enrolled group of persons
manipulation	movement by hand
manipulation or reduction	alignment of a fracture or joint dislocation to its normal position
mastoidectomy	removal of the mastoid bone
Maximum Actual Allowable Charge	MAAC, limitation on the total amount that can be charged by physicians who are not participants in Medicare
meatotomy	surgical enlargement of the opening of the urinary meatus
medial	toward the midline of the body
Medical Volume Performance Standards	MVPS, government's estimate of how much growth is appropriate for nationwide physician expenditures paid by the Part B Medicare program
Medicare Economic Index	MEI, government mandated index that ties increases in the Medicare prevailing charges to economic indicators
Medicare Fee Schedule	MFS, schedule that listed the allowable charges for Medicare services; was replaced by the Medicare reasonable charge payment system
Medicare Risk HMO	a Medicare-funded alternative to the standard Medicare supplemental coverage
melanin	dark pigment of skin
melanoma	tumor of epidermis, malignant and black in color
Ménière's disease	condition that causes dizziness, ringing in the ears, and deafness
M-mode	one-dimensional display of movement of structures
modality	treatment method
Mohs surgery or Mohs micrographic surgery	removal of skin cancer in layers by a surgeon who also acts as pathologist during surgery
monofocal	eyeglasses with one vision correction
multipara	more than one pregnancy
muscle	organ of contraction for movement
muscle flap	transfer of muscle from origin to recipient site
myasthenia gravis	syndrome characterized by muscle weakness
myelography	radiographic recording of the subarachnoid space of the spine

myopia	nearsightedness, eyeball too long from front to back
myringotomy	incision into tympanic membrane
nasal button	synthetic circular disk used to cover a hole in the nasal septum
nasopharyngoscopy	use of a scope to visualize the nose and pharynx
National Provider Identifier	NPI, a 10-digit number assigned to a physician by Medicare
nephrectomy, paraperitoneal	kidney transplant
nephrocutaneous fistula	a channel from the kidney to the skin
nephrolithotomy	removal of a kidney stone through an incision made into the kidney
nephrorrhaphy	suturing of the kidney
nephrostolithotomy	creation of an artificial channel to the kidney
nephrostolithotomy, percutaneous	procedure to establish an artificial channel between the skin and the kidney
nephrostomy	creation of a channel into the renal pelvis of the kidney
nephrostomy, percutaneous	creation of a channel from the skin to the renal pelvis
nephrotomy	incision into the kidney
neurovascular flap	contains artery, vein, and nerve
noninvasive	not entering the body, not breaking skin
nuclear cardiology	diagnostic specialty that uses radiologic procedures to aid in diagnosis of cardiologic conditions
nystagmus	rapid involuntary eye movements
ocular adnexa	orbit, extraocular muscles, and eyelid
olecranon	elbow bone
Omnibus Budget Reconciliation Act of 1989	OBRA, act that established new rules for Medicare reimbursement
oophorectomy	surgical removal of the ovary(ies)
opacification	area that has become opaque (milky)
open fracture repair	surgical opening (incision) over or remote opening as access to a fracture site
open treatment	fracture site that is surgically opened and visualized
ophthalmodynamometry	test of the blood pressure of the eye
ophthalmology	body of knowledge regarding the eyes
ophthalmoscopy	examination of the interior of the eye by means of a scope, also known as fundoscopy
optokinetic	movement of the eyes to objects moving in the visual field
orchiectomy	castration; removal of the testes
orchiopexy	surgical procedure to release undescended testes and fixate them within the scrotum
order	shows subordination of one thing to another; family or class
orthopnea	difficulty in breathing, needing to be in erect position to breathe

orthoptic	corrective; in the correct place
osteoarthritis	degenerative condition of articular cartilage
osteoclast	absorbs or removes bone
osteotomy	cutting into bone
otitis media	noninfectious inflammation of the middle ear; serous otitis media produces liquid drainage (not purulent) and suppurative otitis media produces purulent (pus) matter
otoscope	instrument used to examine the internal and external ear
oviduct	fallopian tube
papilledema	swelling of the optic disc (papilla)
paraesophageal hiatal hernia	hernia that is near the esophagus
parathyroid	produces a hormone to mobilize calcium from the bones to the blood
paronychia	infection around nail
Part A	Medicare's Hospital Insurance; covers hospital/facility care
Part B	Medicare's Supplemental Medical Insurance; covers physician services and durable medical equipment that are not paid for under Part A
participating provider program	Medicare providers who have agreed in advance to accept assignment on all Medicare claims, now termed Quality Improvement Organizations (QIO)
patella	knee cap
pedicle	growth attached with a stem
Peer Review Organizations	PROs, groups established to review hospital admission and care
pelviolithotomy	pyeloplasty
penoscrotal	referring to the penis and scrotum
percussion	tapping with sharp blows as a diagnostic technique
percutaneous	through the skin
percutaneous fracture repair	repair of a fracture by means of pins and wires inserted through the fracture site
percutaneous skeletal fixation	considered neither open nor closed; the fracture is not visualized, but fixation is placed across the fracture site under x-ray imaging
pericardiocentesis	procedure in which a surgeon withdraws fluid from the pericardial space by means of a needle inserted percutaneously
pericardium	membranous sac enclosing heart and ends of great vessels
perineum	area between the vulva and anus; also known as the pelvic floor
peripheral nerves	12 pairs of cranial nerves, 31 pairs of spinal nerves, and autonomic nervous system; connects peripheral receptors to the brain and spinal cord
peritoneal	within the lining of the abdominal cavity
peritoneoscopy	visualization of the abdominal cavity using one scope placed through a small incision in the abdominal wall and another scope placed in the vagina

pharyngolaryngectomy	surgical removal of the pharynx and larynx
phlebotomy	cutting into a vein
phonocardiogram	recording of heart sounds
photochemotherapy	treatment by means of drugs that react to ultraviolet radiation or sunlight
physics	scientific study of energy
pilosebaceous	pertains to hair follicles and sebaceous glands
placenta	a structure that connects the fetus and mother during pregnancy
plethysmography	determining the changes in volume of an organ part or body
pleura	covers the lungs and lines the thoracic cavity
pleurectomy	surgical excision of the pleura
pleuritis	inflammation of the pleura
pneumonocentesis	surgical puncturing of a lung to withdraw fluid
pneumonolysis	surgical separation of the lung from the chest wall to allow the lung to collapse
pneumonostomy	surgical procedure in which the chest cavity is exposed and the lung is incised
pneumonotomy	incision of the lung
pneumoplethysmography	determining the changes in the volume of the lung
posterior (dorsal)	in back of
posterior segment	those parts of the eye behind the lens
posteroanterior	from back to front
postpartum	after childbirth
Preferred Provider Organization	PPO, a group of providers who form a network and who have agreed to provide services to enrollees at a discounted rate
priapism	painful condition in which the penis is constantly erect
primary care physician	PCP, physician who oversees a patient's care within a managed care organization
primary diagnosis	chief complaint of a patient in outpatient setting
primipara	first pregnancy
prior approval	also known as a prior authorization, the payer's approval of care
proctosigmoidoscopy	fiberscopic examination of the sigmoid colon and rectum
Professional Standards Review Organization	PSRO, voluntary physicians' organization designed to monitor the necessity of hospital admissions, treatment costs, and medical records of hospitals
prognosis	probable outcome of an illness
prostatotomy	incision into the prostate
Provider Identification Number	PIN, assigned to physicians by payers for use in claims submission
pyelography	radiographic recording of the kidneys, renal pelvis, ureters, and bladder
qualitative	measuring the presence or absence of

Quality Improvement Organizations	QIO, consists of a national network of 53 entities that work with consumers, physicians, hospitals, and caregivers to refine care delivery systems
quantitative	measuring the presence or absence of and the amount of
rad	radiation-absorbed dose, the energy deposited in patient's tissues
radiation oncology	branch of medicine concerned with the application of radiation to a tumor site for treatment (destruction) of cancerous tumors
radiograph	film on which an image is produced through exposure to x-radiation
radiologist	physician who specializes in the use of radioactive materials in the diagnosis and treatment of disease and illness
radiology	branch of medicine concerned with the use of radioactive substances for diagnosis and therapy
rales	coarse sounds on inspiration, also known as crackles (heard on auscultation)
real time	two-dimensional display of both the structures and the motion of tissues and organs, with the length of time also recorded as part of the study
reduction	replacement to normal position
Relative Value Unit	RVU, unit value that has been assigned for each service
Resource-Based Relative Value Scale	RBRVS, scale designed to decrease Medicare expenditures, redistribute physician payment, and ensure quality health care at reasonable rates
resource intensity	refers to the relative volume and type of diagnostic, therapeutic, and bed services used in the management of a particular illness
retrograde	moving backward or against the usual direction of flow
rhinoplasty	surgical repair of nose
rhinorrhea	nasal mucous discharge
salpingectomy	surgical removal of the uterine tube
salpingostomy	creation of a fistula into the uterine tube
scan	mapping of emissions of radioactive substances after they have been introduced into the body; the density can determine normal or abnormal conditions
sclera	outer covering of the eye
scoliosis	lateral curve of the spine
sebaceous gland	secretes sebum
seborrhea	excess sebum secretion
sebum	oily substance
section	slice of a frozen block
segmentectomy	surgical removal of a portion of a lung
septoplasty	surgical repair of the nasal septum
serum	blood from which the fibrinogen has been removed
severity of illness	refers to the levels of loss of function and mortality that may be experienced by patients with a particular disease

shunt	an artificial passage
sialography	radiographic recording of the salivary duct and branches
sialolithotomy	surgical removal of a stone of the salivary gland or duct
sinography	radiographic recording of the sinus or sinus tract
sinusotomy	surgical incision into a sinus
skeletal traction	application of pressure to the bone by means of pins and/or wires inserted into the bone
skin traction	application of pressure to the bone by means of tape applied to the skin
skull	entire skeletal framework of the head
somatic nerve	sensory or motor nerve
specimen	sample of tissue or fluid
spirometry	measurement of breathing capacity
splenectomy	excision of the spleen
splenography	radiographic recording of the spleen
splenoportography	radiographic procedure to allow visualization of the splenic and portal veins of the spleen
split-thickness graft	all epidermis and some of dermis
spondylitis	inflammation of vertebrae
Staff Model	a Health Maintenance Organization that directly employs the physicians who provide services to enrollees
steatoma	fat mass in sebaceous gland
stem cell	immature blood cell
stereotaxis	method of identifying a specific area or point in the brain
strabismus	extraocular muscle deviation resulting in unequal visual axes
stratified	layered
stratum (strata)	layer
subcutaneous	tissue below the dermis, primarily fat cells that insulate the body
subluxation	partial dislocation
subungual	beneath the nail
superior	toward the head or the upper part of the body; also known as cephalic
supination	supine position
supine	lying on the back
Swan-Ganz catheter	a catheter that measures pressure in the heart
sympathetic nerve	part of the peripheral nervous system that controls automatic body function and nerves activated under stress
symphysis	natural junction
synchondrosis	union between two bones (connected by cartilage)
tachypnea	quick, shallow breathing
tarsorrhaphy	suturing together of the eyelids

Tax Equity and Fiscal Responsibility Act	TEFRA, act that contains language to reward cost-conscious healthcare providers
tendon	attaches a muscle to a bone
tenodesis	suturing of a tendon to a bone
tenorrhaphy	suture repair of tendon
thermogram	written record of temperature variation
third-party payer	insurance company or entity that is liable for another's healthcare services
thoracentesis	surgical puncture of the thoracic cavity, usually using a needle, to remove fluids
thoracic duct	collection and distribution point for lymph, and the largest lymph vessel located in the chest
thoracoplasty	surgical procedure that removes rib(s) and thereby allows the collapse of a lung
thoracoscopy	use of a lighted endoscope to view the pleural spaces and thoracic cavity or to perform surgical procedures
thoracostomy	incision into the chest wall and insertion of a chest tube
thoracotomy	surgical incision into the chest wall
thromboendarterectomy	procedure to remove plaque or clot formations from a vessel by percutaneous method
thymectomy	surgical removal of the thymus
thymus	gland that produces hormones important to the immune response
thyroglossal duct	connection between the thyroid and the tongue
thyroid	part of the endocrine system that produces hormones that regulate metabolism
thyroidectomy	surgical removal of the thyroid
tinnitus	ringing in the ears
titer	measure of a laboratory analysis
tocolysis	repression of uterine contractions
tomography	procedure that allows viewing of a single plane of the body by blurring out all but that particular level
tonography	recording of changes in intraocular pressure in response to sustained pressure on the eyeball
tonometry	measurement of pressure or tension
total pneumonectomy	surgical removal of an entire lung
tracheostomy	creation of an opening into trachea
tracheotomy	incision into trachea
traction	application of pressure to maintain normal alignment
transcutaneous	entering by way of the skin
transesophageal echocardiogram	TEE, echocardiogram performed by placing a probe down the esophagus and sending out sound waves to obtain images of the heart and its movement

transmastoid	creates an opening in the mastoid for drainage antrostomy
transplantation	grafting of tissue from one source to another
transseptal	through the septum
transtracheal	across the trachea
transureteroureterostomy	surgical connection of one ureter to the other ureter
transurethral resection of prostate	TURP, procedure performed through the urethra by means of a cystoscopy to remove part or all of the prostate
transvenous	through a vein
transvesical ureterolithotomy	removal of a ureter stone (calculus) through the bladder
trephination	surgical removal of a disc of bone
trocar needle	needle with a tube on the end; used to puncture and withdraw fluid from a cavity
tubercle	lesion caused by infection of tuberculosis
tumescence	state of being swollen
tunica vaginalis	covering of the testes
tympanolysis	freeing of adhesions of the tympanic membrane
tympanometry	test of the inner ear using air pressure
tympanostomy	insertion of ventilation tube into tympanum
ultrasound	technique using sound waves to determine the density of the outline of tissue
unbundling	reporting with multiple codes that which can be reported with one code
unilateral	occurring on one side
uptake	absorption of a radioactive substance by body tissues; recorded for diagnostic purposes in conditions such as thyroid disease
ureterectomy	surgical removal of a ureter, either totally or partially
ureterocolon	pertaining to the ureter and colon
ureterocutaneous fistula	channel from the ureter to exterior skin
ureteroenterostomy	creation of a connection between the intestine and the ureter
ureterolithotomy	removal of a stone from the ureter
ureterolysis	freeing of adhesions of the ureter
ureteroneocystostomy	surgical connection of the ureter to a new site on the bladder
ureteropyelography	ureter and bladder radiography
ureterotomy	incision into the ureter
urethrocystography	radiography of the bladder and urethra
urethromeatoplasty	surgical repair of the urethra and meatus
urethropexy	fixation of the urethra by means of surgery
urethroplasty	surgical repair of the urethra
urethrorrhaphy	suturing of the urethra
urethroscopy	use of a scope to view the urethra

urography	same as pyelography; radiographic recording of the kidneys, renal pelvis, ureters, and bladder
uveal	vascular tissue of the choroid, ciliary body, and iris
varices	varicose veins
varicocele	swelling of a scrotal vein
vas deferens	tube that carries sperm from the epididymis to the urethra
vasectomy	removal of segment of vas deferens
vasogram	recording of the flow in the vas deferens
vasotomy	incision in the vas deferens
vasorrhaphy	suturing of the vas deferens
vasovasostomy	reversal of a vasectomy
vectorcardiogram	VCG, continuous recording of electrical direction and magnitude of the heart
venography	radiographic recording of the veins and tributaries
vertebrectomy	removal of vertebra
vertigo	dizziness
vesicostomy	surgical creation of a connection of the viscera of the bladder to the skin
vesicovaginal fistula	creation of a tube between the vagina and the bladder
vesiculectomy	excision of the seminal vesicle
vesiculography	radiographic recording of the seminal vesicles
vesiculotomy	incision into the seminal vesicle
viscera	an organ in one of the large cavities of the body
volvulus	twisted section of the intestine
vomer	flat bones of the nasal septum
xanthoma	tumor composed of cells containing lipid material, yellow in color
xenograft	different species graft
xeroderma	dry, discolored, scaly skin
xeroradiography	photoelectric process of radiographs

Combining Forms

abdomin/o	abdomen
acetabul/o	hip socket
acr/o	height/extremities
aden/o	in relationship to a gland
adenoid/o	adenoids
adip/o	fat
adren/o, adrenal/o	adrenal gland
albin/o	white
albumin/o	albumin
alveol/o	alveolus
ambly/o	dim
amni/o	amnion
an/o	anus
andr/o	male
andren/o	adrenal gland
andrenal/o	adrenal gland
angi/o	vessel
ankyl/o	bent, fused
aort/o	aorta
aponeur/o	tendon type
appendic/o	appendix
aque/o	water
arche/o	first
arter/o, arteri/o	artery
arthr/o	joint
atel/o	incomplete
ather/o	plaque
atri/o	atrium

audi/o	hearing
aut/o	self
axill/o	armpit
azot/o	urea
balan/o	glans penis
bi/o	life
bil/i	bile
bilirubin/o	bile pigment
blephar/o	eyelid
brachi/o	arm
bronch/o	bronchus
bronchi/o	bronchus
bronchiol/o	bronchiole
burs/o	fluid-filled sac in a joint
calc/o, calc/i	calcium
cardi/o	heart
carp/o	carpals (wrist bones)
cauter/o	burn
cec/o	cecum
celi/o	abdomen
cephal/o	head
cerebell/o	cerebellum
cerebr/o	cerebrum
cervic/o	neck/cervix
chol/e	gall/bile
cholangio/o	bile duct
cholecyst/o	gallbladder
choledoch/o	common bile duct
cholester/o	cholesterol
chondr/o	cartilage
chori/o	chorion
clavic/o, clavicul/o	clavicle (collar bone)
col/o	colon
colp/o	vagina
coni/o	dust
conjunctiv/o	conjunctiva
cor/o, core/o	pupil

corne/o	cornea
coron/o	heart
cortic/o	cortex
cost/o	rib
crani/o	cranium (skull)
crin/o	secrete
crypt/o	hidden
culd/o	cul-de-sac
cutane/o	skin
cyan/o	blue
cycl/o	ciliary body
cyst/o	bladder
dacry/o	tear
dacryocyst/o	pertaining to the lacrimal sac
dent/i	tooth
derm/o, dermat/o	skin
diaphragmat/o	diaphragm
dips/o	thirst
disc/o	intervertebral disc
diverticul/o	diverticulum
duoden/o	duodenum
dur/o	dura mater
encephal/o	brain
enter/o	small intestine
eosin/o	rosy
epididym/o	epididymis
epiglott/o	epiglottis
episi/o	vulva
erythr/o, erythem/o	red
esophag/o	esophagus
essi/o, esthesi/o	sensation
estr/o	female
femor/o	thighbone
fet/o	fetus
fibul/o	fibula
galact/o	milk
gangli/o	ganglion

ganglion/o	ganglion
gastr/o	stomach
gingiv/o	gum
glomerul/o	glomerulus
gloss/o	tongue
gluc/o	sugar
glyc/o	sugar
glycos/o	sugar
gonad/o	ovaries and testes
gyn/o	female
gynec/o	female
hepat/o	liver
herni/o	hernia
heter/o	different
hidr/o	sweat
home/o	same
hormon/o	hormone
humer/o	humerus (upper arm bone)
hydr/o	water
hymen/o	hymen
hyster/o	uterus
ichthy/o	dry/scaly
ile/o	ileus
ili/o	ilium (upper pelvic bone)
immun/o	immune
inguin/o	groin
ir/o	iris
irid/o	iris
ischi/o	ischium (posterior pelvic bone)
jaund/o	yellow
jejun/o	jejunum
kal/i	potassium
kerat/o	hard, cornea
kinesi/o	movement
kyph/o	hump
lacrim/o	tear
lact/o	milk

lamin/o	lamina
lapar/o	abdomen
laryng/o	larynx
lingu/o	tongue
lip/o	fat
lith/o	stone
lob/o	lobe
lord/o	curve
lumb/o	lower back
lute/o	yellow
lymph/o	lymph
lymphaden/o	lymph gland
mamm/o	breast
mandibul/o	mandible (lower jawbone)
mast/o	breast
maxill/o	maxilla (upper jawbone)
meat/o	meatus
melan/o	black
men/o	menstruation, month
mening/o, meningi/o	meninges
menisc/o, menisci/o	meniscus
ment/o	mind
metacarp/o	metacarpals (hand)
metatars/o	metatarsals (foot)
metr/o	uterus, measure
metr/i	uterus
mon/o	one
muc/o	mucus
my/o, muscul/o	muscle
myc/o	fungus
myel/o	bone marrow, spinal cord
myring/o	ear drum
myx/o	mucus
nas/o	nose
nat/a, nat/i	birth
natr/o	sodium
necr/o	death

nephr/o	kidney
neur/o	nerve
noct/i	night
ocul/o	eye
olecran/o	olecranon (elbow)
olig/o	scant, few
onych/o	nail
oo/o	egg
oophor/o	ovary
ophthalm/o	eye
opt/o	eye, vision
optic/o	eye
or/o	mouth
orch/i, orch/o, orchi/o, orchid/o	testicle
orth/o	straight
oste/o	bone
ot/o	ear
ov/o	egg
ovari/o	ovary
ovul/o	ovulation
ox/i, ox/o	oxygen
oxy/o	oxygen
pachy/o	thick
palat/o	palate
palpebr/o	eyelid
pancreat/o	pancreas
papill/o	optic nerve
patell/o	patella (kneecap)
pelv/i	pelvis (hip)
pericardi/o	pericardium
perine/o	perineum
peritone/o	peritoneum
petr/o	stone
phac/o	eye lens
phak/o	eye lens
phalang/o	phalanges (finger or toe)
pharyng/o	pharynx

phas/o	speech
phleb/o	vein
phren/o	mind, diaphragm
phys/o	growing
pil/o	hair
pituitar/o	pituitary gland
pleur/o	pleura
pneumat/o	lung/air
pneumon/o	lung/air
poli/o	gray matter
polyp/o	polyp
pont/o	pons
proct/o	rectum
prostat/o	prostate gland
psych/o	mind
pub/o	pubis
pulmon/o	lung
pupill/o	pupil
py/o	pus
pyel/o	renal pelvis
pylor/o	pylorus
quadr/i	four
rachi/o	spine
radi/o	radius (lower arm)
radic/o, radicul/o	nerve root
rect/o	rectum
ren/o	kidney
retin/o	retina
rhin/o	nose
rhiz/o	nerve root
rhytid/o	wrinkle
rube/o	red
sacr/o	sacrum
salping/o	uterine tube, fallopian tube
scapul/o	scapula (shoulder)
scler/o	sclera
scoli/o	bent

seb/o	sebum/oil
semin/i	semen
sept/o	septum
sial/o	saliva
sigmoid/o	sigmoid colon
sinus/o	sinus
somat/o	body
son/o	sound
sperm/o, spermat/o	sperm
sphygm/o	pulse
spir/o	breath
splen/o	spleen
spondyl/o	vertebra
staped/o	middle ear, stapes
staphyl/o	clusters
steat/o	fat
ster/o, stere/o	solid, having three dimensions
stern/o	sternum (breast bone)
steth/o	chest
stomat/o	mouth
strept/o	twisted chain
synovi/o	synovial joint membrane
tars/o	tarsal (ankle)
ten/o	tendon
tend/o, tendin/o	tendon (connective tissue)
test/o	testicle
thorac/o	thorax
thromb/o	clot
thym/o	thymus gland
thyr/o, thyroid/o	thyroid gland
tibi/o	shin bone
toc/o	childbirth
tonsill/o	tonsil
top/o	place
tox/o, toxic/o	poison
trache/o	trachea
trich/o	hair

tympan/o	eardrum
uln/o	ulna (lower arm bone)
ungu/o	nail
ur/o	urine
ureter/o	ureter
urethr/o	urethra
urin/o	urine
uter/o	uterus
uve/o	uvea
uvul/o	uvula
vagin/o	vagina
valv/o, valvul/o	valve
vas/o, vascul/o	vessel
ven/o	vein
ventricul/o	ventricle
vertebr/o	vertebra
vesic/o	bladder
vesicul/o	seminal vesicles
vitre/o	glass/glassy
vulv/o	vulva
xanth/o	yellow
xer/o	dry

Prefixes

a-	not
an-	not
ante-	before
audi-	hearing
bi-	two
brady-	slow
de-	lack of
dys-	difficult, painful
ecto-	outside
endo-	in
epi-	on/upon
eso-	inward
eu-	good/normal
exo-	outward
extra-	outside
hemi-	half
hyper-	excess, over
hypo-	under
in-	into
inter-	between
intra-	within
meta-	change, after
multi-	many
neo-	new
nulli-, nulti-	none
oxy-	sharp, oxygen
pan-	all
para-	beside

per-	through
peri-	surrounding
poly-	many
post-	after
primi-	first
pseudo-	false
quadri-	four
retro-	behind
sub-	under
supra-	above
sym-	together
syn-	together
tachy-	fast
tetra-	four
tri-	three
tropin-	act upon
uni-	one

Suffixes

-agon	assemble
-algesia	pain sensation
-algia	pain
-ar	pertaining to
-arche	beginning
-ary	pertaining to
-asthenia	weakness
-blast	embryonic
-capnia	carbon dioxide
-cele	hernia
-centesis	puncture to remove (drain)
-chezia	defecation
-clast, -clasia, -clasis	break
-coccus	spherical bacterium
-cyesis	pregnancy
-desis	fusion
-dilation	widening, expanding
-drome	run
-dynia	pain
-eal	pertaining to
-ectasis	stretching
-ectomy	removal
-edema	swelling
-emia	blood
-esthesis	feeling
-gram	record
-graph	recording instrument
-graphy	recording process

-gravida	pregnancy
-ia	condition
-iatrist	physician specialist
-iatry	medical treatment
-ical	pertaining to
-ictal	pertaining to
-in	a substance
-ine	a substance
-itis	inflammation
-listhesis	slipping
-lithiasis	condition of stones
-lysis	separation
-malacia	softening
-megaly	enlargement
-meta	change
-meter	measurement; instrument that measures
-metry	measurement of
-oid	resembling
-oma	tumor
-omia	smell
-one	hormone
-opia	vision
-opsy	view of
-orrhexis	rupture
-osis	condition
-oxia	oxygen
-para	woman who has given birth
-paresis	incomplete paralysis
-parous	to bear
-penia	deficient
-pexy	fixation
-phagia	eating
-phonia	sound
-phylaxis	protection
-physis	to grow
-plasty	repair
-plegia	paralysis

-pnea	breathing
-poiesis	production
-poly	many
-porosis	passage
-retro	behind
-rrhagia	bursting of blood
-rrhaphy	suture
-rrhea	discharge
-schisis	split
-sclerosis	hardening
-scopy	to examine
-spasm	contraction of muscle
-steat/o	fat
-stenosis	blockage, narrowing
-stomy	opening
-thorax	chest
-tocia	labor
-tom/o	to cut
-tome	an instrument that cuts
-tomy	cutting, incision
-tripsy	crush
-tropia	to turn
-tropin	act upon
-uria	urine
-version	turning

Abbreviations

ABG	arterial blood gas
ABN	Advanced Beneficiary Notice; used by CMS to notify beneficiary of payment of provider services
ACL	anterior cruciate ligament
AD	right ear
AFB	acid-fast bacillus
AFI	amniotic fluid index
AGA	appropriate for gestational age
AGCUS	atypical glandular cells of undetermined significance
AKA	above-knee amputation
ANS	autonomic nervous system
APCs	Ambulatory Payment Classifications, patient classification that provides a payment system for outpatients
ARDS	adult respiratory distress syndrome
ARF	acute renal failure
ARM	artificial rupture of membrane
AS	left ear
ASCUS	atypical squamous cells of undetermined significance
ASCVD	arteriosclerotic cardiovascular disease
ASD	atrial septal defect
ASHD	arteriosclerotic heart disease
AU	both ears
AV	atrioventricular
BCC	benign cellular changes
BiPAP	bi-level positive airway pressure
BKA	below-knee amputation
BP	blood pressure
BPD	biparietal diameter
BPH	benign prostatic hypertrophy

BPP	biophysical profile
BUN	blood urea nitrogen
BV	bacterial vaginosis
bx	biopsy
C1-C7	cervical vertebrae
ca	cancer
CABG	coronary artery bypass graft
CBC	complete blood (cell) count
CF	conversion factor, national dollar amount that is applied to all services paid on the Medicare Fee Schedule basis
CHF	congestive heart failure
CHL	crown-to-heel length
CK	creatine kinase
CMS	Centers for Medicare and Medicaid Services, formerly HCFA, Health Care Financing Administration
CNM	certified nurse midwife
CNS	central nervous system
COB	coordination of benefits, management of payment between two or more third-party payers for a service
COPD	chronic obstructive pulmonary disease
CPAP	continuous positive airway pressure
CPD	cephalopelvic disproportion
CPK	creatine phosphokinase
CPP	chronic pelvic pain
CSF	cerebrospinal fluid
CTS	carpal tunnel syndrome
CVA	cerebrovascular accident, stroke
CVI	cerebrovascular insufficiency
D&C	dilation and curettage
D&E	dilation and evacuation
derm	dermatology
DHHS	Department of Health and Human Services
DLCO	diffuse capacity of lungs for carbon monoxide
DRGs	Diagnosis Related Groups, disease classification system that relates the types of inpatients a hospital treats (case mix) to the costs incurred by the hospital
DSE	dobutamine stress echocardiography
DUB	dysfunctional uterine bleeding
ECC	endocervical curettage

EDC	estimated date of confinement
EDD	estimated date of delivery
EDI	electronic data interchange, exchange of data between multiple computer terminals
EEG	electroencephalogram
EFM	electronic fetal monitoring
EFW	estimated fetal weight
EGA	estimated gestational age
EGD	esophagogastroduodenoscopy
EGJ	esophagogastric junction
EMC	endometrial curettage
EOB	explanation of benefits, remittance advice
EPO	Exclusive Provider Organization, similar to a Health Maintenance Organization except that the providers of the services are not prepaid, but rather are paid on a fee-for-service basis
EPSDT	Early and Periodic Screening, Diagnosis, and Treatment
ERCP	endoscopic retrograde cholangiopancreatography
ERT	estrogen replacement therapy
ESRD	end-stage renal disease
FAS	fetal alcohol syndrome
FEF	forced expiratory flow
FEV_1	forced expiratory volume in 1 second
FEV_1:FVC	maximum amount of forced expiratory volume in 1 second
FHR	fetal heart rate
FI	fiscal intermediary, financial agent acting on behalf of a third-party payer
FRC	functional residual capacity
FSH	follicle-stimulating hormone
FVC	forced vital capacity
fx	fracture
GERD	gastroesophageal reflux disease
GI	gastrointestinal
H or E	hemorrhage or exudate
HCFA	Health Care Financing Administration, now known as Centers for Medicare and Medicaid Services (CMS)
HCVD	hypertensive cardiovascular disease
HD	hemodialysis
HDL	high-density lipoprotein
HEA	hemorrhage, exudate, aneurysm
HHN	hand-held nebulizer

HJR	hepatojugular reflux
H&P	history and physical (examination)
HPV	human papillomavirus
HSG	hysterosalpingogram
HSV	herpes simplex virus
I&D	incision and drainage
IO	intraocular
IOL	intraocular lens
IPAP	inspiratory positive airway pressure
IRDS	infant respiratory distress syndrome
IVF	in vitro fertilization
IVP	intravenous pyelogram
JBP	jugular blood pressure
KUB	kidneys, ureter, bladder
L1-L5	lumbar vertebrae
LBBB	left bundle branch block
LEEP	loop electrosurgical excision procedure
LGA	large for gestational age
LLQ	left lower quadrant
LP	lumbar puncture
LUQ	left upper quadrant
LVH	left ventricular hypertrophy
MAT	multifocal atrial tachycardia
MDI	metered dose inhaler
MI	myocardial infarction
MRI	magnetic resonance imaging
MSLT	multiple sleep latency testing
MVV	maximum voluntary ventilation
NCPAP	nasal continuous positive airway pressure
NSR	normal sinus rhythm
OA	osteoarthritis
OD	right eye
OS	left eye
OU	each eye
PAC	premature atrial contraction
PAT	paroxysmal atrial tachycardia
PAWP	pulmonary artery wedge pressure

PCWP	pulmonary capillary wedge pressure
PEAP	positive end-airway pressure
PEEP	positive end-expiratory pressure
PEG	percutaneous endoscopic gastrostomy
PERL	pupils equal and reactive to light
PERRL	pupils equal, round, and reactive to light
PERRLA	pupils equal, round, and reactive to light and accommodation
PFT	pulmonary function test
pH	symbol for acid/base level
PICC	peripherally inserted central catheter
PID	pelvic inflammatory disease
PND	paroxysmal nocturnal dyspnea
PNS	peripheral nervous system
PROM	premature rupture of membranes
PSA	prostate-specific antigen
PST	paroxysmal supraventricular tachycardia
PSVT	paroxysmal supraventricular tachycardia
PT	prothrombin time
PTCA	percutaneous transluminal coronary angioplasty
PTT	partial thromboplastin time
PVC	premature ventricular contraction
RA	remittance advice, explanation of services
RA	rheumatoid arthritis
RBBB	right bundle branch block
RDS	respiratory distress syndrome
REM	rapid eye movement
RLQ	right lower quadrant
RSR	regular sinus rhythm
RUQ	right upper quadrant
RV	respiratory volume
RVG	*Relative Value Guide*
RVH	right ventricular hypertrophy
RVS	relative value studies, list of procedures with unit values assigned to each
RV:TLC	ratio of respiratory volume to total lung capacity
SHG	sonohysterogram
sp gr	specific gravity
SROM	spontaneous rupture of membranes

subcu, subq, SC, SQ	subcutaneous
SUI	stress urinary incontinence
SVT	supraventricular tachycardia
T1-T12	thoracic vertebrae
TAH	total abdominal hysterectomy
TEE	transesophageal echocardiography
TENS	transcutaneous electrical nerve stimulation
TIA	transient ischemic attack
TLC	total lung capacity
TLV	total lung volume
TM	tympanic membrane
TMJ	temporomandibular joint
TPA	tissue plasminogen activator
TSH	thyroid-stimulating hormone
TST	treadmill stress test
TURBT	transurethral resection of bladder tumor
TURP	transurethral resection of prostate
UA	urinalysis
UCR	usual, customary, and reasonable—third-party payers' assessment of the reimbursement for health care services: usual, that which would ordinarily be charged for the service; customary, the cost of that service in that locale; and reasonable, as assessed by the payer
UPJ	ureteropelvic junction
URI	upper respiratory infection
UTI	urinary tract infection
V/Q	ventilation/perfusion scan
VBAC	vaginal birth after cesarean
WBC	white blood (cell) count

Further Text Resources

ANATOMY AND PHYSIOLOGY

Book Title	Author	Imprint	Copyright Date	ISBN-13
The Anatomy and Physiology Learning System, 4th Edition	Applegate	Saunders	2011	978-1-4377-0393-1
Gray's Anatomy for Students, 2nd Edition	Drake, Vogl, Mitchell	Churchill Livingstone	2010	978-0-443-06952-9
Anthony's Textbook of Anatomy and Physiology, 20th Edition	Thibodeau, Patton	Mosby	2012	978-0-323-09600-3

CODING

Book Title	Author	Imprint	Copyright Date	ISBN-13
Step-by-Step Medical Coding, 2016 Edition	Buck	Saunders	2016	978-0-323-38919-8
2016 ICD-10-CM Hospital Professional Edition	Buck	Saunders	2016	978-0-323-27975-8
2016 ICD-10-CM Physician Professional Edition	Buck	Saunders	2016	978-0-323-27976-5
2016 ICD-10-PCS Professional Edition	Buck	Saunders	2016	978-0-323-28918-4
2016 HCPCS Level II Professional Edition	Buck	Saunders	2016	978-0-323-38983-9
The Next Step: Advanced Medical Coding and Auditing, 2016 Edition	Buck	Saunders	2016	978-0-323-38910-5
Physician Coding Exam Review 2016: The Certification Step	Buck	Saunders	2016	978-0-323-22750-6
Online Internship for Medical Coding 2015/2016 Edition	Buck	Saunders	2016	978-0-323-39250-1
ICD-10-CM/PCS Coding: Theory and Practice, 2016 Edition	Lovaasen	Saunders	2016	978-0-323-38993-8

PATHOPHYSIOLOGY

Book Title	Author	Imprint	Copyright Date	ISBN-13
Pathology for the Health Professions, 4th Edition	Damjanov	Saunders	2012	978-1-4377-1676-4
Essentials of Human Diseases and Conditions, 5th Edition	Frazier, Drzymkowski	Saunders	2012	978-1-4377-2408-0
Pathophysiology for the Health Professions, 4th Edition	Gould	Saunders	2011	978-1-4377-0965-0
The Human Body in Health and Illness, 4th Edition	Herlihy	Saunders	2011	978-1-4160-6842-6
The Human Body in Health and Disease, 6th Edition	Thibodeau, Patton	Mosby	2014	978-0-323-10124-1

MEDICAL TERMINOLOGY

Book Title	Author	Imprint	Copyright Date	ISBN-13
The Language of Medicine, 10th Edition	Chabner	Saunders	2014	978-1-4557-2846-6
Mastering Healthcare Terminology, 4th Edition	Shiland	Mosby	2013	978-0-323-08032-3
Jablonski's Dictionary of Medical Acronyms & Abbreviations, 6th Edition	Jablonski	Saunders	2008	978-1-4160-5899-1
Exploring Medical Language, 8th Edition	LaFleur, Brooks	Mosby	2012	978-0-323-07308-0
Building a Medical Vocabulary (with Spanish Translations), 8th Edition	Leonard	Saunders	2012	978-1-4377-2784-5
Quick & Easy Medical Terminology, 7th Edition	Leonard	Saunders	2014	978-1-4557-4070-3
Dorland's Illustrated Medical Dictionary, 32nd Edition		Saunders	2011	978-1-4160-6257-8

INTRODUCTION TO COMPUTERS

Book Title	Author	Imprint	Copyright Date	ISBN-13
Computerized Medical Office Procedures: A Worktext, 4th Edition	Larsen	Saunders	2014	978-1-4557-2620-2

BASICS OF WRITING/MEDICAL TRANSCRIPTION

Book Title	Author	Imprint	Copyright Date	ISBN-13
Medical Transcription Guide: Do's and Don'ts, 3rd Edition	Diehl	Saunders	2005	978-0-7216-0684-2
Medical Transcription: Techniques and Procedures, 7th Edition	Diehl	Saunders	2012	978-1-4377-0439-6

COMPREHENSION BUILDING/STUDY SKILLS

Book Title	Author	Imprint	Copyright Date	ISBN-13
Career Development for Health Professionals: Success in School and on the Job, 3rd Edition	Haroun	Saunders	2010	978-1-4377-0673-4

BASIC MATH

Book Title	Author	Imprint	Copyright Date	ISBN-13
Using Maths in Health Sciences	Gunn	Churchill Livingstone	2001	978-0-4430-7074-7

MEDICAL BILLING/INSURANCE

Book Title	Author	Imprint	Copyright Date	ISBN-13
Health Insurance Today: A Practical Approach, 4th Edition	Beik	Saunders	2013	978-1-4557-0819-2
Medical Insurance Made Easy: Understanding the Claim Cycle, 2nd Edition	Brown	Saunders	2006	978-0-7216-0556-2
Insurance Handbook for the Medical Office, 12th Edition	Fordney	Saunders	2012	978-1-4377-2256-7
Electronic Health Record "Booster" Kit for the Medical Office, 2nd Edition	Buck	Saunders	2012	978-1-4557-2301-0
ePractice Kit for the Medical Front Office	Buck	Saunders	2012	978-1-4377-2722-7
Practice Kit for Medical Front Office Skills, 3rd Edition	Buck	Saunders	2011	978-1-4377-2201-7

Pharmacology Review

Generic Name	Registered Brand or Trade Name	Therapeutic Use/Medication Action
ANTI-ATTENTION DEFICIT HYPERACTIVITY DISORDER		
atomoxetine	Strattera	Attention Deficit Hyperactivity Disorder (ADHD) therapy
AMNESIC		
diazepam	Valium	amnesic, antianxiety, anticonvulsant, antipain, anti-tremor agent, sedative-hypnotic, skeletal muscle relaxant adjunct
lorazepam	Ativan	amnesic, antianxiety, anticonvulsant, antiemetic, antipanic, anti-tremor, sedative-hypnotic, skeletal muscle relaxant
ANALGESIC		
acetaminophen-codeine	Phenaphen with Codeine	analgesic
acetaminophen-codeine	Tylenol with Codeine	analgesic
celecoxib	Celebrex	analgesic, antirheumatic NSAID
fentanyl	Duragesic	analgesic
fentanyl	Actiq	analgesic, anesthetic adjunct
fentanyl	Sublimaze	analgesic, anesthetic adjunct
hydrocodone	Hycodan	analgesic
hydrocodone-acetaminophen	Lortab	analgesic
hydrocodone-acetaminophen	Vicodin	analgesic
ibuprofen	Advil	analgesic
ibuprofen	Motrin	analgesic
naproxen	Aleve	analgesic, nonsteroid anti-inflammatory, antidysmenorreal, antigout, antipyretic, antirheumatic, vascular headache prophylactic and suppressant
naproxen	Naprosyn	analgesic, nonsteroid anti-inflammatory, antidysmenorreal, antigout, antipyretic, antirheumatic, vascular headache prophylactic and suppressant
oxycodone	OxyContin	analgesic
oxycodone-acetaminophen	Endocet	analgesic
oxycodone-acetaminophen	Percocet	analgesic
oxycodone-acetaminophen	Tylox	analgesic
propoxyphene-acetaminophen	Darvocet-N 100	analgesic
tramadol	Ultram	analgesic
tramadol-acetaminophen	Ultracet	analgesic

Generic Name	Registered Brand or Trade Name	Therapeutic Use/Medication Action
ANTI HIV AIDS		
efavirenz	Sustiva	anti HIV AIDS
emtricitabine	Emtriva	anti HIV AIDS
tenofovir	Viread	anti HIV AIDS
ANTI-IMPOTENCE		
sildenafil	Viagra	impotence, anti-erectile dysfunction
ANTI-PARKINSONISM		
cabergoline	Dostinex	anti-parkinsonism, anti-migraine headache
ANTIPROSTATIC HYPERTROPHY		
finasteride	Propecia	benign prostatic hyperplasia therapy, hair growth stimulant
finasteride	Proscar	benign prostatic hyperplasia therapy, hair growth stimulant
tamsulosin HCL	Flomax	benign prostatic hyperplasia therapy
ANTIACNE		
ethinyl estradiol-norethindrone	Estrostep Fe	antiacne, antiendometriotic, systemic contraceptive, estrogen-progestin, gonadotropin inhibitor
ethinyl estradiol-norethindrone	Femhrt	antiacne, antiendometriotic, systemic contraceptive, estrogen-progestin, gonadotropin inhibitor
ethinyl estradiol-norethindrone	Loestrin Fe	antiacne, antiendometriotic, systemic contraceptive, estrogen-progestin, gonadotropin inhibitor
ethinyl estradiol-norethindrone	Ovcon	antiacne, antiendometriotic, systemic contraceptive, estrogen-progestin, gonadotropin inhibitor
ethinyl estrodiol-norgestinmate	Ortho Tri-Cyclen	antiacne, antiendometriotic, systemic contraceptive, estrogen-progestin, gonadotropin inhibitor
ANTIADRENERGIC		
metoprolol	Lopressor	antiadrenergic, antianginal, antianxiety, antiarrhythmic, antihypertensive, anti-tremor, hypertrophic cardiomyopathy, MI therapy
metoprolol succinate	Toprol XL	antiadrenergic, antianginal, antianxiety, antiarrhythmic, antihypertensive, anti-tremor, hypertrophic cardiomyopathy, MI therapy
propranolol	Inderal	antiadrenergic, antianginal, antianxiety, antiarrhythmic, antihypertensive, anti-tremor, hypertrophic cardiomyopathy, MI prophylactic, MI therapy, neuroleptic-induced akathisia therapy
timolol	Blocadren	antiadrenergic, antianginal, antianxiety, antiarrhythmic, systemic antiglaucoma, antihypertensive, anti-tremor, hypertrophic cardiomyopathy, MI prophylactic
ANTIANGINAL		
diltiazem	Cardizem	antianginal, antiarrhythmic, antihypertensive
diltiazem	Dilacor	antianginal, antiarrhythmic, antihypertensive
felodipine	Plendil	antianginal, antihypertensive
isosorbide mononitrate	Imdur	antianginal
isosorbide mononitrate	Ismo	antianginal
nifedipine	Procardia	antianginal, antihypertensive

Generic Name	Registered Brand or Trade Name	Therapeutic Use/Medication Action
ANTIANGINAL—cont'd		
nitroglycerin	Minitran	antianginal, congestive heart failure (CHF), vasodilator
nitroglycerin	Nitrolingual	antianginal, CHS, vasodilator
nitroglycerin	Nitrostat	antianginal, CHS, vasodilator
verapamil	Isoptin	antianginal, antiarrhythmic, antihypertensive, hypertrophic cardiomyopathy therapy vascular headache prophylactic
verapamil	Verelan	antianginal, antiarrhythmic, antihypertensive, hypertrophic cardiomyopathy therapy vascular headache prophylactic
verapamil	Calan	antianginal, antiarrhythmic, antihypertensive, hypertrophic cardiomyopathy therapy, vascular headache prophylactic
verapamil	Covera HS	antianginal, antiarrhythmic, antihypertensive, hypertrophic cardiomyopathy therapy, vascular headache prophylactic
ANTIANXIETY		
alprazolam	Xanax	antianxiety
buspirone	BuSpar	antianxiety
escitalopram oxalate	Lexapro	antianxiety, antidepressant
paroxetine HCL	Paxil	antianxiety, antidepressant, antiobsessional, antipanic, posttraumatic stress disorder, social anxiety disorder agent
sertraline	Zoloft	antianxiety, antidepressant, antiobsessional, antipanic, posttraumatic stress disorder, premenstrual dysphoric disorder therapy
ANTIARRHYTHMIC		
digoxin	Digitek	antiarrhythmic, cardiotonic
digoxin	Lanoxicaps	antiarrhythmic, cardiotonic
digoxin	Lanoxin	antiarrhythmic, cardiotonic
phenytoin	Dilantin	antiarrhythmic, anticonvulsant, trigeminal neuralgic antineuralgic, skeletal muscle relaxant
ANTIASTHMATIC		
budesonide	Pulmicort	antiasthmatic
fluticasone-salmeterol	Advair Diskus	antiasthmatic, inhalation anti-inflammatory, bronchodilator
ipratropium bromide	Atrovent	antiasthmatic bronchodilator
lipatropium-albuterol	Combivent	antiasthmatic bronchodilator
montelukast sodium	Singular	antiasthmatic, leukotriene receptor antagonist
salmeterol maleate	Serevent	antiasthmatic
zafirlukast	Accolate	antiasthmatic
ANTIBACTERIAL		
amoxicillin	Trimax	systemic antibacterial
amoxicillin-clavulanate	Augmentin	systemic antibacterial
azithromycin	Zithromax	systemic antibacterial
cefadroxil	Duricef	systemic antibacterial
cefdinir	Omnicef	systemic antibacterial
cefluroximine axetil	Ceflin	systemic antibacterial

Generic Name	Registered Brand or Trade Name	Therapeutic Use/Medication Action
ANTIBACTERIAL—cont'd		
cefprozil	Cefzil	systemic antibacterial
cephalexin	Keflex	systemic antibacterial
ciprofloxacin	Ciloxan	ophthalmic antibacterial
ciprofloxacin	Cipro	systemic antibacterial
clarithromycin	Biaxin	systemic antibacterial, antimycobacterial
clindamycin	Cleocin	systemic antibacterial
doxycycline	Vibramycin	systemic antibacterial, antiprotozoal
levofloxacin	Levaquin	systemic antibacterial
metronidazole	Flagyl	systemic antibacterial
minocycline	Minocin	systemic antibacterial
moxifloxacin	Avelox	systemic antibacterial
moxifloxacin	Vigamox	ophthalmic antibacterial
mupirocin	Bactroban	topical antibacterial
nitrofurantoin	Macrodantin	systemic antibacterial
nitrofurantoin monohydrate	Macrobid	systemic antibacterial
ofloxacin	Floxin	systemic antibacterial
penicillin V	Veetids	systemic antibacterial
sulfamethoxazole-trimethoprim	Bactrim	systemic antibacterial, antiprotozoal
sulfamethoxazole-trimethoprim	Cotrim	systemic antibacterial, antiprotozoal
sulfamethoxazole-trimethoprim	Septra DS	systemic antibacterial, antiprotozoal
trimethoprim	Bactrim	systemic antibacterial
ANTICOAGULANT		
dipyridamole/ASA	Aggrenox	anticoagulant
warfarin	Coumadin	anticoagulant
ANTICONVULSANT		
clonazepam	Klonopin	anticonvulsant
divalproex sodium	Depakote	anticonvulsant, antimanic, migraine headache prophylactic
gabapentin	Neurontin	anticonvulsant, antineuralgic
lamotrigine	Lamictal	anticonvulsant
levetiracetam	Keppra	anticonvulsant
oxcarbazepine	Trileptal	anticonvulsant
tiagabine	Gabitril	anticonvulsant
topiramate	Topamax	anticonvulsant, antimigraine headache
zonisamide	Zonegran	anticonvulsant
ANTIDEMENTIA		
donepezil	Aricept	antidementia
galantamine HBr	Reminyl	antidementia-mild/moderate Alzheimer's
rivastigmine tartrate	Exelon	antidementia of Parkinson's

Generic Name	Registered Brand or Trade Name	Therapeutic Use/Medication Action
ANTIDEPRESSANT		
amitriptyline	Elavil	antidepressant
bupropion	Zyban	antidepressant, smoking cessation
bupropion HCL	Wellbutrin	antidepressant, smoking cessation
citalopram hydrobromide	Celexa	antidepressant
doxepin	Sinequan	antidepressant
fluoxetine	Prozac	antidepressant, antiobsessional agent
fluoxetine	Sarafem	antidepressant, antiobsessional, antibulimic agent
mirtazapine	Remeron	antidepressant
trazodone	Desyrel	antidepressant, antineuralgic
venlafaxine HCL	Effexor	antidepressant, antianxiety agent
ANTIDIABETIC		
doxazosin mesylate	Diabinese	antidiabetic
glimepiride	Amaryl	antidiabetic
glipizide	Glucotrol	antidiabetic
glyburide	DiaBeta	antidiabetic
glyburide	Glynase	antidiabetic
glyburide	Micronase	antidiabetic
glyburide-metformin	Glucovance	antidiabetic
insulin	Nolog	antidiabetic
insulin	Novolin	antidiabetic
insulin glargine	Lantus	antidiabetic
insulin lispro	Humalog	antidiabetic
metformin HCL	Glucophage	antihyperglycemic
miglitol	Glyset	antidiabetic
NPH isophane insulin	Humulin N	antidiabetic
NPH regular insulin	Humulin 70/30	antidiabetic
pioglitazone	Actos	antidiabetic
repaglinide	Prandin	antidiabetic
rosiglitazone	Avandia	antidiabetic
ANTIEMETIC		
meclizine	Antivert	antiemetic, antivertigo
promethazine	Phenergan	antiemetic, antihistaminic, H1 receptor, antivertigo, sedative-hypnotic
ANTIENDOMETRIOTIC		
ethinyl estradiol-desogestrel	Cyclessa	antiendometriotic, systemic contraceptive, gonadotropin inhibitor
ethinyl estradiol-desogestrel	Desogen	antiendometriotic, systemic contraceptive, gonadotropin inhibitor
ethinyl estradiol-desogestrel	Kariva	antiendometriotic, systemic contraceptive, gonadotropin inhibitor
ethinyl estradiol-desogestrel	Mircette	antiendometriotic, systemic contraceptive, gonadotropin inhibitor

Generic Name	Registered Brand or Trade Name	Therapeutic Use/Medication Action
ANTIENDOMETRIOTIC—cont'd		
ethinyl estradiol-desogestrel	Ortho-Cept	antiendometriotic, systemic contraceptive, gonadotropin inhibitor
ethinyl estradiol-levonorgestrel	Levlen	antiendometriotic, systemic postcoital contraceptive, systemic contraceptive, estrogen progestin, gonadotropin inhibitor
ethinyl estradiol-levonorgestrel	Nordette	antiendometriotic, systemic postcoital contraceptive, systemic contraceptive, estrogen-progestin, gonadotropin inhibitor
ethinyl estradiol-levonorgestrel	Seasonale	antiendometriotic, systemic postcoital contraceptive, systemic contraceptive, estrogen-progestin, gonadotropin inhibitor
ethinyl estradiol-levonorgestrel	Tri-Levlen	antiendometriotic, systemic postcoital contraceptive, systemic contraceptive, estrogen-progestin, gonadotropin inhibitor
ethinyl estradiol-levonorgestrel	Triphasil	antiendometriotic, systemic postcoital contraceptive, systemic contraceptive, estrogen-progestin, gonadotropin inhibitor
ethinyl estradiol-levonorgestrel	Trivora-28	antiendometriotic, systemic postcoital contraceptive, systemic contraceptive, estrogen-progestin, gonadotropin inhibitor
ethinyl estradiol-norgestrel	Lo/Ovral	antiendometriotic, systemic postcoital contraceptive, systemic contraceptive, estrogen-progestin, gonadotropin inhibitor
ethinyl estradiol-norgestrel	Low-Ogestrel	antiendometriotic, systemic postcoital contraceptive, systemic contraceptive, estrogen-progestin, gonadotropin inhibitor
ethinyl estradiol-norgestrel	Ovral	antiendometriotic, systemic postcoital contraceptive, systemic contraceptive, estrogen-progestin, gonadotropin inhibitor
ANTIFUNGAL		
clotrimazole	Mycelex Cream	antifungal
clotrimazole-betamethasone	Lotrisone	antifungal, corticosteroid
econazole	Sporanox	antifungal
econazole	Spectazole Cream	antifungal
fluconazole	Diflucan	systemic antifungal
griseofulvin	Grifulvin	antifungal
itraconazole	Sporanox	antifungal
ketoconazole	Nizoral	antifungal
miconazole	Monistat Derm	cream antifungal
terbinafine	Lamisil	antifungal
terconazole	Terazol	vaginal antifungal cream, suppositories
ANTIGLAUCOMA		
bimatoprost	Lumigan Ophthalmic	antiglaucoma solution
brimonidine	Alphagan P	antiglaucoma solution
dorzolamide/timolol maleate	Cosopt	decreases ocular hypertension
latanoprost	Xalatan	antiglaucoma
latanoprost	Xalatan Ophthalmic	antiglaucoma, ocular antihypertensive
timolol	Timoptic	ophthalmic antiglaucoma
ANTIGOUT		
allopurinol	Zyloprim	antigout agent

Generic Name	Registered Brand or Trade Name	Therapeutic Use/Medication Action
ANTIHISTAMINE		
cetirizine	Zyrtec	antihistamine, H1 receptor
cetirizine-pseudoephedrine	Zyrtec-D	antihistamine, H1 receptor-decongestant
desloratadine	Clarinex	antihistamine, H1 receptor
fexofenadine	Allegra	antihistamine, H1 receptor
fexofenadine-pseudoephedrine	Allegra D	antihistamine, H1 receptor-decongestant
hydrocodone-chlorpheniramine	Tussionex	antihistamine, H1 receptor antitussive
hydroxyzine	Vistaril	antihistamine
loratadine	Claritin	antihistamine
olopatadine	Patanol	ophthalmic antihistamine, H1 receptor, mask cell stabilizer, antiallergic
promethazine-codeine	Prometh with Codeine	antihistamine, H1 receptor-antitussive
ANTIHYPERCALCEMIC		
furosemide	Lasix	antihypercalcemic, antihypertensive, renal disease diagnostic aid, diuretic
ANTIHYPERLIPIDEMIC		
atorvastatin	Lipitor	antilipidemic, statin
colesevelam	WelChol	antihyperlipidemic
ezetimibe	Zetia	antihyperlipidemic
fenofibrate	TriCor	antihyperlipidemic
fluvastatin sodium	Lescol	antihyperlipidemic
gemfibrozil	Lopid	antihyperlipidemic
lovastatin	Mevacor	antihyperlipidemic
pravastatin sodium	Pravachol	antihyperlipidemic, HMG-CoA reductase inhibitor
simvastatin	Zocor	antihyperlipidemic, HMG-CoA reductase inhibitor
ANTIHYPERTENSIVE		
amlodipine/atorvastatin	Caduet	antihypertensive, calcium channel blocker
amlodipine-benazepril HCL	Lotrel	antihypertensive, calcium channel blocker
amlodipine-besylate	Norvasc	antihypertensive, calcium channel blocker
atenolol	Tenormin	antihypertensive
benazepril	Lotensin	antihypertensive, ACE inhibitor
bepridil	Vascor	antihypertensive, calcium channel blocker
candesartan	Atacand	antihypertensive
captopril	Capoten	antihypertensive, ACE inhibitor
carvedilol	Coreg	antihypertensive
clonidine	Duraclon	antihypertensive
clonidine HCL	Catapres	antihypertensive
doxazosin	Cardura	antihypertensive, alpha blocker
enalapril	Vasotec	antihypertensive, vasodilator, ACE inhibitor
fosinopril sodium	Monopril	antihypertensive, vasodilator, ACE inhibitor

Generic Name	Registered Brand or Trade Name	Therapeutic Use/Medication Action
ANTIHYPERTENSIVE—cont'd		
hydrochlorothiazide	Esidrix	antihypertensive, diuretic, antiurolithic
irbesartan	Avapro	antihypertensive
irbesartan-hydrochlorothiazide	Avalide	antihypertensive
lisinopril	Prinivil	antihypertensive, vasodilator
lisinopril	Zestril	antihypertensive, vasodilator, ACE inhibitor
losartan potassium	Cozaar	antihypertensive, angiotensin II-receptor antagonist
losartan-hydrochlorothiazide	Hyzaar	antihypertensive
perindopril	Coversyl	antihypertensive, vasodilator, ACE inhibitor
prazosin	Minipress	antihypertensive, alpha blocker
prazosin/polythiazide	Minizide	antihypertensive, alpha blocker
quinapril	Accupril	antihypertensive, vasodilator, ACE inhibitor
ramipril	Altace	antihypertensive, vasodilator, ACE inhibitor
spironolactone	Aldactone	antihypertensive, antihypokalemic, hyperaldosteronism diagnostic aid, diuretic, aldosterone antagonist
terazosin	Hytrin	antihypertensive, benign prostatic hyperplasia
trandolapril	Mavik	antihypertensive, vasodilator, ACE inhibitor
travoprost	Travatan	antihypertensive, reducing intraocular pressure
triamterene-hydrochlorothiazide	Dyazide	antihypertensive, antihypokalemia, diuretic
triamterene-hydrochlorothiazide	Maxzide	antihypertensive, antihypokalemia, diuretic
valsartan	Diovan	antihypertensive
valsartan-hydrochlorothiazide	Diovan HCT	antihypertensive
verapamil/trandolapril	Tarka	antihypertensive, calcium channel blocker
ANTIHYPOKALEMIC		
potassium chloride	Klor-Con	antihypokalemic, electrolyte replenisher
ANTI-INFLAMMATORY (NONSTEROID)		
diclofenac	Arthrotec	anti-inflammatory, analgesic
hydroxychloroquine	Plaquenil	systemic anti-inflammatory
mesalamine	Asacol	anti-inflammatory in colon/rectum
piroxicam	Feldene	anti-inflammatory, analgesic
tolmetin	Tolectin	anti-inflammatory, analgesic
triamcinolone	Azmacort	inhalation anti-inflammatory, antiasthmatic
valdecoxib	Bextra	nonsteroidal anti-inflammatory, antirheumatic, antidysmenorrheal
ANTIMETASTATIC		
bicalutamide	Casodex	antimetastatic—used with LHRH-A to treat advanced prostate cancer
ANTIMIGRAINE		
eletriptan HBr	Relpax	antimigraine
sumatriptan	Imitrex	antimigraine

APPENDIX I Pharmacology Review

Generic Name	Registered Brand or Trade Name	Therapeutic Use/Medication Action
ANTINEOPLASTIC		
conjugated estrogen	Enjuvia	antineoplastic, systemic estrogen, osteoporosis prophylactic, ovarian hormone therapy agent
conjugated estrogen	Premarin	antineoplastic, systemic estrogen, osteoporosis prophylactic, ovarian hormone therapy agent
levothyroxine sodium	Synthroid	antineoplastic, thyroid function diagnostic aid, thyroid hormone
levothyroxine T4	Levothroid	antineoplastic, thyroid function diagnostic aid, thyroid hormone
ANTIPSYCHOTIC		
olanzapine	Zyprexa	antipsychotic
quetiapine	Seroquel	antipsychotic
risperidone	Risperdal	antipsychotic
thiothixene	Navane	antipsychotic
ziprasidone	Geodon	antipsychotic
ANTIRHEUMATIC		
meloxicam	Mobic	antirheumatic (NSAID)
ANTISEIZURE		
ethosuximide	Zarontin	antiseizure
ANTISPASMOTIC		
oxybutynin chloride	Ditropan XL	urinary tract antispasmodic
tolterodine tartrate	Detrol	urinary bladder antispasmodic
ANTITHROMBOTIC		
clopidogrel bisulfate	Plavix	antithrombotic, platelet aggregation inhibitor
ANTIULCER		
esomeprazole magnesium	Nexium	gastric acid pump inhibitor, antiulcer
lansoprazole SR	Prevacid	gastric acid pump inhibitor, antiulcer
misoprostol	Cytotec	gastric acid pump inhibitor, antiulcer
omeprazole SA	Prilosec	gastric acid pump inhibitor, antiulcer
pantoprazole	Protonix	gastric acid pump inhibitor, antiulcer
rabeprazole	AcipHex	gastric acid pump inhibitor, antiulcer
ranitidine	Zantac	histamine H2-receptor antagonist, antiulcer, gastric acid secretion inhibitor
ANTIVIRAL		
acyclovir	Zovirax	systemic antiviral
ribavirin	Rebetol	antiviral
ribavirin	Copegus	antiviral
valacyclovir	Valtrex	systemic antiviral
ANTIWRINKLE (TOPICAL)		
tretinoin	Retin-A	antiwrinkle cream

Generic Name	Registered Brand or Trade Name	Therapeutic Use/Medication Action
BRONCHODILATOR		
albuterol	Proventil	bronchodilator
albuterol	Ventolin	bronchodilator
BONE RESORPTION INHIBITOR		
alendronate sodium	Fosamax	bone resorption inhibitor
calcitonin-salmon	Miacalcin	bone resorption inhibitor
raloxifene sodium	Evista	selective estrogen receptor modulator, osteoporosis prophylactic
risedronate sodium	Actonel	bone resorption inhibitor
CATHARTIC		
polyethylene glycol	MiraLax	hyperosmotic laxative
CENTRAL NERVOUS SYSTEM STIMULANT		
dextroamphetamine-amphetamine	Adderall	CNS stimulant, ADHD therapy
methylphenidate	Concerta	CNS stimulant, ADHD therapy
methylphenidate	Metadate	CNS stimulant, ADHD therapy
methylphenidate	Ritalin	CNS stimulant, ADHD therapy
CONTRACEPTIVE		
ethinyl estradiol-drospirenone	Yasmin	systemic contraceptive
ethinyl estradiol-norelgestromin	Ortho Evra	systemic contraceptive
ENZYME		
pancrelipase	Pancrease	pancreatic enzyme replacement
HEMOPOIETIC		
erythropoietin	Epogen	hematopoietic
erythropoietin	Procrit	hematopoietic
HORMONE		
conjugated estrogen-medroxyprogesterone	Premphase	estrogen-progestin, osteoporosis prophylactic, ovarian hormone therapy
conjugated estrogen-medroxyprogesterone	Prempro	estrogen-progestin, osteoporosis prophylactic, ovarian hormone therapy
estrogen conjugated	Premarin	hormone replacement—estrogen
IMMUNE ENHANCER		
pimecrolimus	Elidel	immunomodulator
NEOPLASTIC		
anastrozole	Arimidex	chemotherapeutic-hormone receptor-positive
SEDATIVE		
temazepam	Restoril	sedative-hypnotic
zolpidem tartrate	Ambien	sedative-hypnotic

Generic Name	Registered Brand or Trade Name	Therapeutic Use/Medication Action
SKELETAL MUSCLE RELAXANT		
carisoprodol	Soma	skeletal muscle relaxant
chlorzoxazone	Parafon Forte DSC	skeletal muscle relaxant
cyclobenzaprine	Flexeril	skeletal muscle relaxant
metaxalone	Skelaxin	skeletal muscle relaxant
STEROIDS		
fluticasone	Flonase	steroidal nasal anti-inflammatory, nasal corticosteroid
fluticasone	Flovent	steroidal nasal anti-inflammatory, nasal corticosteroid
methylprednisolone	Medrol	steroidal anti-inflammatory, corticoid, steroid, immunosuppressant
mometasone furoate	Nasonex	nasal steroid anti-inflammatory, nasal corticosteroid
prednisone	Deltasone	systemic steroidal anti-inflammatory, cancer chemotherapy antiemetic, corticosteroid immunosuppressant
tobramycin-dexamethasone	TobraDex	ophthalmic corticosteroid, steroidal anti-inflammatory, antibacterial
triamcinolone	Nasacort AQ	nasal steroid anti-inflammatory, nasal corticosteroid
VITAMIN		
niacin	Niacor	nutritional supplement, vitamin

Index

Page numbers followed by "*f*" indicate figures, and "*b*" indicate boxes.

A

Abbreviations, medical. *See* Medical abbreviations
Abductor group, 36
Ablation, 54*b*–56*b*
Abnormal heart rhythms, 77–78
Abnormal menstruation types, 92
Abortion, 89*b*, 102, 380–381
  with liveborn fetus, 381
  services, 340
Abruptio placentae, 100, 101*f*
Abscess, brain, 204
Absence, 5*b*–7*b*
Absorption atelectasis, 59
Abuse, Medicare, 254
Accessory sinuses, 49, 309
Accounts receivable (AR), 250
Achilles tendon, 36
Acne vulgaris, 17
Acromegaly, 182
ACS. *See* Acute coronary system (ACS)
Actinic keratosis, 23
Acute coronary system (ACS), 70*b*–71*b*
Acute lymphocytic leukemia (ALL), 170
Acute myelogenous leukemia (AML), 170
Acute necrotizing fasciitis, 20
Acute pericarditis, 80
Acute poststreptococcal glomerulonephritis (APSGN), 129
Acute prostatitis, 114–115
Acute pyelonephritis, 127–128, 127*f*
Acute renal failure, 125
Acute respiratory failure, 58
Acute respiratory infection, 377
Addison's disease, 186
Adenoidectomy, 54*b*–56*b*
Adenomyosis, 95–96
Adipose, 5*b*–7*b*
Adjacent tissue transfer, 282–287
Adrenal gland, 118*f*, 175*f*, 176, 178*b*–179*b*
  disorders, 185–187
Adrenal medulla, 187
Adrenocorticotropic hormone (ACTH), 185–186
Adult respiratory distress syndrome (ARDS), 58, 158
Advance beneficiary notice, 257*b*–259*b*
Albinism, 5*b*–7*b*
ALL. *See* Acute lymphocytic leukemia (ALL)
Allergic contact dermatitis, 13
Alopecia, 5*b*–7*b*

Alphabetic index, ICD-10-CM, 363–364
ALS. *See* Amyotrophic lateral sclerosis (ALS)
Alveolar ducts, 50
Alzheimer's disease, 196
Amblyopia, 218
Ambulatory Patient Classification (APC) levels of service, 269–271
Ambulatory Patient Groups (APGs), 233
Ambulatory Payment Classifications (APCs), 233–240
  ambulatory surgery procedures, 239
  -CA modifier, 237
  device-dependent procedures, 238–239
  discounting, 239
  incidentals, 235
  inpatient-only procedures with status indicator "C", 239
  observation status, 239–240
  outlier adjustments, 239
  outpatient code editor (OCE), 240
  pass-through codes, 235, 238*f*
  payment rate and co-insurance, 235, 237*f*
  payment status indicators (SI), 235–240, 236*f*
  structure, 234–235, 234*f*
  transitional pass-through payments for certain devices and items, 237–238
Ambulatory surgery procedures, 239
Amenorrhea, 91
AML. *See* Acute myelogenous leukemia (AML)
Amniocentesis, 89*b*
Amniotic sac, 89*b*
Amyotrophic lateral sclerosis (ALS), 197
Analgesia, 271
  patient-controlled, 271
Anastomosis, 70*b*–71*b*, 140*b*–141*b*
Anatomy and terminology
  cardiovascular system, 63–67
  digestive system, 134–137
  endocrine system, 175–177
  female genital system and pregnancy, 83–85
  hemic and lymphatic system, 162
  integumentary system, 2–8
  male genital system, 104
  mediastinum and diaphragm, 160
  musculoskeletal system, 26–36
  nervous system, 189–191
  respiratory system, 49–51
  senses, 210–212
  urinary system, 118–120
Ancillary service, 257*b*–259*b*
Anconeus, 36

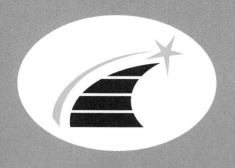
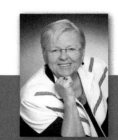
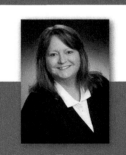

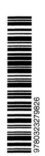